SPIRITUALLY INTEGRATED PSYCHOTHERAPY

SPIRITUALLY INTEGRATED PSYCHOTHERAPY

*Understanding and
Addressing the Sacred*

KENNETH I. PARGAMENT

THE GUILFORD PRESS
New York   London

Paperback edition 2011

No part of this book may be reproduced, translated, stored in a retrieval system,
or transmitted, in any form or by any means, electronic, mechanical, photocopying,
microfilming, recording, or otherwise, without written permission from the Publisher.

Printed in the United States of America

This book is printed on acid-free paper.

Last digit is print number: 9   8   7   6   5

Library of Congress Cataloging-in-Publication Data

Pargament, Kenneth I. (Kenneth Ira), 1950–
 Spiritually integrated psychotherapy : understanding and addressing the sacred /
Kenneth I. Pargament.
   p. ; cm.
 Includes bibliographical references and index.
 ISBN 978-1-57230-844-2 (hardcover : alk. paper)
 ISBN 978-1-60918-993-8 (paperback : alk. paper)
  1. Psychotherapy—Religious aspects. 2. Spirituality. I. Title.
 [DNLM: 1. Psychotherapy—methods—Case Reports. 2. Mental Disorders—therapy—
Case Reports.   3. Spirituality—Case Reports.   WM 420 P229s 2007]
 RC489.S676P37 2007
 616.89′166—dc22

                                                                    2007019485

The following publishers and/or authors have generously given permission to reprint or adapt their original
work:
    American Anthropological Association, for "'Espiritus? No. Pero la Maldad Existe': Supernaturalism,
Religious Change, and the Problem of Evil in Puerto Rican Folk Religion" by G. Jeffrey Jacobson, Jr., in
Ethics, 31, 1–30 (2003).
    Brenda Cole, for *The Integration of Spirituality and Psychotherapy for People Who Have Confronted
Cancer* by Brenda Cole (Unpublished doctoral dissertation, Bowling Green State University, Bowling Green,
OH, 1999).
    Guilford Press, for *Encountering the Sacred in Psychotherapy: How to Talk with People about Their
Spiritual Lives* by J. L. Griffith and M. E. Griffith (New York: Guilford Press, 2002).
    Ideals Publications, for *I'm Thankful Each Day* by P. K. Hallinan (Nashville, TN: Ideals Children's
Books, 1981).
    Jessica Kingsley Publishers, for *Psychotherapy and Spirituality: Integrating the Spiritual Dimension into
Therapeutic Practice* by Agneta Schreurs (London: Kingsley, 2002).
    John Wiley & Sons, Inc., for "Religious-Issues Group Therapy" by N. C. Kehoe in *New Directions for
Mental Health Services, 80*, 45–55 (1998).
    Kluwer Academic Publishers, for *Psychotherapy in a Religious Framework: Spirituality in the Emo-
tional Healing Process* by Rebecca Propst (New York: Human Sciences Press, 1988).
    Lawrence Erlbaum Associates, for *Counseling and Psychotherapy with Religious Persons: A Rational
Emotive Behavior Therapy Approach* by S. L. Nielsen, W. B. Johnson, and A. Ellis (Mahwah, NJ: Erlbaum,
2001).
    Life Inc., for "Here I Was Sitting at the Edge of Eternity" in *Life*, pp. 28–33, 38, 39 (1989).
    Oxford University Press, for *The Spiritual Nature of Man: A Study of Contemporary Religious Experi-
ence* by A. Hardy (Oxford, UK: Clarendon Press, 1979).
    Random House, Inc., for *A Path with Heart: A Guide through the Perils and Promises of Spiritual Life*
by Jack Kornfield (New York: Bantam Books, 1993).
    Random House, Inc., for *Father Joe: The Man Who Saved My Soul* by Tony Hendra (New York: Ran-
dom House, 2004).
    Taylor and Francis Journals, for "Development of a Model for Clinical Assessment of Religious Coping:
Initial Validation of the Process Evaluation Model" by E. A. Butter and K. I. Pargament in *Mental Health,
Religion, and Culture, 6*, 175–194.

To the memory of my mother, Florence,
and to my father, Sol,
who leavened our lives
with music, laughter, and love

About the Author

Kenneth I. Pargament, PhD, is Professor of Psychology at Bowling Green State University, where he has been on the faculty since 1979. He has published extensively on the vital role of religion and spirituality in coping with stress and trauma. Dr. Pargament has been a leading figure in the effort to bring a balanced view of religion and spirituality to the attention of scientists and professionals. He is author of *The Psychology of Religion and Coping: Theory, Research, Practice* and coeditor of *Forgiveness: Theory, Research, and Practice* (with Michael E. McCullough and Carl E. Thoresen). He is a recipient of the William James Award for excellence in research in the psychology of religion, the Virginia Staudt Sexton Mentoring Award for guiding and encouraging others in the field, and the Oskar Pfister Award for his research and practice in religion and mental health. Dr. Pargament is a practicing clinical psychologist who has worked with people from diverse spiritual backgrounds. In 2011–2012, he will serve as Distinguished Scholar in Residence at the Institute for Spirituality and Health of the Texas Medical Center in Houston.

Preface

Several years ago, while driving a rental car in California, I came across my favorite bumper sticker of all time. "Honk if you believe in a unified field theory," it read. I would have honked if I could have found the horn on the car.

For much of my career, I have been searching for the equivalent of a unified field theory in the psychology of religion, a perspective that could lend unity to theory, research, and clinical practice. "Trying to put things together," is the way my mentor Forrest Tyler described it. Much of my initial work in psychology consisted of trying to put religion together with health. Initially, I focused on empirical studies that explored the connections between various aspects of religiousness and positive mental health or psychosocial competence. At the same time, I kept my fingers in clinical work. Once a week I saw clinical cases and, in addition, I supervised graduate students in psychotherapy. No two days were alike, and between teaching, research, and practice, my professional life was always stimulating. Even so, I often felt that I was living separate professional lives. On the one hand, my research colleagues reacted with surprise when they found out that I was a clinical psychologist. On the other, my clients would be equally surprised to discover that I studied religion and health. The problem was that my research on religion had little to do with my clinical practice, and my clinical work had little impact on my research. Of course, I wasn't the only one. The split between science and practice was and is commonplace in psychology. Most clinicians are quite finicky when it comes to consuming research, and it is the rare clinician who conducts research of his or her own. Researchers seem just as reluctant to involve themselves in clinical practice. But I needed to put things together.

In particular, I needed a way to think about and study religion that spoke more directly to the problems people face in their lives. To know that a measure of religiousness correlated .30 with a measure of depression or life satisfaction said little to me about helping the client who was unsure whether her religious faith was calling on her to return to her husband who had been cheating on her. So I began to look for a different research strategy. I focused on the roles that religion plays in the process of coping. The metaphor of "coping" was appealing to me because it challenged the all-too-common psychological stereotype that religion is inevitably passive, defensive, and maladaptive. Instead, it suggested another possibility—that religion could be a positive resource to people in times of stress. Coping also conveyed an appreciation for the interplay of (1) the person (2) facing critical problems (3) in the context of a larger social milieu. In short, the metaphor of coping seemed to come closer to capturing something important about real people confronting real problems. My research on this topic culminated in my book *The Psychology of Religion and Coping: Theory, Research, Practice* (Pargament, 1997).

Now I felt like I was getting somewhere—I was beginning to put some things together. I found that my research on religion and coping was helpful in my clinical work and that my clinical work, in turn, often stimulated new ideas for research. Nevertheless, something was still missing. I needed a larger, more encompassing perspective to guide my work. It wasn't enough to know how religion expresses itself in the process of coping with life stressors. I needed to know more about the heart and soul of religion—spirituality—how it develops and evolves over the lifespan, how it operates in everyday life, how it can be a source of solutions to problems, how it can be a problem in and of itself, and how it can be addressed in psychotherapy.

Over the past 10 years, I have been trying to learn more about these issues. This book is the result. More generally, it is in some sense a culmination of my own, very personal attempt to put things together as a researcher, theorist, and practitioner. Of course, I hope this book has some value to other people too. The field of psychology, I believe, is in need of a unified perspective on human behavior, one that expands the biopsychosocial perspective to a biopsychosociospiritual perspective. In this book, I have tried to bring spirituality more fully into the domain of clinical thought and practice. One of my basic assumptions has been that we can't work with spiritual issues in psychotherapy unless we understand what spirituality is. Thus, I have tried to provide practitioners with an empirically grounded way to think about spirituality as a foundation for clinical practice. I have also emphasized the richness of spirituality, the importance of being able to work with diverse spiritual expressions, both traditional and nontraditional, and the need to draw on diverse theories, research, and clinical methods to capture at least a part of this complex and elusive phenomenon. In addition, I have warned against attempts to "explain spirituality away" by reducing it to seemingly more basic psychological, social, or physical processes. Instead, I have insisted that spirituality be understood and addressed as a legitimate dimension of human experience in itself. And I have avoided the temptation to idealize spirituality, stressing instead the need for clinicians to recognize a basic fact of life: that spirituality can be a part of the solution and a part of the problem.

We haven't arrived at a unified field theory yet. Much more is unknown than known when it comes to the place of spirituality in life. But let's not be too impatient. After all, psychology is still a young field, just a little over a hundred years old. And the study of spirituality is even younger, having been largely neglected by psychologists for many years. My hope is that this work contributes in some way to a more integrated approach to understanding and addressing the spiritual dimension in psychotherapy.

I haven't been putting things together by myself. Over the years, I have been exceptionally fortunate to have many other people teach, support, and challenge me. I am very appreciative of my former graduate students—Drs. Gene Ano, Ethan Benore, Brenda Cole, Erin Emery, Gina Magyar-Russell, Russell Phillips, Mark Rye, Nichole and Aaron-Murray Swank, Nalini Tarakeshwar, and Amy Wachholtz-Ayala—whose own imaginative approaches to psychological change and research helped shape my thinking about spiritually integrated psychotherapy. I am also grateful to my current graduate students—Hisham Abu Raiya, Lisa Backus, Carol Ann Caprini, Maria Gear, Krystal Hernandez, Elizabeth Krumrei, Quinten Lynn, Shauna McCarthy, Meryl Reist, David Rosmarin, and Kelly Trevino—who took the risk of providing me with invaluable critiques of each chapter of this book.

While writing this book, I was able to collaborate with a remarkable group of faculty and graduate students in the Counseling Psychology and Religion Program in the School of Theology at Boston University. My job was to help them develop their program of research, but they also taught me a great deal about the interface between religion, spirituality, and psychotherapy. Special thanks go to Dr. Nancy Devor, Dr. Carol Bohn, Dr. Brian McCorkle, Theresa Hughes, David Kim, Ann Clarke, Peter Rothschild, and Lori Brown-Frankel.

Several colleagues also provided me with guidance, insights, and support. First, I would like to express my deep appreciation to my friend, colleague, and collaborator of many years, Dr. Annette Mahoney. Many of the key concepts (e.g., the sacred, sanctification, desecration) and empirical studies in this book were developed and implemented in partnership with Annette. I have been very fortunate to be able to work with such a talented researcher, incisive scholar, and pioneering figure in the psychology of religion, marriage, and the family. In addition, I thank Dr. Everett Worthington, who gave me the initial advice and encouragement to pursue this book; Dr. James Jones, who helped clarify my thinking about the discovery of the sacred and spiritual dis-integration; and Dr. William Hathaway, who generously shared his knowledge about several topics in the book. Special thanks are also due Dr. Carrie Doehring and her graduate students at the Iliff School of Theology, who provided me with important feedback and recommendations on the first draft. The Fetzer Institute and John Templeton Foundation have also generously supported several of the key studies that contributed to the development of spiritually integrated therapy. I would particularly like to acknowledge Dr. Lynn Underwood and Dr. Arthur Schwartz from Fetzer and Templeton for their visionary and leading roles in stimulating not only my work, but an entire field of scientific spiritual study. I am very grateful to my editor, Jim Nageotte, of The Guilford Press, whose perceptive reading, astute comments, and expert guidance helped sharpen and refine the manuscript. Finally, thanks go to Anna Brackett and Jane Keislar from Guilford for their patience and proficiency in bringing this work to its final form.

I am especially grateful to my clients for their willingness to share their stories with me and the reader. They continue to teach me a great deal about spirituality, the courage it takes to examine one's life with another person, and the capacity to grow in the most difficult of situations. The clinical quotations in this book were drawn from extensive case notes of my sessions with clients. I have changed personal information in these stories that could reveal a client's identity.

This book would not have been possible without the love, support, and encouragement of my two sons, Jonathan and Benjamin, and my wife, Aileen. Aileen was more than gracious in keeping our lives on an even keel while I went through the ups and downs of writing. It's also my good fortune that Aileen happens to be the finest therapist I know. Thus, I was able to rely on her unfailing clinical wisdom and honesty whenever I had questions about material in the book. My greatest satisfaction (and greatest relief) came after Aileen finished the last page of the manuscript, put it aside, and said: "I think it's good."

I would like to dedicate this book to my parents, Sol and Florence. My father continues to serve as a model for how to approach the world with delight, a sensitive ear, a critical eye, and, always, a sense of humor. He and my mother were devoted to each other throughout their marriage of 58 years. While I was writing this book, my mother struggled with a series of illnesses, accidents, and surgeries. In spite of her tenacious spirit, her love of life, and the love and support of my father, family, and friends, my mother lost the battle and died. She lived a life dedicated to her family and community. She loved nothing better than to "kvell" on the accomplishments of her children and grandchildren. It was terribly sad but perhaps not surprising that her final injury occurred when she tried to help a sick friend out of her car. My mother was also an inspirational woman. She taught me that it is possible to commit fully and deeply to a religion, yet remain respectful and open to what other traditions may have to teach us. And she taught us all how to live in even the toughest of times with grace and dignity. She continues to be deeply loved and deeply missed.

Contents

PART IV. CONCLUSIONS

Part I

INTRODUCTION

I

A Rationale for a Spiritually Integrated Psychotherapy

As I held my baby in the delivery room, I looked up. I saw billions of stars, and I heard music I can only describe as celestial. The stars began to form like a fence, like a huge chain. And I knew that I was part of everything.
—"Why We Pray" (1994, p. 62)

When [my partner] first died I felt a very strong presence of him for the first few weeks. I would be sitting somewhere and suddenly get a whiff of him. Just my head down on my arms, and I turned my head and all of a sudden he was there. I know he was just lying on top of me. It was very comforting . . . he's very definitely still there. Sometimes more than others.
—Richards, Acree, and Folkman (1999, p. 117)

Spirituality is an extraordinary part of the ordinary lives of people. From birth to death, spirituality is manifest in life's turning points, revealing mystery and depth during these pivotal moments in time. In crisis and catastrophe, spirituality is often intertwined in the struggle to comprehend the seemingly incomprehensible and to manage the seemingly unmanageable. But this isn't the full story. Spirituality is not reserved exclusively for times of crisis and transition. It is interwoven into the fabric of the everyday. We can find the spiritual in a piece of music, the smile of a passing stranger, the color of the sky at dusk, or a daily prayer of gratitude upon awakening. Spirituality can reveal itself in the ways we think, the ways we feel, the ways we act, and the ways we relate to each other. Paradoxically, the presence of the spiritual dimension can also be felt through its absence, in feelings of loss and emptiness, in questions about meaning and purpose, in a sense of alienation and abandonment, and in cries about injustice and unfairness. Spirituality is, in short, another dimension of life. An extraordinary dimension, yes, but one that is a vital part of ordinary life and what it means to be human. We are more than psychological, social, and physical beings; we are also spiritual beings.

When people walk into the therapist's office, they don't leave their spirituality behind in the waiting room. They bring their spiritual beliefs, practices, experiences, values, relationships, and struggles along with them. Implicitly or explicitly, this complex of spiritual factors often enters the process of psychotherapy. And yet many therapists are unaware of or unprepared to deal with this dimension in treatment. How does the therapist understand spirituality? How does the therapist address the spiritual dimension in psychotherapy? These questions are the focus of this book. In this introductory chapter I consider the peculiar tension between psychology and religion, and discuss several reasons why it makes sense to move beyond this tension to integrate spirituality into psychotherapy. As a prelude to what's to come in the chapters that follow, I briefly characterize the essential features of spiritually integrated psychotherapy. I conclude by making explicit some of my own values and beliefs that underlie this approach to treatment. Let me start with a story.

ALICE'S STORY

Several years ago, I worked with a client named Alice. At first glance, there was nothing remarkable about her, but I was to learn otherwise. She came to my office dressed in formless polyester pants and shapeless sweatshirts, perhaps as a way to conceal her heavy frame. Her hair was clean but cut short and unstyled, and the scattered lines and wrinkles on her face were untouched by makeup. What Alice did convey was a deep sense of sadness. It showed in her slow walk, in the slight bend in her shoulders, and most of all in her eyes. They had the look of a puppy that had been mistreated, fearful of what might come next but still hopeful that something better might come along. It was hard for Alice to tell her story. Her face reddened, she directed her gaze downward, her words seemed to get caught in her throat, and she frequently apologized for her difficulty in speaking with me. At times, though, she offered a small joke that lifted the deep melancholy that had settled in the room. During these moments her eyes would sparkle and her sad face would break into a delightful almost child-like smile.

Alice had experienced emotional pain for most of her 45 years. Overweight as a child, she had been mercilessly teased and taunted by her father until he abandoned the family when she was an adolescent. Convinced of her own unattractiveness, Alice had avoided romantic entanglements. In late adolescence, Alice developed symptoms of bipolar disorder and over the next decades suffered from a terrible roller-coaster of emotional upheavals. Medications had helped her achieve a modest level of emotional stability, but she was still subject to unpredictable and powerful shifts in moods that occasionally resulted in hospitalization.

In spite of her illness, Alice had succeeded in creating a meaningful life for herself, one that centered around other people. She was devoted to the care of her elderly mother. She was a loyal volunteer at both the local hospice and the school for the blind. She was a good friend to several people with serious mental illness and spent many hours helping them through their own emotional crises. In our sessions, Alice showed a genuine interest in how things were going in my life. And yet Alice was unable to derive any satisfaction from the knowledge that she was an exceptionally caring and compassionate person. She described herself in the same language her father had used: "big and stupid." Her contemptuous view of herself was deep-seated. Through our conversations, Alice learned more about the root causes of her self-contempt, but her insights led to minimal change. My other efforts to buoy her self-image were just as unsuccessful.

Over many months, I watched Alice go through the full spectrum of her moods: exuberance tinged with the unsettling recognition of where it was leading her, depression that seemed to wash over her like huge waves plunging her into the sea of despair, and total exhaustion that followed her emotional whirlwinds. Yet, time and again, she emerged from these cycles intact, picking up the pieces of the life that she had created, reconnecting with the people she loved and cared for. How, I wondered, did this remarkable woman manage to sustain herself through her periods of emotional upheaval when she was so weighed down by the added burden of her self-contempt? What could I do to help make her life more bearable?

A pivotal moment in therapy occurred when Alice was in the midst of another deeply depressive period. She had been withdrawing from social contact for a few weeks (always a danger sign for Alice) and was thinking more and more about suicide. In this session, Alice was wracked with pain, sobbing so hard it was difficult for me to follow her. I was about to suggest her need for hospitalization when Alice spoke in a kind of language that was unusual for her. "When will my suffering end?," she cried. The question had a spiritual, almost biblical, sound to me, like a lamentation. Understand that I had talked with Alice about the role of religion and spirituality in her life earlier in therapy. Although she had mentioned that she was a churchgoer, she left it at that and showed no interest in pursuing the subject any further. So I had put the topic aside. But now I was struck by the spiritual tone of her question. I responded in kind with a question of my own: "I've often wondered, Alice, how in the midst of your terrible suffering, you are able to find some consolation?" She didn't seem surprised by the question. Instead, she paused for a long moment and then told me a story.

"When I was first hospitalized," she said, "they put me in restraints and threw me in a seclusion room. I was only 16 at the time and I didn't know what was going to happen to me. I was so frightened. I was so scared. I thought I was going to die. And then, lying on my bed, I felt something warm in the center of my chest. And the feeling spread through the rest of my body."

"How did that feeling affect you?," I asked.

"It calmed me down. I felt comforted."

"Did that feeling speak to you in some way?"

"Yes, I knew that God[1] was speaking to me, God was with me, telling me that He would always be with me no matter how badly I felt. I would be okay."

Alice and I sat quietly in the room. From a corner of my mind, I noticed that her sobbing had stopped.

"Alice," I went on, "have you felt this presence at other times in your life?"

"Oh, yes," she said immediately. "I feel it sometimes when I'm with other people who are going through hard times. And sometimes," she paused, "I feel it with you." She hesitated for a longer period of time, looked down at her feet, and softly asked, "Do you feel it too?"

Every therapist knows that there are some special moments in psychotherapy. I experience them as "sacred moments" when immediate realities fade into the background, when time seems to stand still, when it feels as if something larger than life is happening. In these moments, I believe, a meeting of souls is taking place. This was one of those times.

So I answered Alice, "Yes, I do."

Alice sat quietly and seemed to be at peace with herself—quite a dramatic change from the intense pain she was feeling just minutes earlier. After a while, I said, "I'd like to talk with you some more about this presence in your life. Would that be alright with you?" Alice agreed.

In the following months, Alice and I spoke often about her sense of spiritual connection. It had been, for much of her life, the source of her resilience and strength. We explored ways she could draw more fully on this powerful resource as she went through her emotional ups and down. And we discussed the implications of her spirituality for overcoming her own unmerciful sense of herself. There was no miracle cure. Alice would continue to struggle with her illness and with her own sense of inadequacy. However, armed with a more fully realized spirituality, Alice was far better

---

[1]The term "God" is capitalized and referred to as "He" when used by clients who view the divine as a personal, patriarchal figure. I also capitalize God in this book, though I avoid using gender pronouns to refer to God. In some instances, I use "gods" in lowercase to refer to problematic representations of divinity (e.g., false gods, small gods).

equipped to face her challenges. She became more aware of herself, more confident in her own capabilities, and more hopeful about her future. In the process, her mood swings lost much of their ferocious intensity and her visits to the hospital became rare.

As she was leaving the room that day, I asked Alice whether she had ever mentioned her sense of spiritual presence to the other mental health professionals who had worked with her over the years.

"No," she said.

"Why not?"

Alice gave me a quizzical look as if the answer was only too obvious. "Why would I do that? They already think I'm crazy."

Spirituality is another dimension of the lives therapists encounter in psychotherapy. Yet, oddly enough, as Alice's parting words suggest, psychologists and other mental health professionals are often uncomfortable with spirituality. No decent clinician avoids the most private and sensitive of topics; love, sex, death, jealousy, violence, addictions, and betrayal are grist for the therapist's mill. Questions about spirituality and religion, however, are routinely neglected. Spirituality is separated from the treatment process as if it were an irrelevant topic or a subject so esoteric that it falls outside the bounds of psychotherapy. "Priests should stay out of therapy and therapists should stay out of spirituality" is the way some have put it, as Prest and Keller (1993, p. 139) note. Of course, clients do bring "God," "religion," or "spirituality" into therapy on their own, but when they do many practitioners admit to feelings of irritation ("Damn, we're going to have to talk about this stuff?") coupled with the desire to punch through this language of illusion and magic to get to the stark truths of reality. Not all therapists are so dismissive of spirituality. Many would like to be more responsive, but they feel uneasy when spiritual issues are raised. They fear entering potentially dangerous, uncharted waters, and find themselves at a loss for ways to proceed. This is a strange state of affairs. As Allen Bergin and I. Reed Payne (1991) commented, "It is paradoxical that traditional psychology and psychotherapy, which fosters individualism, free expression, and tolerance of dissent, would be so reluctant to address one of the most fundamental concerns of humankind—morality and spirituality" (p. 201). Why should this be the case?

THE PECULIAR TENSION
BETWEEN PSYCHOLOGY AND SPIRITUALITY

The founding figures of psychology saw no reason to separate spirituality from psychological study and practice. Eminent leaders of the field, from William James to G. Stanley Hall, took the root meaning of the word *psychology*, from *psyche* (soul) and *-logy* (study of), quite seriously and focused their attention on a variety of religious phenomena, most notably conversion and mysticism. In the early 20th century, however, this picture began to change as the attitude of those in the field regarding religion shifted from interest and openness to suspicion and hostility. Under the influence of the positivistic philosophy of the time, psychology moved quickly to ally itself with the natural sciences and thereby distinguish itself from its embarrassingly close disciplinary kin, philosophy and theology. Within the developing field, religion came to be seen as an impediment to the scientific search for enlightenment and a roadblock to rationally based efforts to improve the human condition. Commenting on this transition, David Wulff (1997) writes, "Only the new social sciences, in concert with the physical and biological sciences, might hope to deliver humankind from the fears and suffering that some say inspired the first prayers and magical incantations" (p. 17). Psychology began to attract young people who were disaffected from their religious upbringing; these were "enlightened fundamentalists" (Bellah, 1970), fervently convinced that religious beliefs would go the way of other superstitions with the advance of scientific knowledge.

Out of this context emerged models of personality and psychotherapy that depicted spirituality in oversimplified, stereotypical terms. Consider behaviorism and psychoanalysis, the two major psychological paradigms of the 20th century. B. F. Skinner, the founder of behaviorism, was himself the product of a fundamentalist religion that he later rejected. "God," he wrote, "is the archetype pattern of an explanatory fiction" (1971, p. 201). He believed that religious institutions maintain this fiction by attempting to control behavior, primarily through the use of aversive measures, including punitive laws, fears of hell and damnation, and religious practices that discourage sinful behavior. In his vision of utopia, as presented in his fictional *Walden Two* (1948), the members of the community act out Skinner's own history and gradually leave their religious practices behind. "Religious faith," he writes, "becomes irrelevant when the fears which nourish it are allayed and the hopes fulfilled—here on earth" (p. 165).

Similarly, Sigmund Freud was raised in a moderately Jewish household, but he eventually rejected traditional Jewish beliefs and practices, though he continued to identify himself as Jewish, culturally and ethnically. Freud (1927/1961) held that religion was rooted in the child's sense of helplessness in a world of dangerous forces. Early in life, he theorized, the child is able to find comfort and security in the presence of the father. As the child ages, he or she discovers the limitations of the father, but the child must continue to reckon with the powers of nature, powerful others in the surrounding world, and powerful conflicts that lie within. Out of the child's deep wish for safety and protection from these hostile, overwhelming forces, a psychic transformation takes place; the natural becomes supernatural, the uncontrollable becomes malleable, and, as a result, "we can breathe freely, can feel at home in the uncanny and can deal by psychical means with our senseless anxiety" (p. 20). Yet, Freud maintained, this sense of security is illusory, for the powers that be have not been tamed and the individual's emotional comfort has been purchased at the price of personal mastery and maturity. "Surely infantilism is destined to be surmounted," wrote Freud (p. 63). Painful as it may be, the head-on confrontation with reality offers a far better solution to the problems of existence.

Attracted to and shaped by these forces of positivism and these models of personality and psychotherapy, modern practitioners of psychotherapy have become in some important respects quite different from those they serve and in some ways unprepared to help them. Edward Shafranske (2001) has conducted a number of surveys in which he contrasts the religious beliefs and practices of psychologists with those of the general public in the United States. He finds a clear difference. While 58% of the national sample reports that religion is very important to them, only 26% of clinical and counseling psychologists indicate that religion is very important to them. While over 90% of the U.S. population reports belief in a personal God, only 24% of clinical and counseling psychologists do so. When it comes to religion, therapists and their clients come from different worlds. These statistics suggest that a client who believes in a personal God and sees religion as a salient part of his or her life is likely to work with a therapist who does not believe in a personal God and does not consider religion to be very important personally.

True enough, therapists do not have to be "like" their clients to help them. After all, therapists treat people with depression, anxiety, or addictions without being depressed, anxious, and addicted themselves. However, while therapists receive a great deal of education about a full range of psychological problems, they are taught little or nothing about religion and spirituality. For instance, according to a survey of training directors of counseling psychology programs in the United States, only 18% of the directors indicated that their graduate program offered a course that focused on religion or spirituality (Schulte, Skinner, & Claiborn, 2002). Only 13% of training directors of clinical psychology programs in the United States and Canada reported that their curriculum included a course on religion and spirituality (Brawer, Handal, Fabricatore, Roberts, & Wajda-Johnston, 2002). Most young professionals leave graduate school unprepared to address the spiritual and religious issues that they will face in their work. This state of affairs is a reflection of the deeply seated assumption within the mental health field that spirituality is, at most, a side issue in psychotherapy, one that can be either sidestepped or resolved through an education to reality. I believe this assumption is just plain wrong. There are, in fact, a number of good reasons to take the spiritual dimension of life far more seriously and to integrate it far more fully into the process of psychotherapy.

A RATIONALE FOR A SPIRITUALLY
INTEGRATED PSYCHOTHERAPY

Spirituality Can Be Part of the Solution

Although mental health professionals have often viewed spirituality more as a cause of problems than as a source of solutions, stories like Alice's suggest that this attitude toward spirituality is out of kilter. Of course, any single case could be the exception rather than the rule, but research studies show that Alice's story is not unusual. Many people look to their spirituality for support and guidance in times of stress. In fact, for some groups spirituality is one of the most commonly used methods of coping. For example, Bulman and Wortman (1977) asked people who had been paralyzed in severe accidents how they explained their situation. The most common response to the question "Why me?" was "God had a reason." In a study of black and white elderly women facing medical problems, prayer emerged as the most frequent method of coping (Conway, 1985–1986). Ninety-one percent of the women coped through prayer, more than the number who coped through going to a doctor, resting, using prescription drugs, or seeking information. The United States as a whole sought support and solace from religion following the September 11 terrorist attacks; 90% of a random sample of people drawn from across the United States said they coped with their feelings after the disaster by turning to religion (Schuster et al., 2001). And, it is important to add, many people are supported and sustained not only in times of major stress but in their daily lives by involvement in regular religious practices.

Most people who look to their faith for support find it helpful. In studies of veterans of combat, hospital patients, parents of children with physical handicaps, widows, and physically abused spouses, 50–85% of the studies' participants reported that religion was helpful to them in coping with their difficult situations (Pargament, 1997).

Do the same findings hold true for people experiencing serious psychological problems? Expressions of spirituality among this group have often been seen as symptoms of an illness rather than as signs of a potentially valuable resource for coping with that illness. A few empirical studies have challenged this perspective. For example, in a survey of more than 400 people with serious mental illness, over 80% reported that they used some sort of religious belief or practice to help them cope with their symptoms and daily problems (Tepper, Rogers, Coleman, & Malony, 2001). They had been engaged in religious coping for an average of 16 years. Most (65%) found their religious coping helpful, and 30% indicated that their religious beliefs or practices were the most important things they had to keep them going. Religious coping when symptoms worsened was also tied to fewer hospitalizations. Studies of people with eating disorders have yielded similar findings; spiritual resources are often described by individuals as critical to their recovery (see Richards, Hardman, & Berrett, 2007, for a review).

These findings are clear. Many, if not most, people in the United States draw on their spirituality when they encounter significant problems. The same holds true for people with serious mental disorders. Why might this be the case? In later chapters, I talk about the specific resources of spirituality and what they add to peoples' lives. For now, I would like to make a more general point. There is a deeper dimension to our problems. Illness, accident, interpersonal conflicts, divorce, layoffs, and death are more than "significant life events." They raise profound and disturbing questions about our place and purpose in the world, they point to the limits of our powers, and they underscore our finitude. These are, as theologian Paul Tillich (1952) put it, matters of "ultimate anxiety": the anxiety of fate and death, the anxiety of emptiness and meaninglessness, and the anxiety of guilt and condemnation. These deep questions seem to call for a spiritual response.

The solutions prescribed by modern psychology are insufficient. I have argued elsewhere that U.S. psychology is largely a psychology of control (Pargament, 1997). In spite of their differences, all the major paradigms of psychotherapy share an interest in helping people maximize the control they have in their lives. Within psychodynamic therapy, patients are encouraged to make the unconscious conscious. Behaviorally oriented therapists help their clients unlearn maladaptive reactions and replace them with new skills that provide greater mastery and competence. Cognitive therapists teach their clients how to identify and control irrational and self-defeating thoughts.

This picture has begun to change in recent years. With the rise of positive psychology (Peterson & Seligman, 2004), the development of new treatments, such as acceptance and commitment therapy (ACT; Hayes, Strosahl, & Wilson, 1999), and the introduction of Buddhist thought into Western psychology (Wallace & Shapiro, 2006), a new set of more spiritually friendly terms has begun to enter the psychological lexicon, terms such as "mindfulness," "acceptance," "virtues," "detachment," "being present." Nevertheless, promising as they are, these are recent developments, and our discipline remains largely a psychology of control.

Yet there is a limit to how much we can control. Anthropologist Clifford Geertz (1968) put it this way: "The events through which we live are forever outrunning the power of our ordinary, everyday moral, emotional, and intellectual concepts to construe them, leaving us, as a Javanese image has it, like a water buffalo listening to an orchestra" (p. 101). Spirituality helps people come to terms with human limitations. It offers solutions to problems that are not merely substitutes for secular solutions, including those that psychologists often advocate. In response to the unfathomable and uncontrollable, it speaks a language that is relatively unfamiliar to psychology. We hear strange words such as "forbearance," "faith," "suffering," "compassion," "transformation," "transcendence," "sacredness," "hope," "surrender," "love," and "forgiveness." These terms should not be quickly dismissed as merely soft and sentimental, for they embody deep yearnings, powerful emotions, and more generally a different way of viewing the world. Through the spiritual lens, people can see their lives in a broad, transcendent perspective; they can discern deeper truths in ordinary and extraordinary experience; and they can locate timeless values that offer grounding and direction in shifting times and circumstances. Through a spiritual lens, problems take on a different character and distinctive solutions appear: answers to seemingly unanswerable questions, support when other sources of support are unavailable, and new sources of value and significance when old dreams are no longer viable. Spirituality, then, represents a distinctive resource for living, one particularly well suited to the struggle with human limitations and finitude. By bringing the spiritual dimension into the helping process, psychotherapists could tap more fully into this reservoir of hope and source of solutions to life's most profound problems.

It is important to add one word of caution for those interested in drawing more fully on spirituality in psychotherapy. Spiritual resources are not simply another problem-solving tool. They are, instead, embedded in a larger worldview. As I stress throughout this book, spiritual resources are, first and foremost, designed to facilitate an individual's spiritual journey. Therapists who overlook the larger sacred purpose and meaning of these resources risk trivializing spirituality by reducing it to nothing more than a set of psychological techniques.

Spirituality Can Be Part of the Problem

Freud, Skinner, and other psychologists who have criticized religion haven't been wrong so much as they have been incomplete. They have focused on the dark side of faith to the exclusion of its other qualities. And yet there is, in fact, a "seamy side" to religion, as Paul Pruyser (1977) put it. Several years ago, Lynn came to my office quite distraught, crying, wringing her hands, and repeatedly telling me that she just didn't know what to do. She had recently discovered that her husband of 15 years, a minister in a conservative church, had been having an affair with another church member. Lynn was 35 years old, the mother of four children, and devoutly Christian. She was devastated by her husband's affair. How could he have violated their sacred vows? she asked. What about the commitments he had made not only to her but to God? And what about her own confusion? How could she leave a marriage that she defined as holy? But how could she remain in a marriage that had been desecrated by the actions of her husband? How could she return to the marriage when her husband refused to end his affair? In my initial and, as it turned out, only session with Lynn, I tried to empathize with her feelings of hurt, embarrassment, and anger toward her husband. I reflected on the difficult choice she seemed to be facing and offered her hope that she would be able to come to a resolution for herself. And I let her know I would do all I could to help her through her crisis. We agreed to meet again in a week.

In the middle of the week, I received a call from Lynn. Gone were the tears and turmoil she had been experiencing just a few days earlier. Lynn told me that she had had a dream the previous night. God had come to her and reassured her that if she continued in her marriage, He would soften her husband's heart. (I was thinking a good knock over the husband's head might be more appropriate, but I didn't share that thought.) God, she said, was going to solve their problems for them. I tried to convince Lynn to come back to therapy for another session so we could talk about her dream and her marriage, but she declined. She thanked me for my concern and hung up the phone fully convinced that her problems were a thing of the past. I hung up the phone fully convinced that she was heading for a great deal of trouble.

Spirituality, in this case, was a central part of the problem. It was problematic in two respects. The crisis Lynn was facing was more than marital, psychological, or even existential. It was spiritual. Lynn viewed her husband's actions as a desecration, a violation of something that she held sacred. Life crises that are perceived as spiritual threats, violations, or losses take on a special power and meaning. As Elkins (1995) has written, "Some violations and betrayals . . . wound so deeply that they can only be called abuses to the soul" (p. 91). As we will see in later chapters, these kinds of crises are associated with particularly powerful emotional and physical reactions. Therapists who overlook the spiritual nature of the problem may be neglecting the heart of the matter. In my "postmortem" of my single session with Lynn, I wondered whether I too was guilty of this neglect. Had I failed to acknowledge the fact that Lynn's crisis was as much spiritual as it was marital? And was that one important reason why she turned away from psychotherapy to a more direct religious form of help?

Spirituality, for Lynn, was problematic in a second respect. In her rush to find a resolution of her conflict, she found a religious solution to her problem that, in my view, was likely to make matters worse. In essence, she let God decide for her. We know that sometimes deferral to God or surrender to God is a perfectly reasonable thing to do, particularly in situations that fall outside the realm of our personal control. Lynn's problem, however, called for more personal initiative, interpersonal dialogue with her husband, and collaboration with God. Lynn's solution, spiritual deferral, relieved her of any responsibility she might have shared with God for her life and for her marriage. Because her solution was poorly suited to the demands of the situation, her spiritual solution had become a spiritual problem. It is difficult to imagine how this problem could be ignored or side-stepped in psychotherapy. Had Lynn returned to my office, I would have encouraged her to talk about her relationship with God and, had she been willing, I would have helped her explore how she might become more of a full-fledged partner in this relationship.

Spiritual solutions do, at times, become spiritual problems. As we will see in later chapters, there are several kinds of spiritual problems, including problems associated with spiritual pathways and problems associated with spiritual destinations. These problems reflect a "dis-integrated spirituality," one lacking harmony and balance, and one ill-equipped to deal with the range of critical situations people are likely to confront.

Jung wrote that, of his patients over 35, "there has not been one whose problem in the last resort was not that of finding a religious outlook on life" (1933, p. 264). I think Jung overstated his point: many, but certainly not all, problems are spiritual in nature. Nevertheless, crises, traumas, and the accumulation of hurt and disappointment impact people spiritually as well as psychologically, socially, and physically (Hathaway, 2003). Furthermore, spiritual solutions can lead to trouble in their own right. Practitioners cannot afford to overlook the spiritual dimension of problems. By recognizing that spirituality may serve as a source of solutions or a source of problems, clinicians better equip themselves to address the full range, richness, and complexity of the spiritual dimension in psychotherapy.

Spirituality Cannot Be Separated from Psychotherapy

Unfortunately, many therapists remain uncomfortable about the topic of spirituality, unsure about how to deal with spiritual issues, or fearful of intruding in areas too private even for psychotherapy. As a result, they do their best to avoid the spiritual domain. Of course, this may be about as easy as avoiding a conversation about the 3,000-pound elephant in the therapy room. Even if it goes unmentioned, the proverbial elephant has a way of making its presence known.

Spirituality cannot be separated from psychotherapy, no matter how hard we try. Let me give a few examples. My colleague, Mark Rye, and I were interested in comparing the effects of two forgiveness interventions on women attending a state university who had been wronged in a romantic relationship (Rye & Pargament, 2002). One of the forgiveness interventions was explicitly religious in nature; it drew upon religious models and spiritual beliefs in a program designed to help the participants let go of their anger, bitterness, and resentment. The other forgiveness intervention was explicitly secular in nature; the group leader purposely avoided raising religious or spiritual topics in the forgiveness program. As it turned out, the two groups proved to be equally effective in facilitating forgiveness and well-being.

In our efforts to learn more about their experiences, we asked participants in both groups to describe the strategies that they used to help them forgive their offenders. We were surprised by what the secular group participants had to say. Two of their three top strategies for forgiveness were spiritual in nature: "I asked God for help and/or support as I was trying to forgive" and "I prayed for the person who wronged me as I was trying to forgive." Even though their therapy group was explicitly secular in nature, participants in the secular group were as likely as those in the religious forgiveness group to make use of spiritual resources! Our "secular" group turned out to be something other than purely secular. I suspect that the same process takes place among clients who are receiving ostensibly secular psychotherapy. Spirituality continues to be a relevant resource or a source of problems for people even when it goes unaddressed in psychotherapy.

Secular psychotherapy is not designed to affect people spiritually, and yet spiritual changes are likely to accompany other changes that unfold through the clinical process. Tisdale et al. (1997) illustrated this point in an evaluation of the impact of a psychiatric inpatient treatment program. The treatment was secular in nature and included individual, group, milieu, and psychotropic interventions. Not surprisingly, patients in treatment made significant improvements in their personal adjustment. But Tisdale et al. also included a measure of images of God. They found that the secular inpatient treatment resulted in significant shifts among the patients toward more positive images of God. Once again, I suspect that this is not an unusual finding. The spiritual dimension of life is fully interwoven with other life domains, such that efforts to create change along one dimension are likely to affect the other dimensions as well.

We can try to ignore the elephant, but that doesn't make it go away. Instead, it may lead to problems. "Ignorance of spiritual constructs and experience," Bergin and Payne (1991) write, "predispose a therapist to misjudge, misinterpret, misunderstand, mismanage, or neglect important segments of a client's life which may impact significantly on adjustment or growth" (p. 201). Spirituality is a part of the psychotherapy process; our choice is either to look the other way and proceed with limited vision or to address spirituality more directly and knowingly.

People Want Spiritually Sensitive Help

Certainly, many clinicians might worry about overstepping their bounds by raising spiritual issues in the context of psychotherapy. Some evidence suggests, however, that a good proportion of our potential clients would welcome spiritually integrated treatment. It is important to remember that, although therapists may treat religion as a background variable, for many people religion is part of the foreground (Koltko, 1990). In response to a national survey, two-thirds of the sample agreed that "religion can answer all or most of today's problems" (Smith, 1992). Signs of renewed religious and spiritual interest surround us, from PBS specials and lead articles in *Newsweek* and *Time* on religion to widespread preoccupations with angels, religious visions, and near-death experiences. And it has been hard to ignore the religious roots and significance of recent major traumas, including the September 11, 2001, terrorist attacks, violence in the Middle East, sexual abuse in the ministry, and the moral scandals that have wracked the business world.

An interest in religion is not put aside when people walk through the door to treatment. For example, many people with medical illness seek out alternative forms of therapy that include prayer, exercise, rituals, and traditional healers (Lukoff, Lu, & Turner, 1992). With respect to standard medical treatment, a significant number of patients report spiritual needs and a desire for greater integration of religious and spiritual care into their treatment (Post, Puchalski, & Larson, 2000). In a survey conducted in an inpatient rehabilitation unit, 45% of the patients said that too little attention was paid to their spiritual and religious concerns, and 73% indicated that no one from the staff spoke to them about spiritual matters (Post et al., 2000). According to another national poll, 48% of patients would like their physicians to pray with them, and 64% believe that physicians should pray with their patients if the patients ask (Post et al., 2000).

Do people seeking psychological treatment feel differently? Only a few studies have looked at this question, but they too suggest that people are looking for spiritually sensitive care. For example, in a survey of clients at six mental health centers, Rose, Westefeld, and Ansley (2001) found that 55% reported that they would like to talk about religious or spiritual concerns in counseling. Similarly, two-thirds of a sample of adults with serious mental illness indicated that they would like to discuss spiritual concerns with their therapists, but only half of this group was doing so (Lindgren & Coursey, 1995). My graduate students and I had a very similar experience when we developed a spiritual discussion group for people with serious mental illness who were being treated in a local community mental health center (Phillips, Lakin, & Pargament, 2002). The participants welcomed the opportunity to talk about the role of religion and spirituality in their lives. In their many years of treatment by many practitioners, this was the first chance they had had to talk about spiritual matters. Furthermore, talking about spiritual issues did not, as far as we could tell, trigger any aversive psychological symptoms.

If my own experiences are any guide, many of our clients would welcome us into their spiritual homes if we knocked on the door. It seems that the reluctance to visit is largely ours. And yet I don't believe that we clinicians are a soulless bunch, a collection of well-intended but narrow-minded empiricists who cannot spell "transcendent" let alone integrate it into psychotherapy. In fact, many of us resonate strongly to the spiritual side of life (see Bergin, 1991). In my visits to other universities, I have consistently found that a number of psychology faculty and graduate students had, at one time, studied for the ministry. Many of us, I suspect, were initially drawn into the field of psychology for religious and spiritual reasons. I know that was true for me. And yet my psychological training was not fully satisfying. I didn't enjoy the mechanistic views that seemed to underlie the approaches to treatment that were the bread and butter of clinical training in graduate school. There was something missing. Many practitioners feel the same way: there is something missing in the way we do our work. Thus, it is not only our clients who might welcome the integration of spirituality into psychotherapy; we as therapists may be yearning for the same thing.

There are, in short, several good reasons to integrate the spiritual dimension more fully into the process of psychotherapy. But how do we do that? In this book, I describe a spiritually integrated psychotherapy. Though some readers may be hoping for a short recipe or even a lengthier cookbook, I cannot offer that. There is no typical course of spiritually integrated psychotherapy because spirituality expresses itself in so many ways. There are no definitive guidelines about spiritually integrated psychotherapy because we have only begun to learn about the spiritual worlds of our clients. What I can offer in this book is a perspective on spirituality and psychotherapy, both conceptual and practical. This will not be the final word on the topic. But it will be a start. My hope is that this book will offer some direction and encouragement to practitioners who are interested in understanding and addressing spirituality in treatment. As a prelude to the following chapters, let me highlight the essential features of a spiritually integrated psychotherapy.

ENVISIONING A SPIRITUALLY INTEGRATED PSYCHOTHERAPY

Explicit

Psychiatrist Irvin Yalom (1980) began his book on existential psychotherapy by relating a personal experience. He had taken a cooking class with an expert chef, yet, try as he might, he found himself unable to duplicate the chef's dishes. What special ingredients, he asked himself, was he missing? He came upon the answer one day. As the chef's servant was taking the dish to the oven, Yalom noticed that the chef was walking alongside, throwing in handfuls of varied spices and condiments. These "throw-ins," Yalom realized, "made all the difference" (p. 3). In therapy too, he suggests, the ingredients critical to success may be added when no one is paying attention.

Spirituality is one such critical but hidden ingredient. Spiritual issues often arise in psychotherapy, but without the conscious recognition of clients and therapists. While the explicit content of psychotherapy is focusing on the various causes of and solutions to emotional distress, problems in the home, physical symptoms, or relational conflicts, change may be taking place at a spiritual level. Unbeknownst to the therapist and the client him- or herself, the client may be uncovering sacred losses and violations, identifying and accessing spiritual resources, raising and resolving questions of ultimate meaning, or investing a therapeutic relationship with sacred character. Occasionally, a therapist may have a sense that something deeper is taking place. Consider the comments of Carl Rogers, a humanistic psychologist and the founder of client-centered therapy, who, in a dialogue with theologian Paul Tillich, admitted, "I feel at times when I'm really being helpful to a client of mine . . . there is something approximating an I–Thou relationship between us, then I feel as though I am somehow in tune with the forces of the universe or that forces are operating through me in regard to this helping relationship" (Rogers, 1989, p. 74). And yet, although therapists may sense something going on in the background of psychotherapy, most do not move spirituality from the background to the foreground. Rogers, for one, did not raise spiritual issues in the context of counseling. Similarly, the founders of ACT, a therapy that is embedded in a spiritual matrix strongly influenced by Buddhist thought (see Hayes, 1984), prefer to keep the spiritual dimension of treatment in the background. "ACT," they write, "has an inherent and wordless spiritual quality" (Hayes et al., 1999, p. 273). They caution the therapist that "spiritual and religion as such are discussed only if the client brings these issues into the room" (p. 273).

In contrast, spiritually integrated psychotherapy assumes that clients often bring spiritual issues into the room, and encourages clients to give voice to what may be difficult to express. A spiritually integrated psychotherapy makes the implicit explicit. Within this form of treatment, therapists and clients speak openly to spirituality as a significant dimension in its own right, one that is not reduced to presumably more basic psychological or social processes. Therapists and clients identify more clearly what the client holds sacred. They talk more directly about how spirituality may be a part of the clients' problems, a part of the clients' solutions, or a part of the therapeutic relationship. And in the process of making the implicit more explicit, clients and therapists can make better use of one potentially critical ingredient of success in psychotherapy.

Psychospiritual

Spiritually integrated psychotherapy is both spiritual and psychological in character. How is it spiritual? Spirituality is the central phenomenon of interest in this approach to treatment. As noted above, spirituality receives explicit attention as a dimension that shapes and is shaped by other aspects of life, and as a dimension of significance in and of itself. In working with spirituality, the therapist recognizes that he or she is dealing with sacred matters, that the subjects of conversation will range from timeless truths and unfathomable mysteries to transcendence and the hereafter. The therapist also appreciates that the client is describing what are perceived to be sacred realities in his or her life, realities that express themselves in many forms, be they revelations, divine signs, a sense of calling, healings, mystical experiences, higher standards to live by, or a sense of being in communication with God.

But spiritually integrated therapy is psychological as well as spiritual in nature. What makes this approach to treatment psychological? I want to stress that spiritually integrated therapy is not grounded in religious authority or legitimacy. Unlike the pastoral counselor, the therapist cannot claim to offer absolute truth or to deliver the rituals and sacraments of a religious tradition. From a psychological perspective, the practitioner cannot know in an ontological sense what is true, what (if anything) is actually sacred, or whether there is a divine power and, if so, what is its nature. This is not to say that therapists do not live, personally and professionally, according to truths of their own. Like everyone else, clinicians are guided by their own and a larger professional set of ethical and moral values. Paramount among these values, however, is the commitment to help clients discover and live out the truths of *their* own lives as *they* perceive and experience these truths. Toward this end, spiritually integrated therapy draws upon two psychological resources.

The first psychological resource is theory. Spiritually integrated psychotherapy rests on a systematic way of thinking about spirituality. Being able to think clearly about spirituality is a prerequisite to working with this dimension in treatment. After all, how can we integrate spirituality into psychotherapy if we cannot define what spirituality is? How can we integrate spirituality into psychotherapy if we don't know how spirituality develops and changes over the lifespan? How can we integrate spirituality into psychotherapy if we cannot tell when spirituality is a source of problems and when it is a source of solutions? Existing models of personality, psychopathology, and psychotherapy offer some insights, but they fall far short of providing a conceptual road map capable of guiding us in our work. A spiritually integrated psychotherapy requires the devotion of theoretical attention to concrete problems, concrete solutions, and everyday struggles with the question of how to define a life well lived. One of the major goals of this book is to provide therapists with a way to think about spirituality.

The second psychological resource is research. When it comes to spirituality and psychotherapy, few of us are expert in what we are doing—at least not yet. Questions far outnumber answers. How do we address the spirituality of our clients? How do we address our own spirituality in the context of treatment? What forms of spiritual intervention are most helpful to our clients? What do we do when we believe their faith is misguided, or when we feel their faith is destructive to them or to those around them? We can try to answer these questions solely on the basis of our own instincts, values, and worldviews, or we can put some of our ideas to test and see what the world has to teach us. Psychology takes the latter approach. Fortunately, a number of researchers have begun to examine the links among spirituality, health, and well-being. And a small but growing number of scientists have also begun to evaluate the impact of spiritually integrated psychotherapy on clients from diverse religious traditions. Whenever possible, I draw on the emerging empirical literature in this book.

Of course, a scientific approach to spirituality may sound strange to those who see science in terms of observation, skepticism, and hard facts and spirituality in terms of intangibles, faith, and deeply seated values. Yet these distinctions have been overdrawn (Barbour, 1974). There are places where the scientific sentiment and the religious sentiment come together. As David Bakan (1966) has noted, at their core, both science and religion grow out of an openness to surprise, deep feelings of wonder at the mysteries of the universe, and a desire to make manifest the unmanifest. We have an exciting opportunity now to tap into this common sentiment, drawing on knowledge gleaned from scientific explorations to assist people in their own spiritual journeys.

Pluralistic

The world is becoming increasingly diverse religiously. This point certainly holds true for the United States, which is seeing a sharp increase in the number of spiritual organizations, immigrants that bring with them diverse religious traditions, and alternative spiritualities (Hoge, 1996). Here, "Hindu yogis teach next door to South American shamans, and Congregationalist churches share their space with Buddhist and Taoist communities. Jewish men and women become Zen masters and Catholics priests learn Japanese forms of meditation and purification" (Anderson & Hopkins, 1991, p. 122).

Over the course of their careers, few psychotherapists will find it possible to work entirely with clients from their own or familiar religious traditions. Even when working with clients from their own traditions, therapists will encounter more and more clients who have created their own idiosyncratic religions à la carte (Bibby, 1987), picking and choosing selectively from the menu of options their traditions provide them or experimenting with beliefs and practices that fall outside of their own tradition. To speak of *the* Christian, *the* Jewish, *the* Buddhist, *the* Hindu, or *the* Muslim approach to psychotherapy is a misnomer. The spiritually integrated psychotherapist will need to be spiritually multilingual in years to come.

Admittedly, much of the theory and research on spirituality and psychotherapy has grown out of the context of a Western monotheistic perspective that has shaped our worldview in subtle and perhaps not-so-subtle ways. I too am part of this context and culture, and undoubtedly this book reflects a Western bias. Whenever possible, however, I try to correct this bias by reaching out to the religious and clinical wisdom from other cultures and traditions.

Integrative[2]

Spirituality is not divorced from the psychological, social, and physical dimensions of life—far from it. The power of spirituality lies in the fact that it is fully embedded in the fabric of life. As James Hillman (1975) put it, "Psychology does not take place without religion, because there is always a God in what we are doing" (p. 228). The connections are not always smooth; at times, spirituality clashes with other aspects of life, forcing the individual to make hard choices between competing interests. More often, though, spiritual growth and decline go hand in hand with growth and decline in other spheres of life. Facilitating greater spiritual integration can enhance the well-being of the individual not only spiritually, but also psychologically, socially, and physically. For this reason, it makes little sense to overlook the spiritual dimension in psychotherapy. Yet that is also why it makes no more sense to focus solely on spirituality in psychotherapy, for spirituality cannot be approached in isolation from the client's life as a whole.

Spiritually integrated psychotherapy should not be viewed as a new competitor on the block, a rival to other treatments. It neither competes with nor replaces other forms of help. Spiritually integrated psychotherapy is just that, "integrated." It weaves greater sensitivity and explicit attention to the spiritual domain into the process of psychotherapy. In this book, I hope to show that spirituality can be interwoven into virtually any psychotherapeutic tradition: psychodynamic, cognitive-behavioral, family systems, interpersonal, experiential, humanistic, or existential. However, through this process of integration, I believe the character of each of these forms of psychotherapy will be deepened and enriched, and perhaps psychotherapy as a whole will be transformed, for we will have to discover ways to understand and address the extraordinary dimension that is part of the ordinary lives of people.

---

[2]The term "integration" is often used by conservative Christian psychologists and counselors to describe the process of synthesizing Christian theology and psychotherapy (e.g., Eck, 1996; Worthington, 1994). In contrast, spiritually integrated psychotherapy refers to integration in a broader sense. This form of treatment can draw on the resources of a variety of traditions, depending on the needs and preferences of the particular client. Spiritually integrated therapy can be applied to clients from diverse religious and nonreligious backgrounds by therapists from diverse religious and nonreligious backgrounds.

Value Laden

All forms of psychotherapy rest on values. These values are, in some sense, unprovable. Is human nature basically good or evil? Do people have free will or are they shaped by external and internal forces? How do we define the "good life"? Answers to these questions reflect fundamental assumptions about life that shape all human pursuits, including psychotherapy. Various forms of psychotherapy manifest quite different worldviews. They offer, in the words of Don Browning (1987), different "cultures" of symbols, images, and metaphors of human nature. In Freud, we find a "culture of detachment that sees the world as basically hostile and humans as largely self-absorbed creatures with only small amounts of energy for larger altruistic ventures" (p. 5). Implicit in the humanistic psychologies is a "culture of joy [that] sees the world as basically harmonious [and] human wants and needs as easily reconciled and coordinated in almost frictionless compatibility" (p. 5). Behavioral psychologies provide yet another culture, a culture of control in which humans are viewed "as primarily controlled and controllable by the manipulative power of various environments" (p. 6).

Spiritually integrated psychotherapy is no less value laden than any other form of treatment. Of course, spiritually integrated psychotherapy is also no more value laden than other treatments, though the values of spiritual therapy may be more apparent. This may be more of an advantage than a disadvantage, however, for the danger is not in bringing values to treatment. That is inevitable. As Stanton Jones (1994) noted, "One cannot intervene in the fabric of human life without getting deeply involved in moral and religious matters" (p. 197). The attempt to adopt a therapeutic neutrality may lead only to a psychology lacking in spirit. Presumably value-free, the "neutral" therapist may, in fact, take on and promote the goals of the larger social context even if that context is destructive. When it comes to values, the real danger is not in having values, but rather in *imposing* values, spiritual or secular, knowingly or unknowingly, on clients in the therapeutic setting.

Greater openness is one of the most important antidotes to the risks of value imposition in psychotherapy. In this book, I try to make the underlying assumptions of spiritually integrated psychotherapy as visible as possible by explicitly discussing value-laden topics and by taking explicit stands on these issues: the meaning of spirituality, the criteria of spiritual health and well-being, and the stance therapists should take regarding spiritual issues in psychotherapy.

Values are not only a part of therapeutic orientations, they are also embedded in the lives of individual therapists. Forged over time by personal history, temperament, habits, dreams, relationships, and a larger culture, each of us brings our own deep-seated assumptions about life to psychotherapy. And each of us also runs the risk of imposing our personal views on clients. Again, however, one of the best remedies for this potential problem is greater explicitness about our own values, combined with respect for the client's right to choose. In this spirit of openness, let me conclude this chapter by presenting a bit of personal background as well as some personal beliefs and values that undoubtedly shape my work.

A PERSONAL NOTE

One of the first stories I can remember was about my childhood nextdoor neighbor, Lester. Les was a bear of a man with thick eyebrows set atop a pair of twinkling eyes, a broad nose, and a huge smile that continues to warm me as I recall it now, some 50 years later. Whenever I saw Les in the neighborhood, he would welcome me with a loud "Kenny!," a crushing hug, and a handshake that enveloped my tiny hands in fingers the size of small trees. Les seemed larger than life. One day my parents told me something about Lester's history. He had been raised in a poor Jewish shtetl (village) in eastern Russia, a part of the country in which Jews suffered periodic pogroms (massacres) carried out by peasants from surrounding villages. In hushed tones, my parents described how Lester had hidden himself in the cellar of his barn as one such pogrom swept through his small town. There he watched in silence as his father was caught by the peasants and hanged. Shortly after, Les was able to escape to the United States. It was hard for me to imagine that this seemingly indestructible force had witnessed this terrible scene and come close to death himself. Lester was vulnerable and life was precarious.

This sense of precariousness was imprinted upon me as a child of the Holocaust generation (in which every Jewish family on our block seemed to have its own story of tragedy), and as I came of age in the time of the race riots of the 1960s (when we lost the family business) and the Vietnam War (when my cousin, born a week earlier than me, joined the military after receiving a draft number of 3 in the lottery in contrast to my draft number of 348). Like most families, ours has also been touched by illness, loss, violence, death, and disappointments over the years . . . events that serve as further reminders of life's tenuousness.

I went into psychology in search of firmer ground, a way to make life a little less precarious. Unfortunately, much of the psychology I encountered was disturbing in its own right, offering up bleak, mechanistic views of people driven by unseen forces or shaped by powerful external contingencies. I stayed in the field, but I began to read about religion.

Although I had been born in a Conservative Jewish family, had my bar mitzvah at age 13, and had participated in the regular round of Jewish rituals over the years, not until my 20s did I discover that I had a Jewish soul. Reading Irving Howe's (1976) rich account of the journey of Jews from

Europe to the United States in the 19th and 20th centuries, I came across descriptions of people who could have been (and perhaps were) members of my family: people holding close to loved ones, sheltering them against dangers that never seemed too far off; faces with prominent dark eyes filled with a melancholy about the human condition and a yearning for better times; scholars devoting their lives to study, eager for knowledge, skeptical of sure answers, intensely curious about the workings of the world; introspective minds struggling with moral anxieties about how best to conduct oneself in life; passionate activists, zealots too, committed to bringing about a more equitable society; and always comedians and storytellers offering distance and perspective on the craziness of the world, reminding us not to take ourselves too seriously. "Man plans," we are reminded, "God laughs." Being Jewish, I learned, was more than a label, more than an affiliation, it was a quality of spirit. In reading Howe's stories, I was reading about myself and I discovered that I had a Jewish soul. Totally intrigued by this discovery, I wanted to learn more.

Early on, I decided that if I were to pursue the study of religion and spirituality, I could not focus exclusively on Judaism. I needed to know more about the religions of the world, or at least my part of the world. So I began to broaden my readings. In addition, I started to talk to people from different religious traditions. With time, I began to contemplate a far more difficult step: visits to people in their religious "homes," their churches and other meeting places. This was a scary thought. What business did a Jew have attending the services of other faiths, I asked myself? Was I a traitor to my own tradition? Would I face scorn from members of the church? Was it even safe to walk inside? Catastrophic fantasies arose: I enter a church service in progress, the service comes to an abrupt halt, a silence follows as members slowly turn around in unison, pointing their fingers accusingly at me, and shouting "Jew, Jew." But I went ahead with my plan anyway.

Going to church was one of the smartest decisions of my life. Large, small, black, white, conservative, liberal, Catholic, Protestant, Greek Orthodox—the churches welcomed me, educated me, and challenged me. In the process, I came face to face with my own deep-seated religious stereotypes. In contrast to my preconceptions, I found beauty and power in diverse religious traditions: the deep expressions of emotion in religious testimony, the religious support offered by clergy and members to fellow congregants going through hard times, the transformations people experienced as they took communion. I discovered that I was able to learn from other traditions while remaining true to my own. In fact, my experiences with other faiths enriched rather than diminished my appreciation for Judaism. Today, I continue my process of learning through readings, conversations, visits to different congregations, teaching, research, and clinical practice.

Out of this background of experiences, I have arrived at some basic beliefs. These beliefs are not provable or disprovable; they are pretty well fixed. But they certainly shape my way of looking at the world. Let me highlight a few of my beliefs that have special relevance to this book.

I was a small, slow-growing child. Concerned about me, my mother took me to my pediatrician. He checked me over and announced, "Well, he's healthy, but he'll never be a football player." My pediatrician was right. Much as I loved sports, I was never to be a football player (nor any other type of athlete). Genetics, biology, and the environment certainly limit our possibilities. Even so, powerful as they are, these forces do not limit all possibilities. People are more than reactive. We are also active, volitional beings who strive toward any number of imagined futures. In this process, we are constantly choosing. Choices come in a variety of shapes and sizes: well-thought-out choices that emerge from a judicious weighing of values, goals, pros, cons, and potential consequences; automatic choices that take place with little conscious consideration; and foolish choices that seem to defy logic or reason.

Each of us, I believe, has the capacity to choose and this capacity creates the opportunity to live many possible lives. To take it one step further, I believe each of us has the capacity to commit good or bad acts at any time. The individual who has led a decent life can slip up and, in a single moment, cross a moral and ethical line that destroys the work of a lifetime. Conversely, the individual who has been a source of terrible misery and pain to others and him- or herself can reach a turning point and take a dramatically new and more fulfilling direction. When I speak of good and bad, I am not thinking of a singular trait, action, or quality. I believe the good life has to do with the way we balance and integrate varied and, at times, conflicting visions, desires, pressures, and constraints. What matters is how we put it all together.

Finally, I believe in God. God has never spoken directly to me, as far as I know. My belief in God comes secondhand. It grows out of experiences in which I have sensed larger forces at play in the universe. These experiences have been elicited by a number of triggers: something majestic (my first glimpse into the Grand Canyon), a wondrous human creation (Mozart's *Symphony No. 40*), a personal encounter (my work with Alice)—to name just a few. In these moments, I feel I have encountered something sacred, something transcendent, paradoxically set apart from and yet a part of ordinary life. These experiences are, I believe, manifestations of God in the concrete world.

Of course, mine is not the only way to understand God. Nor is mine the only pathway to the divine. There are, I believe, many worthwhile spiritual roads and destinations. What they share is a concern for things sacred. I believe that whatever its form, the search for the sacred in life is the most distinctively human of all pursuits.

We have good reasons, then, to turn our attention to spirituality, to learn more about it, and to address it as a significant dimension of the lives of our clients. It is time to begin.

In the first half of this book, I suggest a way to think about spirituality. Specifically, I offer a definition of spirituality and introduce readers to the way spirituality works as a natural part of life. Spirituality is not defined as "inherently good." I emphasize the idea that spirituality can lead toward growth or decline. To evaluate the strengths and weaknesses of various approaches to spirituality, I present a framework that centers on the concept of spiritual integration. Building on this understanding, I then shift to how the therapist addresses spirituality in psychotherapy in the second portion of the book, focusing specifically on the challenges of assessment and intervention in the spiritual domain.

Part II

UNDERSTANDING
THE SACRED

2

Spirituality

The Sacred Domain

Sherry, one of my first clinical supervisees, was very nervous about her first case. Recalling my own fears as a novice therapist, I walked Sherry through the first session and then had her role-play with a fellow graduate student serving as the client. Things seemed to be going well. She did a fine job of introducing herself to the client, making him feel comfortable, and encouraging him to talk about his concerns. But at that point Sherry stopped. The silence in the room grew longer and longer. A blush began to creep up Sherry's neck until her face became crimson. She turned around to me and with a look of total bewilderment asked, "What do I do now?" I was about to offer Sherry some more concrete pointers, but stopped myself. The problem went deeper than that. Sherry was lost. She was missing a "map" of psychotherapy that could guide her through the first and subsequent sessions. Before she could "do" psychotherapy, she had to have a way to think about people, problems, and change.

This same point holds true for spiritually integrated psychotherapy. Before we as therapists can address spiritual issues in psychotherapy, we have to have a way to think about spirituality: what it is, how it works, how to evaluate it. Without a way to understand spirituality, practitioners are likely to get lost in the spiritual domain. Like Sherry, we need a map that can guide us through spiritual territory, pointing to the landmarks along the way, the directions to pursue, and the barriers to avoid. Understanding spirituality is not an irrelevant intellectual exercise; it is part and parcel of addressing spirituality in psychotherapy.

In this section of the book, I offer a way to understand spirituality as a foundation for intervention. This chapter focuses on the substantive core of spirituality: the sacred. In subsequent chapters of Part II, I examine the working mechanisms of spirituality: discovery, conservation, and transformation. I emphasize the point that spirituality is a natural, normal dimension of life. Spirituality is, for the most part, a source of health and well-being. Yet spirituality can be a source of problems as well as solutions; it is not inherently positive. I conclude Part II with a framework for understanding the strengths and weaknesses of spirituality in the life of the individual.

PRELUDE: THE EVOLVING MEANINGS OF SPIRITUALITY AND RELIGIOUSNESS

Spirituality has become an increasingly popular construct. Nowadays, bestseller lists frequently include books on enhancing your spiritual well-being, bringing spirituality into your business, or getting in touch with your spiritual self. Since the 1960s the number of empirical studies of spirituality in the health and social scientific literatures has quadrupled (Weaver, Pargament, Flannelly, & Oppenheimer, 2006). Spiritual practices, from meditation and yoga to healing and prayer groups, are also becoming a part of everyday life for many people in the United States. But these changes are relatively recent.

As background for my discussion of spirituality, my readers need to recognize that the meanings of this construct and its close relative, religiousness, have changed dramatically over the past 40 years. Historically, the term "religiousness" encompassed what many people today would define as "spirituality." For instance, many contemporary psychologists would likely be comfortable with William James's (1902/1936) classic definition of religion—"the feelings, acts and experiences of individual men in their solitude, as far as they apprehend themselves to stand in relation to whatever they may consider the divine" (p. 32)—as a definition of spirituality.

In the traditional view, religion was a broad construct, one that included both personal and social expressions, subjective and objective elements, and the potential for both good and bad. More recently, however, a shift in meanings has occurred. Theorists have speculated that these shifts have grown out of broader cultural changes toward greater individualism and greater antagonism to traditional authority and institutions of all kinds (e.g., Hood, 2003). Whatever the cause, the terms "religiousness" and "spirituality" have become increasingly polarized, particularly among mental health professionals and social scientists. Brian Zinnbauer and I (Zinnbauer & Pargament, 2005) have noted that modern definitions of these constructs, at their most extreme, "place a substantive, static, institutional, objective, belief-based, 'bad' religiousness in opposition to a functional, dynamic, personal, subjective, experience-based, 'good' spirituality" (p. 24).

Elsewhere, my colleagues and I have described a number of serious problems with this polarization of religion ("the institutional bad-guy") and spirituality ("the individual good-guy") (Pargament, 1999; Zinnbauer & Pargament, 2005). Let me focus on three of these problems here. First, the tension between these terms that has been described by various theorists does not fit well with the experience of most people. Empirically, a majority of people in the United States do not see any conflict between religion and spirituality. In fact, our surveys have shown that when forced to choose, most people label themselves as both religious and spiritual (74%) rather than as spiritual but not religious (19%), religious but not spiritual (4%), or neither religious nor spiritual (3%) (Zinnbauer et al., 1997). Second, we cannot decontextualize spirituality. This dimension of life does not unfold in a vacuum, but rather in a larger religious context, even if it is a context that has been rejected. Like children who have moved away from their parents, people who have moved away from their original religious traditions continue to be impacted by these traditions as well as by the larger religious cultural context in subtle and not-so-subtle ways. There is no avoiding the fact that religion is part of the air we breathe. Finally, we encounter problems when we romanticize spirituality. Certainly, spirituality has been linked to the best in human nature. However, it is not hard to find examples of destructive acts, both personal and social, perpetrated by people firmly convinced that they are guided by the highest of spiritual motives. We limit the scope and power of spirituality when we build "goodness" into the way we think about this construct. Like the psychological, social, and physical dimensions of life, the spiritual dimension can be both constructive and destructive.

There are, however, some potentially positive consequences to the evolving meaning of spirituality. It could serve as a reminder that the most critical function of religion is spiritual in nature. Although religion serves a host of purposes—providing a sense of meaning and purpose to life, comfort, intimacy, health, and self-development—the most essential of all religious functions is the desire to form a relationship with something we consider sacred. "It is the ultimate Thou whom the religious person seeks most of all," psychologist Paul Johnson (1959, p. 70) wrote. It is unfortunate that social scientists and health professionals have tried to reduce spirituality to purportedly more fundamental human motivations. The new focus on spirituality, though, could remind us that spirituality is a critical part of life that cannot and should not be explained away. Rather than reduce spirituality to more basic drives, the field of psychology could elevate its focus by considering spirituality as a higher dimension of human potential. The new focus on spirituality could also encourage us to look not only at but beyond traditional religious experiences and expressions to understand spiritual phenomena; the sacred can take many forms and people can take many paths to the sacred, both traditional and nontraditional.

I have chosen to focus on spirituality in this book because I believe it deserves attention in its own right. Even though the terms "spirituality" and "religiousness" converge and diverge from each other in important ways (see Pargament, 1999; Zinnbauer, Pargament, & Scott, 1999), for the sake of simplicity and clarity, I will regularly use the term "spirituality" and reserve the use of the terms "religion" and "religiousness" to refer to the larger social, institutional, and cultural context of spirituality. Because religiousness and spirituality have been defined in different ways by different authors, I have also taken the liberty of changing the uses of these terms at times to fit with the conceptualization in this book. I apologize to anyone who may be offended by this license on my part.

The meaning of spirituality has not stopped evolving. Many ideas, studies, values, and practices are now being placed beneath the umbrella of the spiritual concept. Unfortunately, it is not clear how they fit together. Spirituality is, as Spilka (1993) noted, a "fuzzy" construct. Just what is spirituality? This is not purely an academic question. To work with spiritual issues in psychotherapy, practitioners need to know it when they see it, know where it starts and stops, and know how it operates in peoples' lives.

I have defined spirituality as "a search for the sacred" (Pargament, 1999, p. 12). There are two key terms in this definition: "search" and "sacred." Let's begin by focusing on the meaning of "sacred."

THE SACRED DOMAIN

The sacred is the heart and soul of spirituality. For many people, the sacred is equivalent to higher powers or divine beings. Others think of the sacred in a broader sense, one that encompasses any variety of objects, from mountains, music, and marriage to vegetarianism, virtues, and visions. Both perspectives are accurate. Mahoney and I have defined the sacred in terms of concepts of God, the divine, and transcendent reality, as well as other aspects of life that take on divine character and significance by virtue of their association with, or representation of, divinity (Pargament & Mahoney, 2002). Picture the sacred by imagining a sacred core and a sacred ring that surrounds the core (see Figure 2.1). The "sacred core" refers to ideas of God, higher powers, divinity, and transcendent reality. But the sacred is not restricted to concepts of a Supreme Being or greater reality. Surrounding the sacred core is a ring of other aspects of life that become extraordinary, indeed sacred themselves, through their association with the sacred core.

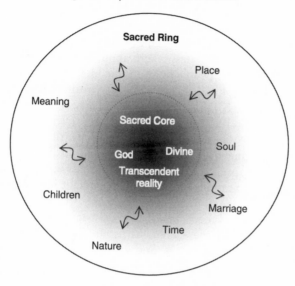

FIGURE 2.1. Picturing the sacred.

The Sacred Core

At the heart of the sacred lies God, divine beings, or a transcendent reality. What do we mean by these terms? It's difficult to imagine a thornier question for the psychologist who prizes clarity in thought, sharpness in concepts, and parsimony in language. The problem is that, according to most religious traditions, the divine or the ultimate reality is inherently mysterious, elusive, and indescribable. Language, symbols, myths, and stories, most religious authorities agree, must always fall short of capturing the essence of ultimate reality. Of course that should not stop us from trying to articulate the meaning of the sacred core. Part of the task of practitioners is to learn about and help clients talk about aspects of life that may be very hard to put into words.

Throughout the world, people have described the core of the sacred in different ways. The monotheistic religions (Judaism, Christianity, Islam) speak of God; Hindus describe Brahman, a mysterious power that sustains all things; Buddhists refer to Nirvana as the ultimate reality; Taoists call the underlying source and ordering principle of everything Tao; and so on. These are not merely different words for the same phenomenon. Between and within religious traditions, people have diverse understandings of ultimate reality. Within monotheistic religions, for instance, God can be addressed by any number of terms: "Lord," "King," "Father," "Mother," "Son," "Friend," "Savior," "Judge," "Spirit," "Creator," "Ground of

Being," "Almighty," "Messiah," "Redeemer," "Merciful," "First Cause," "Truth," "Beloved," and "Hidden One"—to name just some (Armstrong, 1993). Even in the United States, where about 95% of the population reportedly believes in God, people hold diverse images of the divine, images that range from loving, kind, and forgiving to wrathful, strict, and controlling (Spilka, Armitas, & Nussbaum, 1964). Those who reject traditional understandings of God as a figure who watches over them and protects them from harm can also pick and choose from a variety of ways to imagine the divine, ranging from creative power and cosmic energy to Earth Mother and unifying presence (Roof, 1993). Moreover, as we will see, these differences in representations of God have important implications for peoples' lives. But the essential point I wish to make is that, regardless of how they may be understood, concepts of God, divine beings, or transcendent reality lie at the core of the sacred. Christian theologian Thomas Oden (1983) is clear on this point: "It is God whom we worship. We gather not to worship ourselves, our desperate struggle for God, our hungers for God, or our immediate feelings for God, but nothing less than God alone, who awakens our thirst for his presence and who stands at the beginning and end of our struggles, hungers, and feelings" (p. 94).

The Sacred Ring

Though notions of God and ultimate reality are central to the sacred, sacred matters extend beyond these fundamental spiritual constructs to encompass other parts of life (i.e., "objects") that are associated with or represent the sacred core. This is not a new idea. For instance, Mircea Eliade (1957) wrote of the sacred "erupting" into the profane world, saturating it and sanctifying it with ultimate reality, power, and being. Reading Eliade, I imagine an aura radiating out from the sacred core illuminating the surrounding dimensions of life. In less picturesque, more psychological language, Annette Mahoney and I (Pargament & Mahoney, 2005) use the term "sanctification" to refer to this process through which people view seemingly secular aspects of life as holding divine significance and character.[1]

---

[1]The term "sanctification" has specific theological meanings that vary from tradition to tradition (e.g., Dieter, Hoekema, Horton, McQuilken, & Walvoord, 1987; Miethe, 1988). For example, within Christianity, sanctification is an inherently mysterious process through which God transforms profane objects into sacred entities. The sacrament of marriage in the eyes of the Roman Catholic Church is said to transform a heterosexual relationship into an indissolvable holy union. My approach here, however, is not theological. Sanctification is defined as a process of perceiving seemingly secular aspects of life as having divine character and significance (Pargament & Mahoney, 2005). As it is used here, sanctification is a "psychospiritual" construct. It is spiritual because it focuses on sacred matters. It is psychological in two ways: first, it focuses on perceptions of what is sacred, and, second, the methods of studying sacred matters are social scientific rather than theological in nature.

Sanctification may be best understood as a different way of perceiving the world. Ronald Rolheiser (1994) captures this perceptual difference in describing the language of contemplative and noncontemplative people:

> Where the contemplative (of past generations) might refer to his erotic aching as "immortal longings," the non-contemplative is more prone to speak of "being horny"; where the contemplative speaks of a "providential meeting," the non-contemplative is more likely to speak of "an accident"; where the contemplative speaks of finding a "soul-mate," the non-contemplative is more prone to speak of "great chemistry"; where the contemplative speaks of "being caught up in a painful romance," the non-contemplative is more likely to speak of "obsessional neurosis." (p. 49)

Rolheiser may have overdrawn this contrast—after all, many people have a bit of both the contemplative and the noncontemplative in them. But I believe he is correct in pointing to the different languages, sacred and nonsacred, that can be applied to everyday experiences.

To put it another way, when people sanctify, they look at life through a sacred lens (Pargament & Mahoney, 2005). Through this lens, the visual field shifts and changes. What once appeared monochromatic, unidimensional, and ordinary becomes multicolored, multilayered, mysterious, rich, unique, awesome, alive, and powerful. I like the way Elkins (1998) describes it:

> In one sense a painting by Van Gogh is really nothing but a bunch of multicolored smudges on an old piece of canvas. Similarly, music is nothing but the sounds that come from plucking string, beating drums, and blowing through hollow objects. Yet, when those smudges or sounds are arranged in a certain pattern, our soul goes forth to meet a Van Gogh masterpiece or the sounds of a symphony, and in that meeting something happens, and we are transported into the realms of exquisite beauty. (p. 95)

Transcendent perception, according to Elkins, is the ability to see "the more" (p. 97).

Mahoney and I have described two ways in which sanctification may take place (Pargament & Mahoney, 2005).

Manifestations of God

People can perceive an aspect of life as an expression of their images, beliefs, or experiences of God. Through religious readings, education, and ritual, adherents to religions across the world are taught that God is manifest in life. Consider a few examples. In religious services, Jews regularly recite the blessing "Holy, holy, holy is the Lord of hosts! The whole earth is full of His glory" (Isaiah 6:3). Jews are expected to share in the holiness of God by following His laws. These laws wrap virtually every action within a sacred shroud. Theologian Abraham Heschel (1986) writes, "All mitzvoth [good deeds] are means of evoking in us the awareness of living in the neighborhood of God, of living in the holy dimension. . . . Every act of man is an encounter of the human and the holy" (p. 273). By adhering to the Ten Commandments, the individual is said to elevate him- or herself from the animal-like to the God-like.

Within Hinduism, Brahman is described as a power that pervades all of existence. Some see this power as personal, others see it as impersonal. From the Upanishads, the Hindu Scriptures concerned with the knowledge of Brahman, Hindus learn that this divine power dwells in the visible and the invisible:

> Filled with Brahman are the things we see,
> Filled with Brahman are the things we see not,
> From out of Brahman floweth all that is:
> From Brahman all—yet he is still the same.
> —Upanishads (1975, p. 80)

Among Christians, Jesus is the ultimate symbol of the incarnation of the sacred in earthly life ("though he was in the form of God, did not count equality with God a thing to be grasped, but emptied himself, taking the form of a servant, being born in the likeness of men" [Philippians 2:6–7]. Each believer's actions can also reflect the presence of God through the gift of the Holy Spirit ("Now there are varieties of gifts, but the same Spirit; and there are varieties of services, but the same Lord; and there are varieties of working, but it is the same God who inspires them all in every one" [Corinthians 12:4–6]. The Christian sacraments also provide a point of connection between the sacred and the human. The ritual of baptism, for instance, reenacts the blessing of Jesus in which the individual is recognized as a beloved "child of God" imbued with the Holy Spirit. The sacraments can also be more broadly understood and experienced, as we hear in the words of Andrew Dubus (2001), a man who had been crippled nine years earlier:

> It is limiting to believe that sacraments occur only in churches. . . . I know that when I do not go to Mass, I am still receiving Communion, because I desire it; and because God is in me, as He is in the light, the earth, the leaf. . . . I am receiving sacraments with each breath . . . with each movement of my body as I exercise my lower abdomen to ease the pain in my back . . . as I perform crunches and leg lifts. (p. 157)

Although dissatisfied members of various traditions often accuse their religions of irrelevance, the God of most religions is not removed from the workings of the world. However the sacred core may be defined, it is said to be concerned with earthly as well as heavenly matters. Teaching people to see this truth, the manifestations of God in their lives, is one of the central jobs of the religions of the world.

Of course, in an age when faith has become increasingly privatized, more a matter of personal choice than simple acquiescence, many people do not necessarily accept the teachings of their particular religious tradition. Dupre (1976), for one, was skeptical about the degree to which people experience the sacred in the modern age. "Today," he wrote, "most of our Western contemporaries are totally unacquainted with the religious awe and irresistible attraction which are supposed to have manifested the sacred presence in the past. . . . Modern [men and women] frequently can claim no direct experience of the sacred at all, either in the world or in themselves" (p. 23). In support of his argument, he cited the words of one college student: "Nowhere in my world and at no time in my experience is there anything that I can point to as a manifestation of the sacred. I'm not even sure that the notion of the sacred can be meaningful to modern man. I doubt, at any rate, that I have a conception of it" (p. 23).

Is this typical or atypical? Certainly, we can find examples that contrast with the college student above, examples of people who see God as manifest in life. Listen to the words of one of my graduate students, Shauna McCarthy (personal communication, May 24, 2006), who perceives God in the people who surround her:

> God has a deep raspy voice—God is a jazz singer. She is plush, warm and rosy—God is a grandmother. He has the patient rock of an old man in a porch rocker. He hums and laughs, he marvels at the sky. God coos babies—she is a new mother. He is the steady, gentle hand of a nurse, has the cool reassurance of a person pursuing his life's work and a free spirit of a young man wandering only to live and love life.

Which experience is more commonplace today? Are perceptions of the sacred no longer relevant, or do many perceive God to be present in their lives? To answer this question, my colleagues and I (Doehring et al., in press) recently conducted a national survey in which we asked participants to indicate how often they saw God as manifest in various aspects of their lives. As Table 2.1 reveals, the majority of the population reported that they frequently experience God to be present in themselves, their relationships with others, nature, and all of life. God, as perceived by this national sample, was not restricted to a limited sphere of involvement; instead, the influence of the divine extended into the larger circle of their lives. If these findings are to be believed, then perceptions of sacredness in the world are not a thing of the past; they continue to be a part of modern times.

TABLE 2.1. Percentage of People Who Report God as Manifest in Life

Item	Percentage report often/very often
I see God's presence in all of life.	75
I see evidence of God in nature and creation.	78
I experience a sense of God's transcendence in my life.	59
I sense God's presence moving in my relationships with others.	56
I sense that my spirit is part of God's spirit.	68

Note. N = 113.

Sacred Qualities

Perceiving aspects of life as manifestations of God is the most direct form of sanctification. But people can also sanctify objects indirectly by attributing *qualities* to them that are associated with the divine. It is not hard to find examples of this indirect form of sanctification in our culture. Sacred qualities are often used to describe ostensibly secular objects. People speak of "sacred vows," "holy wars," "hero worship," "hallowed ground," "everlasting love," "saintly figures," and so on. These phrases hint at the presence of a deeper process, one through which various aspects of life are instilled with godly qualities.

Here is a personal example. Several years ago, my 12-year-old son joined me in Albuquerque for a long-awaited father–son trip to the Grand Canyon. Driving through New Mexico and Arizona, we were treated to wonderful, constantly changing scenery. Over the next hill or around a gentle sweep of curve, a majestic butte would be waiting or a desert panorama would unfold in front of our eyes. As the sun set, our focus shifted to a sky that seemed to envelope us in rich shades and hues that I had never seen before. The drive had been unforgettable. Spectacular as it was, though, it had not prepared us for our visit to the Grand Canyon the next morning.

Coming up to the Grand Canyon from the south, we drove for miles along a narrow road surrounded by tall pines and unremarkable flat, high plains countryside. The only sign that we were approaching the Grand Canyon was the toll booth that marked our entry into the national park. We drove on, parked our car in a narrow lot, walked over to the end of the lot—and then the earth gave way. I saw something I had never seen before, something I could never have fully imagined. The earth opened before me into a huge chasm, indescribably deep. The canyon itself seemed to stretch out to the horizon, well beyond the limits of my vision. I felt as though I had stepped outside of my own world and entered a more profound reality, one of far greater force and power. Peering into the depths, I experienced a strange mix of feelings: there was fear that my son and I could easily be swallowed up without a trace of us left behind; there was goose-pimpled, jaw-dropping astonishment at the immense beauty all around us; and there was a tremendous sense of gratitude that I had been fortunate enough to live to see such a wonderful sight with my son. For me, the Grand Canyon was more than a great view, spectacular scenery, or even a natural wonder. It was something sacred.

What made the Grand Canyon sacred? I believe it contained qualities that are often used to describe the divine by theologians, philosophers, psychologists, and artists. They include attributes of transcendence, boundlessness, and ultimacy. The first sacred quality, transcendence, speaks to the perception that there is something out of the ordinary in a particular object or experience, something that goes beyond our everyday lives and beyond our usual understanding. At the Grand Canyon, I experienced this sense of "extraordinariness," of entering a dimension that transcended my limited world. Where did this incredible chasm come from? How could it be so vast, I wondered? It seemed incomprehensible, a mystery that defied any rational understanding. Rudolf Otto, the 19th-century theologian, is perhaps best known for his description of the transcendent, mysterious quality of the holy. There is, he said, an "otherness" to religious experience. It is "wholly other . . . quite beyond the sphere of the usual, the intelligible and the familiar, which therefore falls quite outside the limits of the 'canny' " (1917/1928, p. 26).

The second sacred quality, boundlessness, involves a perception of endless time and space. In the Grand Canyon, I also felt this vastness in time and place extending beyond all normal boundaries. The sense of boundlessness is not restricted to nature at its grandest. It can be perceived in something as small as a grain of sand, as we hear in the poetry of William Blake (1977): "To see a World in a grain of Sand; And Heaven in a Wild Flower; Hold Infinity in the palm of your hand; And Eternity in an Hour" (p. 506). The perception of boundlessness is nothing new. A few thousand years ago, Plato captured the timeless element of this sacred quality in the ideal of Beauty. "Beauty," he wrote, "is first of all eternal; it neither comes into being nor passes away, neither waxes nor wanes; next it is not beautiful in part and ugly in part, nor beautiful at one time and ugly at another" (1951, p. 93). In our own era, David Elkins (1998) describes this same quality succinctly: "Eternity breaks in, limitedness falls away, and we find ourselves in an eternal present" (p. 126).

Ultimacy is the third sacred quality. Although my experience in the Grand Canyon was unusual for me, it felt anything but artificial. Beneath the surface of the rocks, cliffs, and sand, I perceived something vibrant and alive, something basic and elemental. As Tillich (1957) describes it, ultimacy lies at the very center of existence. It refers to the essential and absolute ground of truth, the foundation for all experience. Similarly, Jones (1991) notes that the sacred evokes the most primary and fundamental of our experiences, "those constituting its creation and re-creation" (p. 116).

Ultimacy is not simply an abstraction; it has to do with what is perceived as "really, real" (Geertz, 1966).

The qualities of transcendence, boundlessness, and ultimacy are usually assigned to the divine, but they can also be seen within other aspects of life. I need to emphasize that although people perceive sacred qualities as *lying within* various aspects of life, these objects are not disconnected from their perceivers. As we will see in the next chapter, once imbued with divine qualities, objects in the sacred ring take on a power to elicit strong emotional responses, actions, and motivations. Thus, the sacred is not "out there," remote or disconnected from us; it is instead linked to us through thought, feeling, behavior, and motivation. "The quality of sacredness," Jones says, "refers to the potential to resonate with the deepest recesses of ourselves" (1991, p. 116). In short, we have relationships *with* the sacred.

How relevant is this discussion about sacred qualities and our relationships to the sacred to people today? To what extent do people actually perceive sacred qualities in their lives? We have conducted several studies that address this question. For example, as part of a larger study, our research team led by Annette Mahoney administered a measure entitled Sacred Qualities to 97 couples from the Midwest (Mahoney et al., 1999). Sacred Qualities consists of a variety of sacred adjectives that could be used to describe a marriage. These adjectives include "holy," "inspiring," "blessed," "mysterious," "everlasting," "awesome," "heavenly," and "spiritual." Our couples were not at all averse to describing their marriages in terms of these sacred qualities. Eighty-four percent of the couples reported that these adjectives were at least "somewhat" descriptive of their marriages. Our findings were not unusual. Using variants of the Sacred Qualities scale, we have found that many people perceive sacred qualities in other domains, such as parenting, nature, strivings, sexuality, and life in general. Overall, this line of study underscores the point I made earlier: perceptions of sacredness are not a thing of the past. Many people continue to perceive their lives in sacred terms.

Before I move on, I should stress that none of the items on the Sacred Qualities scale makes any explicit reference to higher powers, divine beings, or God. These items speak only to qualities of the sacred. Conceivably, then, people who do not hold strong beliefs in God or do not believe in God at all could still perceive aspects of their lives to be sacred in a less theistic or nontheistic sense. Listen, for example, to the sense of timelessness one woman, an atheist from Sweden, experiences in nature: "Whatever happens in the world for me or others, nature is still there, it keeps going. That is a feeling of security when everything else is chaos. The leaves fall off, new ones appear, somewhere there is a pulse that keeps going. . . . It is a spiritual feeling if we can use this word without connecting it to God, this is what I feel in nature" (Ahmadi, 2006, p. 134). This example may not be all that unusual. Eliade (1957) suggests that vestiges of the sacred can still be found in the thoughts and actions of nonreligious people, even though they are unaware of their spiritual heritage. Generally, however, we have found that people tend to experience both forms of sanctification: they perceive aspects of life as manifestations of God and they perceive that those aspects of life contain sacred qualities. My own experience at the Grand Canyon is a case in point. I did not consciously perceive the Grand Canyon to be a manifestation of God. However, my son reminded me that throughout our experience at the precipice, I repeatedly exclaimed "Oh, my God. Oh, my God."

There is a paradoxical quality to sanctification. The sacred object is not to be confused with God, the divine, or any other element of the sacred core. Indeed, when the connection between the sacred object and the divine is lost, and the sacred object is viewed and treated as if it were divine in and of itself, we call that idolatry (Tillich, 1957). However, if the sacred object is not to be confused with God, it should not be confused with a simple object either. Because sacred aspects of life symbolize, contain, or point to something that lies beyond themselves, they are more than simple objects. Once instilled with some of the qualities that are associated with the sacred core, objects of many kinds are transformed from ordinary to extraordinary.

The Varieties of the Sacred

If people defined and experienced the spiritual domain in similar ways, our task as practitioners might be a little easier. However, in an age when spirituality has become increasingly personalized, people see the sacred quite differently. Conceptions of God and transcendent reality vary from tradition to tradition, culture to culture, and person to person. The elements that make up the sacred ring can be just as diverse. Complicating matters is the fact that people are capable of instilling virtually any aspect of life with spiritual significance and meaning. Sociologist Emile Durkheim (1915/ 1965) wrote: "By sacred things one must not understand simply those personal beings which are called gods or spirits; a rock, a tree, a pebble, a piece of wood, a house, in a word anything can be sacred" (p. 52). Similarly, Tillich (1967) noted that "the encounter with the holy, in its essence, is not an encounter besides other encounters. It is within the others" (p. 128). To create some order out of the potentially vast and complex realm of the sacred, it may be useful to consider the ways three different classes of objects—the self, relationships, and place and time—can be perceived as manifestations of God and take on sacred qualities.

The Self

Mention of the self as sacred may bring to mind images of narcissistic figures who worship the ground they themselves walk on. In fact, it is not hard to find individuals who have made religions of themselves. As Robert Bellah and his colleagues (Bellah, Madsen, Sullivan, Swidler, & Tipton, 1985) have noted, the tradition of self-reliance in our culture, whose exemplars include Thomas Jefferson ("I am a sect myself") and Thomas Paine ("My mind is my church"), has created fertile soil for the growth of a self-centered religiousness. They cite the case of Sheila Larson, a young nurse (now famous within sociological and psychological circles) who says, "I can't remember the last time I went to church. My faith has carried me a long way. It's Sheilaism. My own little voice." Caring for a dying woman, Sheila describes an experience in which she felt that "if she looked in the mirror" she "would see Jesus Christ" (p. 235).

Most religious traditions have harsh words for this form of self-centeredness. Indeed, confusing the self with the sacred or placing the self above the sacred is seen as the dynamic that drives the Seven Deadly Sins: pride, avarice, lechery, envy, gluttony, anger, and sloth. I will have more to say about self-worship later in this book when I consider the topic of idolatry. But for now, it is important to note that although the religions of the world do not encourage self-worship, neither do they see the self as antithetical to the sacred.

Many traditions hold that God is manifest in the self. Within Hinduism, we hear that "the Lord God, all-pervading and omnipresent, dwells in the heart of all beings" (Upanishads, 1975, p. 122). Christians are told that "the kingdom of God is within you" (Luke 17:21). Jews learn that "God created man . . . in the image of God" (Genesis 2:27).

The idea that there is something of the sacred within ourselves is not foreign to people. In his work with Carl Rogers, Jared Kass (1991) held lengthy discussions with 40 well-functioning individuals to learn about their process of personal growth. Content analysis of these conversations revealed two patterns in the ways these adults described themselves. First, almost all of the participants described their inner core in transcendent terms; they felt they were made up of something "greater than themselves." Second, most of the participants found it hard to articulate the character of their inner selves in everyday language. Instead, they called upon metaphors. Kass found that although these metaphors were different in content, they shared an underlying meaning: "These participants experienced themselves as drawing water from wells connected to a vast underground sea" (p. 2). The individuals in Kass's study felt a greater power in the world. They did not confuse this power with themselves, but they did not experience this power as disconnected from themselves either. Rather, it was perceived as part of the "fundamental ground of being within the person, a spiritual core" (p. 2).

Theologians and spiritually minded psychologists have described the sacred character of the self in numerous ways, referring to virtues, a divine spark, and the soul. According to one perspective, we find the sacred in the highest of human potentials. Acts of justice, courage, creativity, compassion, forgiveness, honesty, and hope are not merely exemplary or noble behaviors; they are "signals of transcendence," signs of a reality that goes beyond the empirical situation (Berger, 1969). Even humor can signal the transcendent, says Peter Berger. Humor acknowledges the tragic nature of the human condition, but humor refuses to give tragedy the last word; laughter signals that the "imprisonment of the human spirit . . . is not final but will be overcome" (Berger, 1969, p. 70).

Moral and virtuous behaviors represent signals of transcendence, but they can be more than that. Many theologians assert that standards of right and wrong, good and evil, fairness and injustice are not human constructions, but are instead woven into our essential being. Referencing Charles Darwin, who wrote that "man is the only animal that blushes," Kushner (1989) suggests that this distinctive human characteristic is a reflection of a self-consciousness that "we are being watched and held to standards" (p. 79). From his point of view, a virtuous life is more than a matter of morality and more than a life well lived, it is a way to respond to what God expects of us and it is a way to experience the divine. "Where is God?" Kushner asks. In courage, determination, love, and hope, he answers. "God is found in the incredible resiliency of the human soul, in our willingness to love though we understand how vulnerable love makes us, in our determination to go on affirming the value of life even when events in the world would seem to teach us that life is cheap" (p. 178).

The sacred character of the self has also been depicted as a divine spark or treasure. For instance, in some traditions people are said to contain a "spark of God" (Steinberg, 1975, p. 70). Similarly, Zimmer writes, "The real treasure is never very far; there is no need to seek it out in a distant country. It lies buried in the most intimate parts of our own houses; that is, of our own being" (cited in McCready, 1975, p. 69). This view of the self has far-reaching implications, for if the self contains a divine spark, then people are obligated to locate and care for that spark, protecting and nurturing it so that it can become a source of illumination and warmth. Understood in this way, people who are trying to develop themselves and find meaning in their lives are not engaging in secular pursuits; they are involved in spiritual quests. Not long before he died, the Hasidic rabbi Susya said that when he gets to heaven, God will not ask him "Why were you not Moses?" Instead, God will ask him "Why were you not Susya? Why did you not become what only you could become?" (cited in Yalom, 1980, p. 278).

Finally, no dimension of the self is more fully identified with the sacred than the soul. On the face of it, this term should be easy to define. After all, psychology itself refers to the "study of the soul." But the meaning of "soul" is difficult to pin down, perhaps because it refers not to a "thing" but to a "quality" of ourselves and our experiences (Moore, 1992). These qualities are sacred in character. For instance, the soul has been described as "the infinite depth of a person . . . comprising all the many mysterious aspects that go together to make up our identity" (Moore, 1992, p. 268). The soul has also been depicted in terms of ultimacy, as the essential animating dimension of living things, and as the overarching force that links and reconciles disparate aspects of our lives: thought and feeling, mind and matter, inner and outer, dark and light (Hillman, 1975). The soul has both transcendent and immanent qualities. As Hillman (1975) writes, "Soul enters into all of man and is everything human . . . [but it] extends beyond the nature of man. The soul has inhuman reaches" (p. 173). In this sense, the soul can be seen as a point of connection between individuals and God.

The Relational

Many people look for the sacred beyond themselves as individuals. As one woman put it, "I'm tired of hearing from people who let me know how holy *they* are. Find me women who let me know how holy *we* are" (Anderson & Hopkins, 1991, p. 209). The sacred can be located in relationships—not in any relationship, but in relationships of a particular kind. This was the point philosopher Martin Buber (1970) made so eloquently in his classic book *I and Thou*. Buber distinguished between two types of relationships: "I-It" relationships in which an individual approaches an object as separate from the self, something to be acted upon; and "I-Thou" relationships that involve a meeting between two subjects who complete each other. Spirituality, as Buber viewed it, is essentially relational. "Man lives in the spirit when he is able to respond to his Thou. He is able to do that when he enters this relation with his whole being. It is solely by virtue of his power to relate that man is able to live in the spirit" (p. 87). Although people can respond to any aspect of life as a "Thou," Buber believed that God is most fully encountered in relationships with people. "The relation to a human being," he wrote, "is the proper metaphor for the relation to God—as genuine address here is accorded a genuine answer" (p. 151).

Love is perhaps the most critical emotional ingredient of I-Thou relationships. Through experiences of love and compassion, many people feel they come closest to an encounter with the divine. Here is how one young woman described it: "The things that make me feel as if I could touch the face of God are times when I am overwhelmed by love and friendship. The last time I went to a family reunion, I was touched by the level of love and caring everyone showed me. There's nothing like the feeling of being loved. I would say that love is the one thing in life that can truly take a person to another level in life, because the source behind love . . . is God" (Rosenberg, 2002, p. 8).

This woman is not alone in her feelings. Followers of the world's religious traditions learn that love is sacred in character. Christians are told that God is manifest in love: "God is love; and he who dwells in love dwells in God" (1 John 4:16). Jews are taught that love is the highest religious obligation: "Above all, the Torah asks for love: Thou shalt love thy God: thou shalt love thy neighbor. All observance is training in the art of love" (Heschel, 1986, p. 256). Buddhists learn that loving-kindness is one of the highest spiritual perfections: "As water quenches the thirst of the good and the bad alike, and cleanses them of dust and impurity, so also shall you treat your friend and your foe alike with loving-kindness" (Gaer, 1958, p. 12). Even those who reject organized religion or belief in God may imbue love with sacred qualities. For example, avowed atheist Bertrand Russell demonstrated his fluency in the language of the sacred when he spoke of his quest for love: "I have sought [love] because in the union of love I have seen, in a mystic miniature, the prefiguring vision of the heaven that saints and poets have imagined" (Russell, cited in Mahoney, 2000, p. 54).

The products of love—marriage, sexuality, and family—can also be perceived in sacred terms. For example, within Judaism and Christianity, a marriage is much more than a contract; it is a covenant based on sacred vows that join the couple not only to each other, but to God in a "three-fold cord" (Ecclesiastes 4:9–12). In our own research, we have found that many people experience God as a third presence in their marital relationship (Mahoney et al., 1999), a presence that transforms the marriage from an intimate bond into a transcendent union. One spouse said, "To me, it would be like being inside a room with no air, not to have God in a marriage" (Robinson, 1994, p. 211). People who are not a part of a traditional religious system or nontheists may also attribute sacred qualities to the marital relationship. Elkins (1998) puts it this way: "Marriage is not sacred because the church says so or because a clergyman performed the ceremony. Marriage is sacred because it involves the joining of two hearts and souls for life—an awe-inspiring commitment that has 'sacred' written all over it" (p. 143).

Although sexuality has often been viewed as anathema from some religious perspectives, the sexuality that grows out of love can be understood and experienced in sacred terms. This point is nicely illustrated in a qualitative study by Chuck MacKnee of 10 practicing Christians who had had a profound event in which "sexual arousal and orgasm was simultaneously experienced with the presence of God" (MacKnee, 2002, p. 235). Many of the participants felt God to be manifest in the sexual experience. Some perceived God as a peaceful loving presence. Others described God as if He were another person in the room: "I couldn't believe that it was taking place. What is going on? I'm praying and God is talking to me and we're having sex at the same time" (p. 237). Still others experienced God in the sexual act itself; they felt " 'full of God,' 'stroked by God,' or 'penetrated by Him' " (p. 238). The descriptions of the sexual encounters were also filled with sacred qualities. For instance, one man spoke of his sexual experience in terms of transcendence: "In our intense union with one another there's a sense there is something beyond us, a transcendence, not just the two of us" (p. 239). A woman spoke of her experience in terms of reverence and holiness: "Sex became a holier thing. I felt reverence. My body was a holy sanctuary that night" (p. 239). Are these people and their experiences rarities? Probably not. In a survey of college students, Nichole Murray-Swank and colleagues found that it was not unusual for people to sanctify sexual intercourse in loving relationships (Murray-Swank, Pargament, & Mahoney, 2005). These studies begin to challenge common stereotypes of religion and spirituality as forces that restrict or inhibit sexuality, and they illustrate how even the most intimate of acts can be imbued with sacred character and significance.

Various aspects of family life are also sources of sacred meaning, from the "miraculousness" of childbirth and the day-to-day role of being a parent to the treatment of one's own parents and family as a whole (Mahoney, Pargament, Murray-Swank, & Murray-Swank, 2003). The sacredness of the family is central to major religious traditions. "Without exception," Zimmerman (1974) writes, "[the religions] are concerned with the sanctity of family relations more than any other mundane object" (p. 6). "Being religious," he goes on to note, "is tantamount to being a good husband, a good wife or a good parent, child, or kinsman" (p. 6). Within Judaism and Christianity, the bonds among family members, as with the marital bond, are likened to the covenant between God and Israel for Jews, and between Christ and the Church for Christians. Within Hinduism, dharma (divine righteousness and morality) is said to be enhanced by fulfilling family obligations. And in Confucianism, filial piety is a cardinal virtue that can be expressed at both lower ("Don't Let Your Parents Starve") and higher levels ("Do Nothing Which Will Bring Dishonor Upon Your Parents") (Zimmerman, 1974). Are these theologies, in fact, "lived by people"? Certainly, we can find examples of people who describe their families in spiritual terms. Consider the comments of one mother of two young children: "To see my kids is to realize that they are—well, godlike . . . not because they are particularly unusual children, but because I could not with my own two hands have created anything as wonderful or amazing as they are. . . . Just tickling their feet and hearing them giggle—that's cosmic, that's divine" (Fitzpatrick, 1991, p. 2). On the other hand, family life may not always be so divine (most of us have had family episodes that come closer to hell than to heaven). Nevertheless, empirical study suggests that many individuals do perceive family life in spiritual terms (e.g., Murray-Swank, Mahoney, & Pargament, 2006).

Finally, it is important to note that, according to most religious traditions, the love derived from the love of a Supreme Being is not limited to one's immediate network of relationships; it encompasses all of God's children, "far as well as near, unattractive as well as attractive, lost as well as found, outsider as well as insider" (Pope, 2002, p. 169). Nontheistic religions have their own sacred equivalents, as we hear in this Buddhist verse: "Let all-embracing thoughts for all that lives be thine—an all-embracing love for all the universe in all its heights and depths and breadth, unstinted love, unmarred by hate within, not rousing enmity" (Burtt, 1982, p. 47). At least theoretically, the sacred ring can go beyond immediate family relationships to include the larger human family of neighbors, communities, institutions, nations, and, indeed, all of life. How well people do, in fact, succeed in extending the scope of the sacred is certainly arguable. Yet we can find promising signs. For example, a female rabbi from Oakland, California, felt a strong spiritual kinship with other Jewish women throughout history who had offered wisdom and leadership but were largely forgotten (Anderson & Hopkins, 1991). She said, "Many of them did not have children, others' descendants were killed in the holocaust, so they have no one to say prayers for them. I want to reclaim their memories and connect to them in the world of prayer" (p. 207). On religious holidays, this rabbi recites the names of female ancestors of the congregation and, in the process, she widens the sacred ring to include people from other places and times.

Place and Time

Several years ago, I gave a workshop on spirituality and health to a group of hospital chaplains. These were a remarkable group of women, mostly in their 40s and 50s, who had gone into chaplaincy on the heels of successful careers as accountants, lawyers, and educators. Most were involved in pediatric work, ministering to children suffering from cancer, respiratory diseases, burns, and physical abuse. As they shared story after story filled with terrible sadness, loss, and frustration, I wondered how they were able to sustain themselves in their difficult jobs. One chaplain who worked with children on a burns unit answered my question for me. "Thank God," she said, for her "sacred garden." It was nothing extravagant. About the size of a closet, it sat on a small corner of her backyard, and held flowers, shrubs, colored stones, a fountain, and a chair. But it was a special place; this otherwise gentle woman had made it clear to family and friends that she would shoot anyone who crossed into her sacred space. She had created her garden because she needed a place just for her, a place she could control, a place where she could "no longer smell the flesh of burned children." There, she could breathe freely again, draw on her spiritual sources of nourishment, and replenish herself.

As Eliade (1957) noted, not all places are alike. Some lie closer than others to the "Center of the World" (p. 43), the core of the cosmos that is saturated with power, creativity, and timelessness. By virtue of their proximity to the sacred core, these places take on sacred significance of their own. They can be found in the natural world—the Himalayas and the Ganges River for Hindus, the hill on the plains of Arafat where Muhammad preached a sermon on the way to Mecca for Muslims, or the *pilal* tree under which Siddhārtha Gautama received his spiritual enlightenment for Buddhists (Mazumdar & Mazumdar, 1993). Sacred places can also be created almost anywhere: in a corner of a backyard, as we saw above; within a home, as is common among Hindus who create *pooja* areas to house the family shrine; or within mosques, temples, and cathedrals in which believers feel that the doorways are particularly open to God (Mazumdar & Mazumdar, 1993). Indeed, some people may sanctify the entire universe:

> I am connected to everything else. Who I am does not stop at my skin, but extends outward through a complex matrix of interconnectedness to encompass the entire universe. I interact with and interpenetrate my environment as I inhale and exhale, drink water, and eat food. . . . The stars are made of carbon, and so am I. The same God that hurled the stars into the vast darkness of space also bent over my body and sprinkled "star stuff" into my bones and flesh. Thus, I am a sibling of the stars, the suns, and the galaxies. We have the same parent, the same origins, come from the same womb. (Elkins, 1998, p. 216)

Time too can be sanctified. The religious calendar is punctuated with sacred moments in time when the divine order of the world is most manifest, when the windows into the transcendent are clearest. These may be special holy days in which pivotal religious events and divine actions are reenacted through ritual, or regular holy days, such as the Sabbath when time itself is celebrated. Listen to the sacred qualities Heschel (1986) perceives in the Sabbath: "Six days a week we live under the tyranny of things of space; on the Sabbath we try to become attuned to holiness in time. It is a day on which we are called upon to share in what is eternal in time, to turn from the results of creation to the mystery of creation; from the world of creation to the creation of the world" (p. 304). Life transitions such as birth, coming of age, marriage, retirement, and death can also be seen as sacred in character, for they may reveal the underlying transcendent dimension of existence. Indeed, every moment of time may hold sacred potential. One woman put it this way: "We are on earth for a finite time. Every day is blessed, and I want to live that day fully . . . the sacred moment provides a stopping place, a listening post, where the preciousness of immediate experience and the living-in-the-now unite" (Lynn, 1999, p. 61).

In this section, we have considered the variety of objects that make up the sacred domain and the ways they can be perceived as manifestations of God and take on sacred qualities. Although we delineated three different classes of sacred objects—the self, relationships, and place and time—the sacred domain is not partitioned so neatly within individuals' lives. Instead, people generally see the world in terms of a pattern of sacred objects that cut across the self, relationships, and place and time. Thus, one person perceives the sacred largely in terms of nature, music, and an inner soul. Another sees the sacred most clearly in loving relationships and efforts to make the world a more compassionate place. Still another perceives the sacred in terms of church, special religious celebrations, and a very personal God. What distinguishes one person from another, then, is not the presence or absence of one particular sacred object, but rather each individual's configuration of sacred objects.

FURTHER QUESTIONS AND CONCLUDING THOUGHTS ABOUT THE SACRED

We have focused on one particular question that is key to understanding spirituality: Where does spirituality start and stop? Spirituality starts and stops with the sacred. In this chapter, we have explored the sacred domain. At the core of the sacred lie concepts of God, the divine, and transcendent reality. However, the sacred does not stop there; the domain of the sacred extends beyond to a ring that encircles the self, relationships, and place and time. In fact, virtually any aspect of existence can be seen through the sacred lens as a manifestation of God or as the container of sacred qualities. Even experiences of great pain and suffering, our darkest nights of the soul, can be perceived in terms of a deeper transcendent dimension. In Tillich's (1957) words, "No piece of reality is excluded from being a bearer of the holy" (p. 58). This was the same conclusion Frederick Buechner (1992) came to after living on Rupert Mountain:

> There is no event so commonplace but that God is present within it, always hiddenly, always leaving you room to recognize him or not to recognize him, but all the more fascinatingly because of that, all the more compellingly and hauntingly.
> . . . Listen to your life. See it for the fathomless mystery that it is. In the boredom and in the pain of it, no less than in the excitement and gladness: touch and taste your way to the holy and hidden heart of it because in the last analysis all moments are key moments, and life itself is grace. (p. 2)

No discussion of spirituality and the sacred is likely to be satisfying to everyone. Topics as deeply personal and as emotionally based as this one do not generate consensus among any group of people, let alone mental health professionals, social scientists, and the spiritually minded. Here, I have presented only one of several possible ways to understand the special meaning of spirituality, one that certainly raises questions of its own. Before concluding, let's consider some of these questions.

First, if *anything* can be sacred, then does it follow that *everything* is sacred? If that were the case, then the term "sacred" would lack boundaries. Whether anything or everything is sacred in the ontological sense is a question that cannot be answered through the methods of science; there are no scientific proofs when it comes to the divine. However, science can help us determine whether people, in fact, perceive everything as sacred. The answer appears to be "No." Empirical studies indicate that most people are particular in the aspects of their lives they sanctify. As Geertz (1966) remarked, "No one, not even a saint, lives in the world religious symbols formulate all of the time, and the majority of men live in it only at moments" (p. 35). Similarly, religious groups tend to be selective in what they delineate as the profane and what they define as the sacred, and differences in their views of the sacred help define the unique character of each group. This point was brought home to me a few years ago when I was invited to consult with an international group of physicians who had been asked by the World Health Organization to arrive at a common definition of spiritual well-being. The physicians came from all over the world and represented diverse religious traditions. After many hours of lively debate and dialogue, a Christian physician from Europe attempted to reach a consensus:

"I think we can all agree," he proposed, "that the essence of spiritual well-being is love. Love is the most sacred of all attributes." He glanced around the room expecting nods of agreement and murmurs of assent, but he was disappointed.

A Buddhist physician from Asia offered a counterproposal: "I would suggest that we can agree that the essence of the sacred is detachment from all things temporal."

The Christian physician and others in the room appeared startled. "But surely you're not saying that we should detach from love?," one physician asked.

"Of course," the Buddhist answered, equally surprised by the question. "People can attach themselves too greatly to love as they can to any human emotion."

The attempt to reach consensus failed, at least in part, because the members of these different traditions saw the sacred in different ways. It was as if they were looking at the sacred through lenses with different prescriptions and, as a result, they were seeing different worlds. There is a critical lesson here for practitioners. An essential clinical task is to understand how our clients view the sacred, for the sacred domain, whatever it holds, speaks to their deepest personal values and helps define who they are as individuals and as members of communities.

This leads to a second question: Isn't the sacred simply another way of talking about what is most important to people? I don't think so. Certainly our sacred concerns refer to matters of greatest importance to us. However, the reverse isn't necessarily true. Matters of great importance are not necessarily sacred. Only when they are invested with divine qualities (e.g., transcendence, boundlessness, ultimacy) or are perceived to be manifestations of the divine do important matters become sacred matters. And once sanctified, these aspects of life become unique, set apart from other human symbols and values, important though they may be. In our study of marriage and the sacred, we conducted some additional unpublished analyses that spoke to this point (Mahoney et al., 1999). We compared spouses who viewed their marriages as sacred to spouses who viewed their marriages as very important but not sacred on measures of marital satisfaction and commitment. Couples who sanctified their marriages reported significantly greater marital satisfaction and commitment than couples who perceived their marriages as very important but not sacred. Sacred matters are, in short, distinctive and irreducible to other phenomena, even phenomena of great significance. Tillich (1957) underscores this point nicely: "Symbols of faith cannot be replaced by other symbols, such as artistic ones, and they cannot be removed by scientific criticism. They have a genuine standing in the human mind, just as science and art have" (p. 53). The sacred is what distinguishes spirituality from other phenomena. It lends clarity to an otherwise "fuzzy" construct. Nevertheless, it is capable of taking many different shapes and forms, nontraditional as well as traditional. I believe this approach to the meaning of the sacred extends the boundaries of spirituality to encompass the full range of human experience, from the most exalted to the most mundane, from heaven to earth.

Another question deserves consideration: Isn't the sacred simply another word for the good? Once again, I believe the answer is "No." Shortly, we will see that the process of sanctification can have a number of psychological, emotional, and spiritual benefits. However, the ultimate value of perceiving aspects of life as sacred rests on other factors as well. We will consider these complex and thorny evaluative issues in a later chapter. For now, let me simply note that the value of sanctification depends in part on what is being sanctified. Over the course of history, people have sanctified many objects, including, in Tillich's words, "false absolutes" that are destructive to their own well-being and the well-being of others. As Tillich (1967) reminds us, "We saw it in some of the Nazis who committed atrocities with good consciences because 'the voice of God,' for them identical with the voice of Hitler, commanded them" (p. 101).

One final question grows out of this discussion: In describing the meaning of sacred, haven't I offered a rather static view of spirituality? If this were the last word on spirituality, then I believe the answer would be "Yes." However, this chapter focused on only one of the critical elements of spirituality: the sacred. Spirituality involves more than a substantive content area. It is not a static, frozen set of beliefs or practices. It is instead a process of searching, a search for the sacred. What does it mean to *search* for the sacred? We turn our attention to this important question in the next three chapters.

3

Discovering the Sacred

Having discussed the meaning of the sacred, I now focus on what it means to *search* for the sacred. Of course, the idea that individuals are involved in a process of "searching" rests on a critical, even radical, assumption: the assumption that people strive. Before plunging into the search for the sacred, this assumption deserves some attention.

HUMANS AS STRIVING BEINGS

What is radical about the idea of people striving for goals in their lives? It conflicts with the major psychological theories of our time: psychodynamic, social learning, and biological. Different as these theories are, they do have one thing in common: a reactive view of human nature. Be it unconscious forces, the learning environment, or the power of evolution, genetics, and physiology, each of these paradigms assumes that people are products of internal and/or external forces. "Genes 50 percent, Environment 50 percent" is the way one psychologist puts it in explaining the variance in human behavior (Pinker, 2002, p. 380).

There are two major problems with reactive views of human nature. First, they are incomplete. Human nature is reactive, but that is not the full story. As any parent struggling to keep up with an infant or child can attest, we come into this world equipped with a propensity to explore and master the environment. The capacity to investigate, look ahead, think about a future, and imagine and implement ways to achieve goals is a critical ingredient of human nature. "Human beings," Robert Emmons (1999) writes, "are by nature goal oriented" (p. 15). A growing body of theory and research on goals, incentives, self-direction, competence, and volition makes clear that the ability to strive is fundamental to understanding human motivation and behavior (Austin & Vancouver, 1996; Tyler, 2001; White, 1963). This research also challenges many widely held reactive views about human nature.

Take, for example, the old adage "The best predictor of behavior is past behavior." Like many old sayings, this one is incorrect. Actually, the best predictor of behavior, at least in the immediate future, is intentions (Fishbein & Ajzen, 1975). For instance, I can make a very accurate prediction about what you (the reader) will do after you finish this chapter by asking you one simple question: What do you plan to do after you finish reading this chapter? Note that I am able to achieve this prognostic wizardry without knowing anything about your genetics, physiology, unconscious, learning history, or social environment. This example may seem silly, but the underlying point has important clinical implications. Most practitioners are well aware of the single most critical question to ask a client contemplating suicide: "Tell me, are you intending to kill yourself?" Intentions have power.

Psychologists who hold to a reactive view of human nature would counterargue that intentions and, more generally, the human capacity to strive are themselves determined by the forces of genetics, learning, and the unconscious. In this vein, psychologists Kirsch and Lynn (1999) assert that all behaviors, including intentions, are automatic. Undoubtedly, the ability to plan, set goals, and strive is conditioned by a variety of internal and external forces, but does the story end there? I don't believe so, for people also have a degree of freedom to choose.

Though limited by contexts and conditions, choices remain available to people even in the most adverse conditions. Psychiatrist Irvin Yalom (1980) writes, "When all else fails, when the coefficient of adversity is formidable, still one is responsible for the attitude one adopts toward the adversity—whether to live a life of bitter regret or to find a way to transcend the handicap and to fashion a meaningful life despite it" (p. 272). The capacity to choose lends unpredictability to behavior. It may help to explain why research studies using the best deterministic models of physiology, genetics, past experience, environment, and temperament to predict behavior generally leave most of the variability in behavior unexplained. Even if the "50% genetics, 50% environment" rule is accurate, it explains 100% of only a portion of human behavior. Pinker (2002) himself gives a joking nod to the freedom to choose, even among animals, when he recounts the "Harvard Law of Animal Behavior" formulated by B. F. Skinner's students: "Under controlled experimental conditions of temperature, time, lighting, feeding, and training, the organism will behave as it damned well pleases" (p. 177).

There is a second problem with reactive views of human nature: they interfere with change, including the change that is encouraged in psychotherapy. After all, how can practitioners assist people in changing the stories of their lives if they believe that the stories are preordained? Autobiographies cannot be written in advance (Heschel, 1986). The assumption that people strive is certainly optimistic; embedded in it is the possibility of turning away from destructive habits and meaningless goals to new dreams and new directions in life. Of course, the freedom to strive and to choose is no panacea, for it also contains the possibility of foolish choices that make a mess of things, undoing the accomplishments of a life well lived. Nevertheless, by assuming that people have the capacity to act as well as to react, strive for a future as well as respond to a past, choose mindfully as well as automatically, therapists are in a better position to offer the hope to their clients (and themselves) that fundamental, transformational change is indeed possible, even in the midst of a sea of unconscious, biological, and environmental forces.

Perhaps no choice holds more far-reaching implications than the decisions people make about their goals and destinations in life. Elsewhere, I have noted that people search for significance (Pargament, 1997). By "significance," I am referring to things that matter. There is no shortage of potential "objects" of significance. They may be material (e.g., food, money, drugs), physical (e.g., health, appearance, fitness), psychological (e.g., comfort, meaning, self-esteem), or social (e.g., intimacy, social justice). Significant objects are great motivators of behavior; people are drawn to whatever they hold significant. And in the pursuit and attainment of significant objects, people gain feelings of value, worth, and importance; in short, significant objects yield a "sense of significance."

Social scientists have long debated the object of greatest significance to people. The candidates have ranged from tension reduction (Freud) and personal growth (Fromm), to meaning in life (Geertz) and social solidarity (Durkheim). Empirical studies, however, suggest that the search for a common motivational denominator may be misleading (e.g., Davis, Wortman, Lehman, & Silver, 2000). People are drawn to a variety of significant objects (e.g., Ford & Nichols, 1987). Indeed, what makes an individual relatively distinctive may be his or her particular configuration or hierarchy of significant objects.

Oddly enough, in the midst of the large body of theory and research on significant objects, one significant object has been largely neglected: the sacred. Yet for many people the sacred is the focal point of their striving, the object of significance that lends order and coherence to all their other goals. These people are involved in a sacred quest, I believe. In this and the next three chapters, I focus on what it means to *search* for the sacred. Let's start with an example.

CINDY'S SPIRITUAL JOURNEY

Cindy is a 40-year-old, married woman, with four children. She agreed to be interviewed by a member of our Spirituality and Psychology Research Team as part of a study on spirituality and coping. Though she dressed youthfully in jeans and T-shirt and wore her hair long and straight, she had more than her rightful share of wrinkles and a sadness to her eyes that said she had seen hard times. Even so, she spoke directly, laughed easily, and communicated a sense of warmth and vitality.

From her earliest years, Cindy said, she felt a hunger for God. She recalled her first spiritual encounter, at the age of 4 or 5: "I was sitting in a field behind our house, and the sun was going down, and I just felt like God had His arms around me." This experience was, she felt, "a present, a gift, something to hold, to keep, because I think He knew . . . that I would need that to carry me through some of the hard times." However, the God who held her in His arms did not fit well with the God Cindy came to know through her family and her church. Her mother kept a Bible at home but neither talked to her children about religion nor encouraged them to go to church. Her father, embittered by what he felt was rejection from his church, would ridicule Cindy when she attended a small Protestant church with neighbors. These harsh experiences found their way into Cindy's view of God. She recalled thinking that "God was sitting up on a throne someplace, and all He ever really did was throw fire balls down on people . . . because my dad was like that." Her image of God as distant and critical was reinforced by experiences at church. She recalled attending a church service at the age of 10 that was led by a visiting evangelist. Cindy was deeply affected by his call for repentance: "The whole concept of sin really hit me between the eyes. And I felt very, very convicted of that, very guilty, and didn't really know what I felt bad about. I was all upset and crying. It was the first time I realized about sin, and that I was a sinner, and that somehow I was separate from God. And that bothered me. I didn't want that separateness. I wanted to be close to Him."

Discouraged by her parents from any further church involvement, Cindy moved into adolescence with little in the way of religious guidance and the strong belief that her relationship with God depended on her ability to avoid sins. She recalls: "I didn't have anybody to give me any kind of training. I didn't have any idea of where to go for a church, and I thought that when I became a Christian, when I asked the Lord into my heart, that I just wouldn't do anything wrong again." The stage seemed set for failure. "And so the first time I screwed up, I thought, 'That's it,' I blew it, and had nobody to tell me any different. What happened after that was my life really took a downward spiral."

Feeling that she had missed her chance to be with what she described as "the Christian God," Cindy began to look for God elsewhere. Over the years that followed, she experimented with Eastern mysticism, Native American religions, astrology, tarot card reading, palmistry, witchcraft, and the occult. During this period of experimentation, she married four times, gave birth to four children, became addicted to cocaine, and moved out of town leaving her children behind.

The turning point in Cindy's life occurred 10 years ago when her mother died. Upon her return home to attend the funeral, she was surprised to learn that several friends and family members had become Christians over the years. Confused by this turn of events, Cindy asked one friend how she had become "saved." The friend went on to tell the story of a man that has become popularized in the "footprints poster": "He's having a dream and in his dream he sees that in the hardest moments of his life, there was only one set of footprints. And he said, 'Lord, I thought that you said that when things are rough you would never leave me.' And the Lord said, 'Well those were the times that I carried you, and that's why you only saw one set of footprints.' " Cindy was deeply moved by this story: "I felt like that was written for me. And when she told me that, I just thought, my God, He's been there with me this whole time. He never left. Jesus has been standing right by me. And when I thought of the places I had taken Him, and the things I'd made Him see, it was just too much."

Over the next few years, Cindy made dramatic changes in her life. She became sober, returned to her hometown, regained custody of her children, and "rededicated [her] life to the Lord." In this process, Cindy developed a very different understanding of God and the sacred. "God," she said, "accepts you just the way you are. You don't have to attain a level of perfection ever. He doesn't expect that from you." Like the force that had embraced her as a young child, this was a God that Cindy could trust and rely on. So she began to "let go." "I had never fully turned over complete control of my life to the Lord," Cindy said. "I never really said to Him, 'Okay, I'll just relax and let you drive.' I mean we say we want God to take care of things, but we only let Him have so much control, then we take it back. . . . I thought, I'm not gonna do this any more. . . . I just felt very strongly that I needed to let go, and let God do whatever He wanted to do with my life." Cindy's perception of the sacred also widened from a focus on God and Jesus to a sense that the sacred is manifest in people and relationships: "Now I see [God] more in people and how He affects people's lives." Similarly, Cindy began to view her marriage in spiritual terms: "I feel like this marriage is a marriage. This is the first time I've ever [really] been married in my whole life. And the other [marriages]—I don't know what that was. But this one's the real McCoy, because God's at the center of it."

Today, Cindy recognizes that, in spite of her changes, she remains vulnerable to falling back into old patterns. To maintain and strengthen her faith, she has broken off relationships with friends from the past who continue to "party like maniacs." She comments: "When you try to put light and darkness together, it seems like the darkness always kind of gobbles up the light. And so, because I know how I am, it's better for me to keep the distance." In the place of old friends, Cindy has become part of a new church and has formed a new circle of friends who share and support her faith. She has also taken a job as a counselor to chemically dependent women, and sees herself gaining strength by offering spiritual strength to others. "I know how it feels to feel like you've done something that's totally irreversible and unforgivable. I really have an empathy with these women, you know, who need to know God. They need to meet Jesus. They need to know that it's not the end of the line." Cindy is also sustained by her daily prayer life which no longer seems a duty to her but a way of continuing to connect to the Lord. Undoubtedly, the most important source of support and security to Cindy is her relationship with God. "I feel probably the most secure that I've ever felt in my life. I've always felt kind of shaky when I was a kid and growing up. But I don't feel that any more. . . . I really feel that no matter what would happen to me, I could deal with it, because I know I'm not alone. I know that Jesus is right beside me." These resources have given Cindy a new sense of rootedness and stability: "My feet are more firmly planted, in a Christian sense, than they've ever been in my life."

Cindy's spiritual journey is not over. Looking to the future, she comments, "It's an ongoing process that happens your whole life. You're constantly being saved, if that makes any sense at all. . . . God's not done with me, He's still working with me." Cindy's spiritual life is not entirely smooth. She continues to have questions about God and the role of God in her life. "I'd like to know why God let me fall down the shaft with the drugs and the occult and all that. I don't understand why He didn't send anybody into my life at that point. There was nobody, and I don't understand why." The sharp edge to these questions is blunted, though, by a positive faith. "[Maybe] He thought I needed the experience to make me a more capable counselor now. It's hard to tell. I mean, you're dealing with God. He's a big guy. He knows what He's doing." Thus, in spite of her questions, Cindy remains true to her faith. The sacred continues to be the core of her life, guiding her everyday activities, supporting her emotionally, and providing an overarching vision for her life. When asked about the most important thing she would like to pass on to her children, Cindy said, "I'd want them to realize that they're not alone . . . that we don't walk this walk ourselves. Once we reach out, Jesus grabs your hand. He's always right there with you. I think that's such an important thing to hang onto. Because we can fall into all kinds of traps. We're just flesh and bones and blood, and anything can happen to us. But to know that He's there is comforting, you know, that you're not there by yourself. I think that's probably the most important thing."

THE SACRED AS A MOTIVATING FORCE

There is drama in Cindy's story. It is filled with the restlessness and tension of a woman who is on an odyssey, a journey marked by crisis and resolution, confusion and clarity, tragedy and renewal, and exhilaration and despair. Hers is not a one-act play, but rather a series of episodes that unfold over decades. Nor is it a one-person play. Cindy is one among a cast of characters involved in their own dramas who come together to assist each other and, at other times, to create added hardships for each other. And like any drama, this one has a background. It is set against the larger backdrop of social and cultural forces, most notably in this case the context of conservative Christianity in the United States.

No drama, however, is complete without a plot—the overarching force that directs and lends coherence to the whole story. It is not difficult to discern Cindy's guiding force. From her earliest memory of feeling embraced by God to the sacred dreams she now wants to pass on to her own children, Cindy's life has been directed toward the sacred. Her "hunger for God" led her on a search in many directions, some destructive and others more fruitful. Yet God consistently was and remains the most powerful magnetic force in Cindy's life—in the words of Tillich (1957), her most passionate concern.

Not so fast, though, many psychologists would counter. Is the sacred really the key here? On the surface, what appears to be a search for the sacred may, in actuality, be something else. Perhaps Cindy was really hungering for the intimacy and closeness she never experienced with her distant mother. Maybe she was actually looking for the protection and security she was unable to receive from her critical father. This is an important argument, one that raises serious questions about the legitimacy of spiritually integrated psychotherapy. After all, why take spirituality seriously if it is merely a reflection of more basic motivational processes? Doesn't it make more sense to cut through spiritual superficiality and get to the heart of the matter?

Certainly, we know that motivation is multilayered; motivations at one level can mask deeper-seated needs. The point holds true for motivations of all kinds, including spiritual ones. Yet spiritual motives have been assigned particularly superficial status within psychology; in comparison to physiological, psychological, and social motives, spiritual motives have less legitimacy within the field perhaps because psychologists have greater doubts about the ontological validity of spiritual phenomena. Are spiritual motives especially superficial? In Cindy's case, was her search for the sacred simply a smokescreen that masked the more significant motivating forces in her life?

I don't think so. There are some good reasons to treat Cindy's spiritual motivation seriously. First, spiritual strivings were central to her journey.

Failing to attend to Cindy's "spiritual hunger" would leave us with a story devoid of plot, coherence, and "soul." More practically, regardless of a clinician's personal views about the truth of spiritual claims, how could he or she get to know Cindy or develop a working relationship with her without an appreciation for what *she perceived* as a spiritual search? Second, while other motivating forces certainly played a role in Cindy's journey, they do not fully explain many of the critical choices in her life. Why, for instance, did she seek protection and security from God? Why did she look for meaning from a religious system of beliefs? Why did she seek closeness with others from a church? Other options were available to her throughout her life. Like many other people, she could have sought and found comfort, meaning, and intimacy from nonreligious sources. Yet Cindy did not. Her search centered on the sacred. She demonstrated a spiritual persistence that was made all the more striking by the lack of encouragement she received from her mother and father as a child. Without the concept of spiritual motivation it is difficult to explain the course of Cindy's life. Third, going beyond the case of Cindy, there are good empirical and theoretical grounds to view spiritual motivation as an important type of human motivation. We will look more closely at some of these reasons shortly.

From a clinical standpoint, it is important to take the search for the sacred seriously as a directing force in its own right. Just as people enter the world with physical, social, and psychological potentials, they are born with spiritual potential, the potential to seek out the sacred. In this sense, everyone is a spiritual being. Obviously, not everyone has as strong a spiritual motivation as Cindy. I believe people vary in the strength of their spiritual potential. What determines that strength? Psychologists have been especially interested in understanding the forces that shape the strength and character of spirituality. We will take a look at some of this work shortly. However, in the effort to understand these shaping forces, we have to be careful not to "explain spirituality away" by reducing the yearning for the sacred to purportedly more basic phenomena. Regardless of its roots, spiritual motivation is a part of what makes people unique.

This is not to say that spiritual motives work independently from other motivational forces. The relationships among different motivations can be complicated. At times, spiritual motives can be superficial and even disingenuous, offering a sanctimonious cover for less desirable motivations. Spiritual motives can also be intertwined with other needs. It may be difficult to disentangle spiritual motives from a search for intimacy, meaning, or comfort, particularly since any of these motives can take on sacred power and significance. The point I want to stress is not that the sacred is the whole story when it comes to motivation, but rather that the sacred is one among many important elements within the individual's configuration of significant objects. Spirituality is, in short, a critical and distinctive dimension of human motivation.

Cindy's is only one story. Many people are engaged in a search for the sacred, but their stories unfold in different ways, with different leading figures, a different cast of characters, a different backdrop, and a plot driven by a different understanding of the sacred. In contrast to Cindy's journey, some journeys are less explicitly focused on the sacred. Some are smoother and gentler. Some grow out of easier childhood and adolescent experiences. Some occur within other religious contexts or outside of an organized religious system of belief and practice. Some have endings less happy. There is, in short, tremendous variety to the search for the sacred. How can we make sense out of this diversity? What, if anything, does every spiritual journey have in common?

Let me provide a brief overview of the search for the sacred. I elaborate on this process in this chapter and the three chapters that follow (see Figure 3.1 for a simple diagrammatic representation). Every search for the sacred is dynamic rather than static, evolving rather than fixed. The search begins with the individual's discovery of something sacred. Once he or she finds the sacred, the individual takes a spiritual path to sustain and foster his or her relationship with the sacred. Changes from within or outside of the individual's world, however, can violate, threaten, harm, or point to the limits of the sacred. The individual must then cope to preserve and protect the sacred as best he or she can. At times, though, in spite of the person's best efforts to sustain the sacred in the coping process, internal or external pressures can throw the individual's spiritual world into turmoil. Spiritual struggles can be short-lived experiences, followed by a return to established spiritual pathways. However, struggles can also represent a fork in the road that leads to permanent disengagement from the search for the sacred, temporary disengagement from the search followed by rediscovery of the sacred, or fundamental transformations in the character of the sacred. Following a transformation, the individual shifts again to conservation and the effort to hold on to the sacred. The search for the sacred is not time-limited; it continues over the lifespan, unfolding in a larger field of situational, social, cultural, and psychological forces that both shapes and is shaped by the nature of the search. Within this ongoing pursuit, we can identify three important processes: discovery, conservation, and transformation. In the remainder of this chapter, I focus on the process of discovery.

THE DISCOVERY OF THE SACRED

The Experience of Discovery

People experience the discovery of the sacred at different times and in different ways. Some experience it as children. "I used to talk to angels all the time," one woman says. "I began hearing them when I was three years old. They told me how flowers grew and about all the things that went on in the

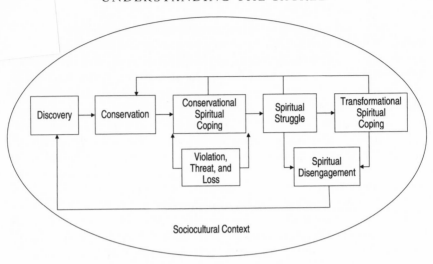

FIGURE 3.1. The search for the sacred.

garden and about relationships" (quoted in Anderson & Hopkins, 1991, p. 28). This isn't an unusual story. Another 8-year-old child recounted her experience of discovery outdoors: "At the foot of our garden was a very old large pear tree, which at the time was crammed with white blossoms and at its summit a blackbird was singing, while beyond the tree a meadow sloped up to a marvelous sunrise. As I looked at this, someone or something said to me: 'That is beautiful,' and immediately the whole scene lit up as though a bright light had been turned on, irradiating everything. . . . A curious thrill ran down my spine" (Hardy, 1979, p. 39).

Although the process of discovery can begin at an early age, it is not limited to childhood. For example, Cindy first felt God reaching out to her and cradling her in his arms when she was 4 or 5. However, without the support of her family and religious community, she lost touch with this experience of God. For many years she pursued the sacred in ways that proved to be fruitless. Only after many wrong turns, the death of her mother, and the support of her family and friends did she rediscover the God she had lost as a child.

"The Bible," Abraham Heschel (1987) notes, "speaks not only of man's search for God but also of God's search for man" (p. 136). Heschel is pointing to a second important difference in the way people can experience the discovery of the sacred. The sacred may come upon people, as we hear in the stories above; their experiences are, in the words of Eliade (1957), "hierophanies," perceptions that a divine presence has erupted into the world. "It is as if God were unwilling to be alone, and He had chosen man to serve Him," says Heschel (1987, p. 136). In contrast, other people experience the process of discovery in a more proactive fashion. One child reaches out to God through a letter: "Dear God, How is it in heaven? How is it being the Big Cheese?" (Heller, 1986, p. 31). Another 10-year-old describes how he tries to find the place where God lives: "It's a planet, like you need special glasses to see it. First, you need to get past the sun and then you have to get past the planets, and then you have to have enough power to get out of the galaxy. . . . And then, and only then, you might find it" (Heller, 1986, p. 58). And still others feel that God has come to them, but only after they have issued an invitation. One woman who had left her religion behind at an early age described the prayer that preceded her discovery of the sacred: "So I made my first prayer in years and years, and I said a very simple thing. I said, 'God, if you exist, get me out of this, cause I can't do it by myself. I am a lost woman here' " (Miller & C'de Baca, 2001, p. 31). Thus, the discovery of the sacred can be experienced as revelation (the sacred reveals itself to the individual), an accomplishment (the individual succeeds in finding the sacred), or both (the individual opens the door and the sacred enters).

Finally, the process of discovery can unfold from "inside to outside" or from "outside to inside." Many people first perceive a direct encounter with the sacred core and then begin to experience sacredness from this core radiating out to the wider ring of life. Listen, for example, to Parker Palmer's description of this process:

> One night, in the middle of one of my depressions, I heard a voice I'd never heard before, and haven't heard since. The voice said, "I love you, Parker." This was not a psychological phenomenon, because my psyche was crushed. It was "the numinous." It was "mysterium tremendum." But it came to me in the simplest and most human way: "I love you, Parker." That rare experience taught me that the sacred is everywhere, that there is nothing that is not sacred, therefore worthy of respect. (1998, p. 26)

Other people undergo a more inductive process of discovery, moving from encounters with sacred aspects of life in the outer ring to a greater understanding of divinity within the sacred core. Smith (1962) captured the flavor of this inductive approach to discovery when he said, "Handel was able to write 'The Messiah' in part because he had the faith that he had. I have the faith that I have in part because Handel wrote 'The Messiah' " (p. 186). Similarly, Anderson and Hopkins (1991) describe a Chumash Indian woman, isolated from her mother and father as a very young child, who first found the sacred in a tree. Asked who raised her, she responded:

> You really want to know who raised me? It was a peppertree with a short trunk. . . . It had a great nest inside that was like a womb. . . . You could sit in that womblike space and look out at the world without the world

seeing you. . . . I felt safe and loved and protected in that tree. It was my link with God/creation—with what was stable and real . . . that tree was a sacred presence in my life, and it taught me more about God and love than I ever learned in all the years I went to Sunday school. (pp. 35, 37)

As these examples suggest, people come to the sacred in different ways.

The Roots of Discovery

External Factors

The process of discovery is often described as a very private affair, an encounter between the individual and the sacred that takes place outside of any social and situational context or within contexts that have been personally chosen and created. In his book, aptly titled *A Generation of Seekers: The Spiritual Journeys of the Baby Boom Generation*, Wade Clark Roof (1993) describes this trend toward the individualization of the spiritual quest. One of his interviewees, Mollie, articulated her view of spirituality as a highly personalized journey, unencumbered by external constraints:

> INTERVIEWER: Religious and spiritual are two different things?
>
> MOLLIE: Yes, they are. With religion you have to choose one, you have to be locked in, which I don't want to be.
>
> INTERVIEWER: Is spiritual more open?
>
> MOLLIE: Uh huh. It's like an individual definition of your relationship to God and nature and religion and family and humanity. (p. 80)

Important as the personal experience of spirituality is, it would be a mistake to view the search for the sacred as "noncontextual." The processes of discovery, conservation, and transformation occur within the contexts of life events, family, community, institutions, and culture. This wider environment may be supportive of the individual's search for the sacred, or it may become the force that the individual *reacts against*. In either case, context plays an important part in determining whether the individual discovers, fails to discover, or rejects the sacred. The context also influences the nature of the sacred the individual comes to know.

It is no accident that a child born in Iran comes to believe in *jinns* (heavenly beings that fall somewhere between humans and angels), that a child raised in India sees Krishna as a personal form of Brahman (the underlying reality of all), that a child born in Brazil perceives God as a Trinity, and that a child who comes of age in the United States may see the sacred in mountains, self-awareness, or efforts to create a new global community. Every child is born into a religious context that provides a way of seeing who and what is sacred. This is the "foundational reality" of every faith tradition (Hood, 1995), a reality that is imparted to its children through religious stories, through religious practices and rituals, and through model religious figures who demonstrate by their actions what aspects of life hold sacred value. But religious traditions are not the only bearers of sacred knowledge. The larger culture also teaches children where to find the sacred. For example, Hallinan's (1981) popular children's book *I'm Thankful Each Day*, which can be found in most public libraries, encourages children to feel a sense of reverence and gratitude for the gifts of life:

> I'm thankful each day for the blessings I see and for all the
>   gifts that are given to me.
> And counting the stars at the edge of the sea, I can't help
>   but feel they were put there for me . . .
> Each breeze in the trees is a promise come true.
> Each evening's a wonder where beauty abounds.
> I'm thankful for friends for laughing and sharing . . .
> I'm thankful for family for loving and caring.
> I'm thankful for all the kindness I see . . .
> I'm thankful for peace and for pure harmony.
> My body's a present of perfect design . . .
> My mind is a power as endless as time . . . .
> Each hour is laden with infinite love . . .
> Each second brings comfort and joy from above. (pp. 1–21)

Although its language is not explicitly theistic, this book is essentially spiritual, designed to teach young child to see the sacred in nature, relationships, human virtues, body and mind, time, and the skies above. Secular institutions, like religious institutions, also create their own rituals and practices that convey a sense of the sacred to children. For instance, almost every child in the United States learns to associate flag and country with God through the Pledge of Allegiance. Other ideas about the sacred come to children by witnessing the actions of family, friends, and television and movie personalities. In short, institutional and cultural forces, religious and nonreligious, present children with a variety of sacred images. Of course, as children mature, they may reject these sacred symbols, but it is not because they are unaware of them. As Jones (1991) has noted, even those who do not believe in God have a very clear idea about the God they do not believe in.

Parents play a particularly important role in the discovery of the sacred. Mother and father are the child's first divine-like figures. The mother, Berger (1969) writes, is the "high priestess of protective order. It is she (and, in many instances, she alone) who has the power to banish the chaos and to restore the benign shape of the world. And, of course, any good mother will do just that. She will take the child and cradle him in the timeless gesture of the Magna Mater" (p. 55). According to psychodynamic theory, the infant's relationships with his or her parents create a model or template for subsequent relationships, including the child's understanding of and relationship with God. In support of this perspective, empirical studies indicate that children who perceive their mothers and fathers as loving and protective generally report more loving and protective images of God (see Spilka, Hood, Hunsberger, & Gorsuch, 2003). Conversely, children who experience more difficult relationships with their parents generally perceive God in more negative terms (e.g., Smith & Exline, 2002). Freud himself may illustrate this point. Applying the psychoanalytic method to explain Freud's own atheism, Rizzuto (1998) attributes Freud's religious antipathy to troubled relationships with his primary caregivers, including the loss of his much-beloved nanny at age 2; his possessive, demanding, yet emotionally unavailable mother; and the disappointment he felt in the weaknesses he observed in his father. Because he lacked strong parental models, Rizzuto (1998) concludes, Freud was unable to generate or discover an "exalted" God for himself.

The sacred is discovered in a situational as well as in a social context. Though the sacred can be found in any aspect of life, some objects and situations seem to have greater sacred power than others. For instance, McReady (1975) surveyed a national sample of Americans and found that a wide range of situations elicited connections to a powerful spiritual force, from the aesthetic (listening to music, the beauties of nature, creative work) to the religious (prayer, church services, listening to sermons) to the sexual (intimacy, lovemaking). These situations seemed to carry their own extraordinary, transcendent qualities that helped open the doors to a spiritual connection.

Major transitions and life crises have similar properties. The critical turning points of the lifespan—birth, puberty, marriage, death—are set apart from everyday experience. They are hinges in time, "holy days," not simply "holidays," that reveal the deepest dimension of life. Similarly, loss, accident, injury, trauma, and disaster can push people to confront the finitude and precariousness of their lives and direct them to look beyond their immediate worlds. As theologian John E. Smith (1968) wrote, "The crisis times fill us with a sense of the finitude and frailty of man, of our creatureliness, of our dependence upon resources beyond our own, and of our need to find a supremely worshipful reality to whom we can devote ourselves without reserve" (p. 59). Perhaps, then, it should come as no great surprise that Cindy rediscovered the loving God she had experienced as a child only after the death of her mother. Her story is not unusual. Kirkpatrick and Shaver (1990) documented this dynamic in a study of a sample of adults. Participants who described their mothers as cold, distant, and nonresponsive to them prior to adolescence were more likely to report a sudden religious conversion in adolescence or adulthood. Furthermore, in the large majority of cases, these conversion experiences were precipitated by a crisis, such as a divorce or a marital or family problem.

In sum, people discover the sacred not in isolation, but within a web of social and situational forces that create commonalities among subgroups of people facing similar situations. Conversely, raised in different contexts and subject to different pressures and constraints, members of varying ethnic, gender, age, and socioeconomic groups are likely to have distinctive perceptions of the sacred. Important as these forces are, though, they cannot fully explain the process of discovery—who will discover the sacred, when it will be discovered, and what form it will take. What is missing from this discussion is what the individual brings to the search.

Internal Factors

Cindy is only one of many people who describe a yearning for the sacred at an early age. On the face of it, accounts such as hers show clear signs of spiritual motivation. Yet social scientists have often been skeptical about spirituality as a motive in and of itself. Instead, they understand spiritual interests as expressions of something other than what they appear to be. At their most critical, theorists maintain that spirituality serves base human needs. Most notably, Freud (1927/1961) asserted that religiousness is, at root, child-like and defensive in nature, unconsciously designed to reduce anxiety and guilt and keep the terrors of nature and our own instincts at bay.

Other theorists also look beneath the spiritual surface to find the motivation driving spiritual experience, but in less critical fashion. Instead, they link spirituality to more elevated human pursuits, such as the needs for meaning (Geertz, 1966), intimacy and social solidarity (Durkheim, 1915/1965), confrontation with human mortality (Greenberg, Porteus, Simon, Pyszczynski, & Solomon, 1995), desire to know the world (Loewald, 1978; Rizzuto, 1979), and cohesion of the self (Kohut, 1984). Consider the thoughts of Hans Loewald and Heinz Kohut.

Hans Loewald (1978) maintains that people come into the world with a spiritual capacity that is basic to human character, not simply a defense mechanism. Spiritual qualities, he argues, are embedded in the unconscious or primary process. There we find experiences marked by a sense of unity and a sense of timelessness. These experiences are not indications of immaturity or pathology. In contrast to Freud, who encouraged people to move beyond their childish reliance on regressive experiences, Loewald asserts that the primary process offers an important way of knowing the world that can add vitality and freshness to the usual modes of rational processing. "To be an adult," he writes, "does not mean leaving the child in us behind" (1978, pp. 21–22). Instead, it involves an openness to both rational and primary forms of knowing. Religion, he states, has a "genuine validity" and a powerful capacity to enrich and enliven human experience (p. 73). Similarly, several object relations and psychodynamic theorists have spoken of spirituality as one of many potentially mature, creative "transitional" experiences (e.g., music, literature, scientific theories) through which people build bridges between their internal worlds and external reality (see Jones, 1991, for an excellent review). I like the way Ana-Maria Rizzuto (1979) puts it:

> [Religion] is an integral part of being human, truly human in our capacity to create nonvisible, but meaningful realities capable of containing our potential for imaginative expansion beyond the boundaries of the senses. Without these fictive realities human life becomes a dull animal creature. Without unseen atoms, imaginary chemical formulas, or even such fictive entities as id, ego, and superego, the entire domain of culture becomes a flat, irrelevant world of sensory appearance. (p. 47)

Heinz Kohut (1984) also rejects the instinctual drive theory of Freud and replaces it with a motivation centered on interpersonal relationships (i.e., object relations). People are born into relationships, he believes, and it is out of this matrix of relationships that people maintain, strengthen, and integrate themselves. Kohut asserts that relational needs direct behavior from birth to death. These relational motives include the need for recognition and acceptance, the need for experiencing that other people are like us, and a third need closely tied to spirituality: the need for connection to a greater, ideal reality, one that can uplift and inspire the individual. Jones (1991) captures the essence of Kohut's approach: "God is needed to ground our sense of who we are: the child who feels secure grounds that security in a caring God; the child who feels guilt and terrible grounds that sense of self by reference to a wrathful God; the child who feels estranged envisions a distant deity or dreams of a compensatory, warm, and tender . . . God" (p. 63).

Although Loewald and Kohut move spirituality closer to the center of human motivation, they do not elaborate on the sacred as a significant end in itself; rather, they focus primarily on the role of the sacred in facilitating the individual's understanding of the world and the development and cohesion of the self. Loewald and Kohut offer a more humane and respectful perspective on religion than that of Freud, but it retains the flavor of reactivity, a spirituality in service of psychological needs.

A few theorists have taken issue with reductionistic views of spirituality. They maintain that the search for the sacred is part and parcel of human motivation rather than an expression of other presumably more basic motivations in disguise. Jung (1938), for example, insisted that there is something of the sacred buried deeply within the self. The most fundamental of all drives, he maintained, is not sexual gratification but rather the recovery and integration of the various levels of the self, including the spiritual dimension. Jones (2002) suggests that we do not need to restrict our analysis to the psychological and social purposes of the sacred. We can start with the sacred as a primary desire that "lures us forward" and as a foundation to the way we experience and know the world (p. 111). Gordon Allport (1950) elaborated on this important point. True, he said, the discovery of the sacred can be rooted in a variety of organic, psychological, and social forces. Yet, with maturity, religion can become "functionally autonomous" of these original fears, hungers, and wishes. This mature faith "behaves no longer like an iron filing, twisting to follow the magnet of self-centered motives; it behaves rather as a master-motive, a magnet in its own right by which other cravings are bidden to order their course" (p. 64). Thus, Allport saw the religion of maturity as an irreducible, dynamic, and intrinsically life-directing force.

Elsewhere, I have suggested that Allport drew too sharp a distinction between spiritual and other motives (Pargament, 1997). Every aspect of life, including human needs and desires, can take on sacred character and meaning. Within the great religious texts of the world, the spiritual quest is woven into the search for other ends. The Muslim hears that "He who honours the learned, honours me" (Gaer, 1958, p. 238). The Christian is told: "Blessed are the peacemakers; they shall be called God's children" (Matthew 5:9). And in the Book of Psalms, Jews find expressions of deep longing for God that go hand in hand with pleas for wisdom, comfort, safety, and forgiveness. Through their association with the sacred, very human goals become elevated to greater meaning. Consider the words of one woman who challenges the split between the sacred and the profane: "When I'm nice to you, it's not just because I'm a nice person. I get to connect somebody to a much bigger picture. One, I'm nice to you because for thousands of years, that's my tradition, and also by being nice to you, I get to create something. . . . I get to create a light, and I also get a window to connect to the force of God" (Porpora, 2001, p. 281). What may seem to be a secular motive can, in fact, have transcendent value. In this sense, it is possible to turn spiritual reductionism on its head. Although the search for the sacred may, in actuality, reflect a search for the strength and comfort of a parent or loved one, the search for a loved one may also, in actuality, reflect a search for the ultimate strength and comfort that comes from the sacred.

In short, many internal factors may lead people on the path to spiritual discovery. Psychologists have been particularly interested in probing the psychological, social, and physical roots of spirituality. While these studies have often been quite illuminating, I have tried to inject a note of caution in these analyses: in the effort to understand the roots of the search for the sacred, we have to be careful not to explain this dimension of life away, for spirituality is a significant motivation in and of itself.

People come into the world with their own intrinsic propensity to seek out and experience the sacred (see also Pargament, Magyar, & Murray-Swank, 2005). The external world can support and encourage this capacity, neglect it, or discourage its development, but even when they are discouraged people may tenaciously pursue their search for the sacred, as we heard in Cindy's story. Thus, both external and internal factors are needed to understand the process of discovery. One half of "God's stuffing," Rizzuto (1979) writes, comes from "the primary objects the child has 'found' in his life. The other half of God's stuffing comes from the child's capacity to 'create' a God according to his needs" (p. 179).

Perhaps it should not be surprising that the sacred takes on such different appearances, given its roots in diverse relationships, situations, cultures, dreams, fears, and desires. As a result of this same matrix of forces, the sacred that is "found" and "created" by the individual can also be deceptively complex. Like an onion, the sacred can generate both sweetness and tears, and like an onion it may be multilayered. Attributes of divine omnipotence and powerlessness, lovingness and wrathfulness, and compassion and detachment can coexist within the same person. Of course, the individual may be unaware of some of these layers of attributes. In times of stress, the individual may be surprised to find that the God who is deeply felt (or deeply missed) in the bones is quite unlike the God who is understood (or rejected) in the mind. Freud himself may have manifested some ambivalence about his avowed atheism. According to Rizzuto (1998), Freud's interests in the collection of antiquities following the death of his father, frequent citations from the Bible, personal superstitions, and lifelong albeit antagonist fascination with religion all represented an effort to satisfy spiritual longings, though disguised and sublimated.

The Consequences of Discovery

Regardless of its roots, the discovery of the sacred has powerful consequences.

The Sacred Elicits Spiritual Emotions

The encounter with the sacred evokes a wave of emotions. These emotions, Rudolf Otto (1928) argued, are what make religious experience most distinctive. In fact, he believed that existing language could not adequately describe the feelings that surround the holy. The new term he coined, *mysterium,* is a complex of emotions. Like a magnet, it has a negative pole, the *mysterium tremendum,* made of feelings of repulsion, fear, and dread, the kinds of feelings we experience when we watch a horror movie. But like a magnet, the *mysterium* has a positive pole, the *mysterium fascinans*, consisting of strong feelings of attraction, including emotions of gratitude, humility, and reverence. Although my trip to the Grand Canyon took place many years ago, I still recall the magnetic feelings of repulsion and attraction I experienced as I stood at the edge of this chasm: the sense of personal insignificance and awe in the face of a power that seemed to dwarf everything around it, on the one hand, and the feelings of deep fascination and gratitude, on the other.

In the words of Abraham Maslow (1968), this would qualify as a "peak experience." Maslow (1968) was not interested in spirituality per se, but his work sheds light on the spiritual emotions and other rich changes in perception and cognition that accompany the peak experience. Maslow asked a group of people to describe how they felt during the "happiest moments, ecstatic moments, [and] moments of rapture" in their lives (p. 71). He analyzed their responses and reached a conclusion that echoes the words of Rudolf Otto: "The emotional reaction in the peak experience has a special flavor of wonder, of awe, of reverence, of humility and surrender before the experience as before something great" (pp. 87–88). And, like Otto, Maslow noted that these emotions are not purely positive: "The experience may have a certain poignancy and piercing quality which may bring either tears or laughter or both, and which may be paradoxically akin to pain, although this is a desirable pain which is often described as sweet" (p. 88). The consequences of peak experiences, Maslow maintained, are neither trivial nor temporary. Instead, they often signal profound and more or less permanent changes in the individual's view of him- or herself, other people, and the world.

More recently, psychologists have begun to follow Maslow's lead and explore spiritually related emotions more systematically. For example, Ralph Hood has developed an important program of research on mystical experiences (Hood, 1995, 2005; Spilka et al., 2003). Mystical experiences, he notes, are commonplace. Though they vary somewhat from person to person, mystical experiences are generally marked by powerful emotions, consisting of feelings of numinous consciousness and feelings of unity. "Numinous consciousness" refers to the individual's feeling that he or she is in the presence of a sacred object. The object is perceived to be absolutely real—"a foundational reality," in the words of Hood. Mystical experience is also characterized by feelings of unity, either a sense of oneness and totality with other objects in the world or a sense of unity with pure consciousness itself in which the individual feels a "no-thing-ness," a consciousness devoid of discrete perceptual objects. Because of their tremendous emotional power, Hood finds, mystical experiences can have long-lasting, life-altering effects.

Jonathan Haidt and Dacher Keltner (2003) have studied another type of spiritual emotion. They propose that people have a "built-in" emotional responsiveness to beauty, remarkable talent, and acts of virtue and morality. Because these stimuli are so vast and so difficult to accommodate, they often elicit feelings of awe. These situations also evoke feelings of being uplifted or elevated. Awe and elevation are not simply subjective experiences; they are objectively identifiable and distinctive emotions. For example, Haidt (2003) conducted research in which he induced emotions of elevation in a laboratory by showing participants video clips about the life of Mother Teresa. Other participants watched video clips from an emotionally neutral documentary and a comedy sketch. The participants were then asked to describe their physical feelings and motivations. Compared to participants in the other two conditions, elevated participants reported more warm, pleasant, or "tingling" feelings in their chests as well as greater desires to help others, to improve themselves, and to connect with other people.

Robert Emmons and Michael McCullough examined yet another spiritually based emotion. In response to the discovery of the sacred, people often feel a sense of gratitude, an emotion of appreciation and thankfulness for the spiritual gift they have received (Emmons, 2000; McCullough, Emmons, & Tsang, 2002). The gift is also accompanied by feelings of indebtedness that may be allayed in part through expressions of gratitude and commitments to pass the gift on to others. We can hear many of these expressions in the prayers of thanksgiving for God's gifts and God's presence in the world that are a major part of the sacred texts, teachings, and worship services of the great monotheistic religions. "The common thread" to all of these prayers, Emmons and Hill (2001) note, "is an overwhelming recognition of the need always, in all circumstances, to remember the source from which we come" (pp. 37, 39).

These prayers may have more power than a perfunctory "thank you." Emmons and McCullough (2003) found that emotions of gratitude were linked to significant emotional and physical benefits. Over a 10-week period, undergraduates completed weekly records of their emotions, physical symptoms, and health behaviors. The students were assigned to one of three conditions: one group recorded the major events that affected them during each week, a second group described the minor stressors they had experienced in the past week, and the third group wrote about the aspects of their lives they were grateful for during the week. Compared to the other two groups, the participants in the gratitude group had fewer physical complaints, exercised more frequently, felt more optimistic about the week to come, and felt better about their lives overall.

Most of the emerging research in this area has focused on the positive spiritual emotions. Yet to be explored are the negative spiritual emotions, the fear and the dread that are a part of the *mysterium tremendum*. Though there is much more to learn about spiritual emotions, we now know that the discovery of the sacred is more than a matter of the mind; it is deeply felt. These emotions should not be dismissed as mere sentiment. As research is beginning to show, spiritually based feelings have effects that ripple out beyond the affective realm to other dimensions of life.

The Sacred Becomes an Organizing Force

Wars can be fought within as well as between people. This is not a new idea to the religious or psychological world. Two thousand years ago, St. Paul the Apostle expressed some of his own personal conflicts: "For the good that I would I do not: but the evil which I would not, that I do" (Romans 7:19). Almost a hundred years ago, William James (1907/1975) pointed out that "our different purposes are . . . at war with each other" (p. 70). The discovery of the sacred, however, can begin to offset some of these forces of fragmentation. As the source of powerful emotions, the sacred becomes a passion and a priority. People feel drawn to, experience a thirst for, or are even grasped by the sacred, and as a result they begin to invest more and more of themselves in sacred pursuits. We have been able to document this process of sacred investment in our research. In one study, we found that people who hold the environment as sacred are more likely to invest their personal funds in environmental causes (Tarakeshwar, Swank, Pargament, & Mahoney, 2001). Another study revealed that college students who perceive their bodies to be sacred place greater priority on physical fitness in their everyday lives and eat more sensibly (Mahoney, Carels, et al., 2005). In yet another investigation, we learned that people spend more of their time on and place more of their energy into their highly sanctified goals and strivings than their less sanctified strivings (Mahoney et al., 2005).

As people begin to build their lives around the sacred, the sacred can begin to lend greater coherence to disparate thoughts, feelings, actions, and goals by superseding all other values, integrating competing aspirations into a unified life plan, and providing direction and guidance from day to day. Again, this is not a new idea to theologians or social scientists (see Emmons, 1999, for an excellent review). Ultimate concerns, Tillich (1957) said, serve as the "ground of everything that is" and the "integrating center of the personal life" (p. 108). Similarly, anthropologist Geertz (1966) wrote that sacred symbols "function to synthesize a people's ethos—the tone, character, and quality of their life, its moral and aesthetic style and mood—and their worldview—the picture they have of the way things in sheer actuality are, their most comprehensive ideas of order" (p. 3). Indeed, the world's religious traditions offer their adherents overarching spiritually based perspectives on how life should be lived. "Look forward and be hopeful, look backward and be thankful, look downward and be helpful" is illustrative of the succinct yet profound words of wisdom that can be found in every tradition (Krauss & Goldfischer, 1988, p. 1).

Anecdotal accounts and empirical studies also point to the organizing power of the sacred. For example, one businessman described his life as a "combination of disjointed events" before he discovered Jesus Christ. After, he testified, "I got my personal Christian relationship with Jesus and that has sort of been the on-going thing that has tied together a whole bunch of different things" (Bellah, Madsen, Sullivan, Swidler, & Tipton, 1985, p. 156). This is not a unique case. Emmons, Cheung, and Tehrani (1998) asked a sample of community members to list their personal strivings ("the things that you typically or characteristically are trying to do in your every-day behavior" [p. 9]). The researchers classified the strivings into various categories including spiritual strivings, such as "trying to discern and fol-low God's will," "teach my children spiritual truths," and "bring my life in line with my beliefs." Participants who reported a higher proportion of spiritual strivings also voiced less conflict among their goals, greater pur-pose in life, and greater goal integration. Similarly, Piedmont (1999) pro-posed that spirituality represents another organizing element of personality. To test his hypothesis, he developed a measure of spiritual transcendence and conducted a factor analysis of this scale along with the traditional five-factor measure of personality (neuroticism, extraversion, openness, agree-ableness, conscientiousness). In support of his argument, he found that the spirituality scale emerged as a sixth factor of personality. Moreover, the spirituality scale predicted a variety of psychological outcomes above and beyond the effects of the traditional five-factor model.

For many people, then, the discovery of the sacred lends order and co-herence to their lives. Not for everyone, though. As we will see in later chapters, depending on the nature of the sacred and the approach people take toward it, the sacred can also be a force for disorder, disharmony, and disintegration.

The Sacred Becomes a Resource

Once discovered, the sacred also takes on rare value. Sacred objects become the most precious of all commodities, the assets people turn to for strength and solace, the aspects of life people reach for in the most dire of times. In 1989, *Life* magazine interviewed survivors of a plane crash that resulted in the deaths of more than 100 passengers. An engine had exploded, the hydraulic system was destroyed, and the plane plunged toward the earth carrying passengers who believed they were about to die. On the brink of catastrophe, many passengers drew upon their sacred resources. One 44-year-old survivor described his harrowing experience this way:

> The plane was moving more erratically. I knew it wasn't good by the in-crease in activity of the stewardesses. . . . The guy next to me at minus four minutes said, "We ain't going to make it." . . . I noticed the nun across

from me had been praying on her rosary. I remembered I had a cross in my pocket. I pulled it out and held it in my hand for the rest of the ride. ("Here I Was . . . , " 1989, p. 32)

Another said:

After the flight attendant explained emergency landing procedures, we were left with our thoughts. That's when I began praying. I closed my eyes and thought, "Dear Lord, I pray that you'll guide the pilot's hands." (p. 29)

Still another survivor spoke about the first few moments after the crash:

The plane smelled like a house of fire. I was exhilarated to be alive but deeply grieved when I could see and smell death. It was like being at the doorstep of hell. I pulled my Bible out of my bag. That's all I wanted. (p. 31)

Far from inert, sacred objects are filled with energy and potential. They are "vital objects" (LaMothe, 1998) that have the capacity to soothe and comfort, inspire and empower (see Greenberg et al., 1995). They can also place life in a context of greater meaning, connect the individual to the past and the future, and link people together in communities with common understandings of the sacred and its symbols. Upon discovery, the sacred becomes a resource that can be accessed throughout life.

Our research group has conducted a number of recent studies that support this point: couples who sanctify their marriages to a greater degree report that they derive greater personal benefits and satisfaction from their marriages (Mahoney et al., 1999); college students who view the act of sexual intercourse as sacred experience greater pleasure and satisfaction from the sexual act (Murray-Swank, Pargament, & Mahoney, 2005); and people who sanctify their strivings in life perceive their strivings to be more meaningful, report greater joy and happiness in the pursuit of these strivings, and feel greater support from family, friends, and God (Mahoney et al., 2005).

CONCLUSIONS

A few years ago, I met an immunologist at a meeting. Our talk turned to the topic of religion and spirituality, and my colleague asked rhetorically, "Isn't religion just a bunch of hormones?" His question reflected two biases in the medical and social sciences: the tendency to view human behavior as largely reactive—a response to genetic, physiological, unconscious, or environmental forces; and the tendency to view religion and spirituality as expressions of presumably deeper, more basic, more "real" processes. I disagreed with my colleague, arguing that people are more than reactive beings and that religion and spirituality are more than a bunch of hormones. In this chapter, I have elaborated on this different set of assumptions.

To paraphrase Gordon Allport (1950), people are guided as much by interest as they are by instinct. As goal-directed beings, people actively shape and direct their lives to attain whatever they hold to be significant. It is important to recognize that this search for significance unfolds in a field of forces with powers of their own to shape and direct, but no understanding of human nature would be complete without an appreciation for the capacity to imagine and move toward a future.

One destination many people strive toward is a connection with the sacred. I believe it is important to resist the tendency to treat spiritual motivation as "nothing but" something else, be it hormones, unconscious drives, genes, or the environment (Pargament, 2002a). Certainly, the search for the sacred has its biological, psychological, and social roots. However, this is not the full story. "From early on human beings are naturally spiritual" is the way Johnson and Boyatzis (2006, p. 220) put it. There are good reasons to view the search for the sacred as a distinctive motive in and of itself, one that can affect as well as be affected by other motives.

This chapter also elaborated on the process of discovery: the way it is experienced, its roots, and its consequences. Discovery, however, does not signal an end to the search for the sacred. Imbued with the qualities of transcendence, boundlessness, and ultimacy, wrapped in powerful emotions, centered in the individual's core, and esteemed as the most precious of resources, the sacred is not to be experienced, enjoyed, and then discarded. Instead, it becomes "the place to be." People want to reexperience, participate, and remain as long as possible in the sacred realm (Eliade, 1957). Thus, upon discovery, the search for the sacred shifts to conservation, and people embark on spiritual pathways that build, sustain, and enhance their relationship with the sacred. In the following chapter, we turn our attention to the process of conservation of the sacred.

4

Holding On to the Sacred

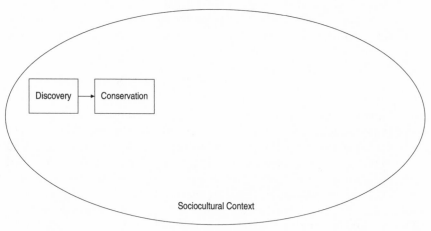

Discovery → Conservation

Sociocultural Context

The Search for the Sacred

After many hours spent closely observing the development of his own children, psychologist Jean Piaget (1954) reached an important conclusion. Children, he said, are by nature conservative; they resist change until it is absolutely necessary. Though Piaget focused his attention on children, his conclusion may apply to people more generally, for the tendency to hold on to significance does not end in childhood. Even in his last days, Bob Hope continued to play the part of the comedian, the role that had defined his life for almost a century. Bob Hope's wife reportedly asked him when he was near death where he would like to be buried. His response was, "Surprise me." In their final words, many people display similar devotedness to their sources of deepest value and meaning. Thus, Wolfgang

Amadeus Mozart asked, "Let me hear once more my solace and delight"; Revolutionary War patriot Nathan Hale regretted that "I have one life to lose for my country"; and Anne Frank persisted in her search for growth and self-discovery: "And finally, I twist my heart round again, so that the bad is on the outside and the good is on the inside, . . . and keep on trying to find a way of becoming what I would so like to be" (Last Words Browser, 2007). From birth to death, people cling tenaciously to whatever they find significant in their lives.

We enter the spiritual domain when the sacred becomes the ultimate destination in the individual's search for significance. In the previous chapter, I described how people discover the sacred. But the search does not end there. Once they discover the sacred, people try to hold on to and enhance (i.e., conserve) their relationship with it. Of course, people are not left totally to their own devices in this quest. Over thousands of years, religious traditions have developed pathways to assist individuals in their attempts to hold on to the sacred. People can construct their own nontraditional pathways as well. This chapter focuses on the rich and varied routes people create and follow as they try to conserve their relationship with the sacred.

PATHWAYS TO CONSERVING THE SACRED

The idea of the path is central to most religious traditions (Schmidt et al., 1999). For example, Buddhism speaks of the "Eightfold Path" that leads to enlightenment. The "Five Pillars of Islam" refer to the pathways that lead the adherent to submission to the will of Allah. Within Taoism, the word *Tao* literally means "the Way." The religions of the world differ in the specific paths they encourage their followers to take, but most religions prescribe various combinations of ways of knowing, ways of acting, ways of relating, and ways of experiencing. Ultimately, then, the pathway that a religious adherent follows is often constructed out of different raw materials joined together to form an overarching way of life.

Of course, not everyone chooses to fully embrace a particular religious way of life. In our pluralistic culture, many people approach religion as they would a meal in a cafeteria, picking and choosing from the "menu" of their own tradition the particular beliefs, practices, relationships, and experiences that they find most "appetizing" (Bibby, 1987). More and more today people are also sampling from the offerings of other religious traditions in designing their religious "meals." Nowadays it is not unusual to find Christians participating in a Passover seder, Jews practicing Buddhist forms of meditation, Buddhists engaging in dialogue with diverse faiths, and mixed-faith couples creating new combinations of rituals and practices. And many people today are completely turning away from existing religious traditions and seeking out their own innovative ways to conserve the sacred in their lives. There is, then, no shortage of pathways that people take to hold on to the sacred. The words of religious scholar Martin Marty, written in the 1960s, still resonate today:

> In search of spiritual expression, people speak in tongues, enter Trappist monasteries, build on Jungian archetypes, go to southern California and join a cult, become involved "where the action is" in East Harlem, perceive "God at work in the world," see Jesus Christ as the man for others, hope for liberation by the new morality, study phenomenology, share the Peace Corps experience, borrow from cosmic synthesis, and go to church. (cited in Roof, 1993, p. 241)

Below we review some of the pathways to conserving the sacred. We will see that, even though these spiritual pathways are constructed out of very human materials—thoughts, behaviors, relationships, and experiences—they are distinctive because they take on sacred form and content and because they lead toward sacred destinations (Jones, 2004). To the spiritually minded, the sacred is neither a temporary resting place nor an occasional source of strength and inspiration. It is a universe in itself, filled with power, being, and reality. It is a place people long to be, it is our most basic habitat.

The Pathway of Knowing

Recently, I took a flight to California. It was shortly after the New Year's celebration, and the flight was long and late in the day, so most of the passengers seemed only too happy to turn off their lights and sleep through the trip. But the fellow sitting next to me pulled a New Testament from his pocket along with a Bible study guide and spent most of the next 4 hours concentrating on a few pages of Scripture. From an outside perspective, his behavior seems hard to understand. Why, when he could have been chatting, sleeping, or watching a movie, did he devote so many hours to studying stories that took place over 2,000 years ago? As with so many questions about spirituality, the answer to this one calls for a look beneath the surface.

The stories of the Bible are more than stories. They speak to fundamental questions about life: how the world was formed, how people were created, the purpose of our lives, what is sacred and what is profane, how to explain tragedy, and what happens to us when we die. The answers to these questions are not written in the language of science. They take the form of epic accounts, parables, myths, allegories, and poetry that respond to the questions of mystery with mysterious answers of their own. We hear of strange events, amazing places, and unusual people: universes created out of a void, hellish landscapes of molten metal and bubbling liquid, messiahs born of virgins, men wrestling with angels, people caught up in an endless series of rebirths, worlds flooded and renewed, prophetic dreams that change the course of civilizations, people swallowed by whales or rising from the dead, the sun standing still. And yet, puzzling as they may be, these stories are said to be containers of divine truth. To some they are the literal word of God. To others their truth is embedded in symbol and metaphor. In either case, study and interpretation are needed to discern the spiritual wisdom within the sacred literature. Not that this search for truth ever ends. From most religious perspectives, the human attempt to decipher divine wisdom must always be incomplete, for God's ways are not necessarily our ways and "we are not the final arbiter of meaning" (Heschel, 1973, p. 295).

Spiritual study, then, is not merely an intellectual exercise. Neither is it merely a way of understanding or making sense of life. To the spiritual mind, the answers to the profound questions raised in these stories *reveal* the world in its most basic, most real sense; they offer a way of *knowing* the world and living more closely to and consistently with the mind of God (Paden, 1988). These stories are not to be viewed from a distance. The readers of the Hebrew Bible, the New Testament, the Koran, or the Upanishads are invited to put themselves into the shoes of the major protagonists, experience the events as if they were actors in the dramas themselves, and apply the lessons from these stories to life today. Thus, the Christian passenger who shared my flight to California was not engaged in idle reading. While others were asleep, he may have been reexperiencing the creation of the world, rejoining the Hebrew people as they wandered in the desert in search of the Promised Land, or reimagining the last moments of Jesus Christ.

Scripture is one source of knowing for many people, but as Carrie Doehring (2006) has pointed out, there are several ways of gaining scriptural knowledge. Approximately 77 million people in the United States believe that the Bible is the literal word of God (Thurston, 2000). Like those in ancient and medieval communities of faith, they believe that God can be known through the plain meanings of the sacred texts. This way of knowing has been described as "premodern." Then there are those who use modern approaches to understand sacred texts, drawing upon methods of scriptural interpretation that highlight their historical context, their literary forms, and their bases in the oral tradition. Nowadays, a third way of knowing, called "postmodern," assumes that all knowledge is socially constructed, with the meanings of any text dependent upon the social context of the reader.

In the United States, people who distrust any religious authority, including the authority of religious texts, live alongside people of faith who view sacred texts through premodern, modern, and postmodern lenses. Those who distrust religious authority are not necessarily spiritually disengaged. For them, reason and intuition rather than religious authority are the pathway to ultimate wisdom. As Wuthnow (1998) notes in his study of spirituality in the United States, today many people are engaged in constructing their own truths through personal soul-searching or by drawing on the perspectives of modern spiritual writers, such as James Hillman, Thomas Moore, or M. Scott Peck, whose works may be perceived as more compelling than the classic religious texts. Still others may search for ultimate answers through use of the systematic tools of reason—that is, science. Einstein (1988) himself wrote that "the path to genuine religiosity [is found] through striving after rational knowledge" (p. 96).

Of course, we have to be careful about distinguishing too sharply between faith and reason. Many notable theologians from Aquinas and Tillich to Maimonides and Spinoza did not hesitate to use reason as a tool for uncovering the divine truths of the sacred texts. And the search for ultimate knowledge through reason rests on a faith not unlike that of the more traditionally religious, the faith that there are indeed ultimate answers. Again, Einstein (1988) put it well: "To know that what is impenetrable to us really exists, manifesting itself as the highest wisdom and the most radiant beauty which our dull faculties can comprehend only in their most primitive forms—this knowledge, this feeling, is at the center of the true religiousness. In this sense, and in this sense only, I belong in the ranks of the devoutly religious men" (p. 95).

Whether their knowledge grows out of reason, intuition, or revelation, many people take the path of study so that they may come to know life's greatest truths and live more fully and consistently within that sacred realm.

The Pathway of Acting

Important as knowledge and wisdom are to many people, they may not be enough to sustain a relationship with the sacred unless they are translated into action. According to a Jewish saying, "Anyone whose good deeds exceed his wisdom, his wisdom will endure; but anyone whose wisdom exceeds his good deeds, his wisdom will not endure" (Ethics of the Fathers, 3:12). To live most fully within the realm of the sacred, individuals must enact their spiritual understandings of the world through ritual and practice.

Religious rituals come in a variety of shapes and sizes. They include rituals that mark certain times of the week or year, such as the Sabbath or harvest festivals; those that celebrate an event in the life of a deity, such as the birthday of the Buddha or Jesus Christ; those that facilitate a cleansing or purification of the spirit, such as the fasting that occurs during Ramadan by Muslims and during Lent by Catholics; and those that reenact critical historical moments within a tradition, such as the ritual of communion with Christ in the Eucharist or the festival of Diwali within Hinduism that commemorates the destruction of a demon by the deity Krishna.

Rituals can be understood, in part, as methods to reduce anxiety, create meaning in life, encourage emotional expression and emotional control, foster personal identity, and promote group cohesiveness (see Jacobs, 1992). From a spiritual perspective, though, this type of psychological and social analysis is incomplete, for rituals are first and foremost ways of connecting to the sacred, ways of bringing another world into existence that can be entered and experienced again and again. Listen, for example, to how one woman describes the ritual lighting of candles to welcome the Sabbath:

> "The rituals turn me on inside. It happens physically. Each Friday at sunset when I light the candles for Shabbat, I have an experience of shedding the weekday and opening up to sanctity. Suddenly the room is filled with something else. The indwelling presence, the femaleness of God, the Shekhinah, awakens. There is a simple, deep sense of connectedness—a linking of the indwelling with the transcendent God." (Anderson & Hopkins, 1991, p. 162)

Rituals are not to be confused with a simple set of repetitive actions; rituals have power. Indeed, some would say they *unleash* sacred power. Rituals unfold in a symbolic context of special objects, colors, smells, shapes, sounds, touch, and places that engage people at many levels. These symbols help to fashion a sacred world and usher the individual into that realm. There, a creative process is reenacted in which the person shifts from the role of distant bystander to that of actor, vitally engaged in replaying life's ultimate dramas (Clothey, 1981). And there the individual experiences a transcendent connection. Thus, in the ritual of communion we see Christians reexperiencing Jesus's sacrifice on their behalf and receiving spiritual nourishment through the gifts of his body and spirit. Similarly, in the Passover seder, we hear Jews retelling the story of the Exodus of the Hebrew people from slavery to freedom, not as historians looking back on an ancient event, but as participants who were and continue to be a part of this sacred tale of redemption. These rituals are ways of "reactualizing sacred history" that keep people "close to the gods—that is, in the real and the significant" (Eliade, 1957, p. 202).

Rituals are only one type of spiritual action. Other spiritual practices are not necessarily limited to certain times and places. Virtually every religious tradition prescribes a set of ethics, virtues, commandments, and practices that extend the reach of the sacred to many if not every sphere of life—from the most appropriate ways to wash, eat, and use the bathroom to the proper handling of money, animals, and personal appetites. These spiritual practices speak not only to what the individual should do, but, just as importantly, to what the individual must avoid doing. Many religious traditions offer their adherents a long list of "don'ts." Certainly, a number of these prohibitions (e.g., against gluttony, incest, avarice) have great value for the health and well-being of individuals and the community. But to the spiritual mind, these practices are condemned primarily because they separate the individual from the sacred. By avoiding vices and engaging in positive spiritual practices, people foster and conserve a world in which even the most mundane of activities takes on an aura of divinity.

Although many spiritual practices are prescribed by religious traditions, people are free to construct their own spiritual practices that enable them to live more fully within the sacred dimension. They may apply traditional spiritual practices in new ways. For instance, following the death of his mother, one man modified the family practice of putting a ceramic angel on the Christmas tree: "[The angel] belonged to her—my dad gave it to her their first Christmas. They always put it on the tree after Midnight Mass. It meant Christmas had come. I haven't gone to Midnight Mass myself for years, but every December 24 at midnight, I put that angel on the tree, and I think of my parents, and just that angel brings back all the Christmases in my mind" (Imber-Black & Roberts, 1992, pp. 129–130). Other spiritual practices may develop outside of a religious tradition. Listen to the sacred qualities one woman imbues into the act of quilting: "By simple definition, quilting is merely sewing pieces of fabric together into a whole. But as spiritual discipline, it is a careful attention to the details of my life. Quilting as spiritual discipline is entering the sensual richness of the universe, creating order out of chaos, beauty out of the simple, wholeness from the scraps, and in the midst, being transformed" (Bushbaum, 1999, p. 236).

In the broadest sense, spiritual practices encompass whatever people do to preserve and protect the sacred in their lives, including those activities that may not be perceived as spiritual in nature. Annette Mahoney, several other colleagues, and I have conducted empirical studies that are relevant to this point. In one study of Presbyterian Church members, elders, and clergy, we found that people who perceive the environment as sacred were more likely to act in environmentally friendly ways (Tarakeshwar et al., 2001). Similarly, we found that spouses who view their marriages as sacred were less prone to verbal aggression and other destructive ways of resolving marital conflicts (Mahoney et al., 1999). Thus, many seemingly secular behaviors—from separating recyclable materials from trash to avoiding the temptation to lash out at a loved one in the heat of the moment—may be practices that are, in fact, laden with spiritual value and meaning.

It would be a mistake, then, to restrict our understanding of the spiritual pathway of action to a few practices that are disconnected from everyday experience. As Wuthnow (1998) notes, "The point of spiritual practice is not to elevate an isolated set of activities over the rest of life but to electrify the spiritual impulse that animates all of life" (p. 198).

The Pathway of Relating to Others

According to Buddhist tradition, Siddhārtha Gautama was born to wealth, power, and prestige (Smith, 1958). Sheltered from ugliness by his father, Siddhārtha Gautama was shaken in his twenties by his encounter with three disturbing scenes: one with a decrepit old man, another with a diseased man, and a third with a corpse. Thus, he discovered the painful realities of aging, illness, and ultimately, death. Unable to return to his life of pleasure and indulgence with these visions in mind, Siddhārtha Gautama left his home and family behind and took off in search of enlightenment. His search was not easy. Over the course of the following 6 years, he traveled some roads that proved to be dead ends, such as the paths of self-indulgence and self-mortification. Ultimately, he experienced what is now known as the "Great Awakening." After sitting beneath a fig tree for 49 days, Siddhārtha Gautama experienced deep rapture and transformation into the Buddha. Having found enlightenment, Buddha confronted the question of what to do with it. Here he faced his last and greatest temptation. He could have remained apart from others, immersed in his private rapturous state, but the Buddha instead chose to return to the world, where he spent the remaining 45 years of his life sharing his truths with others, counseling the afflicted and distressed, and founding an order of monks.

Distinctive as it is, the story of the Buddha is paralleled by the epic stories of other great religious figures, from Moses to Muhammad, who received revelations of their own and also proceeded to build relationships, communities, indeed, nations, to share their wisdom. The same dynamic holds true today. Despite the powerful stream of individualism in Western culture, few people practice their faith in total isolation. The large majority come together to share their ways of knowing the world and enact their truths through shared rituals and practices. For example, more than two-thirds of people in the United States belong to a church, synagogue, or mosque (Hoge, 1996). This figure has been relatively constant since the 1940s. Within these religious organizations, members can choose from varied forms of spiritual relationship, including shared worship, prayer groups, Bible study, religious education, and counseling with religious leaders. Many people who are not members of religious institutions also take part in other spiritual groups, such as spiritual retreats and meditation, healing, and yoga groups (Spilka et al., 2003).

Spiritual relationships are not limited to religious institutions or spiritual groups. Spirituality can also unfold in daily relationships with family, friends, and others in the community. It may grow out of acts of love and compassion. "Love," Thomas Moore (1992) writes, "releases us into the realm of divine imagination, where the soul is expanded and reminded of its unearthly cravings and needs" (p. 81). It may emerge from regular conversation or rituals in the home. Or it may come from witnessing the actions of others. For example, Anderson and Hopkins (1991) introduce the idea of a "resonator" as a spiritual model. A resonator, they say, is someone who is true to his or her own inner reality and, in turn, inspires others to identify and live more faithfully according to their own deepest values. One woman put it this way: "I think if I can remain true to my inner sounding, to my tuning fork, I can set up a harmonic in which your tuning fork will begin to vibrate, and you, in turn, will set up a resonance in someone else" (p. 209).

It is important to remember that spiritual ties are not simply vehicles for sharing, disseminating, and living out spiritual truths. They have a sacred value of their own, for God may be seen as manifest in relationships or relationships may be seen as the containers of sacred qualities. Within Christianity, for example, Christ is said to be present in the church and the members of the church, in turn, are said to be incorporated into Christ. Similarly, many traditions hold that people are children of God and, as a result, we are called to relate to each other with caring and compassion. This is the message of the Golden Rule. People may be surprised to know that variants of the Golden Rule can be found in traditions other than Judaism and Christianity, including Hinduism ("Do not to others what you do not wish done to yourself; and wish for others too what you desire and long for, for yourself"), Islam ("Do to all men as you would wish to have done unto you; and reject for others what you would reject for yourselves"), and Confucianism ("Do not to others what you do not want done to yourself") (Peterson, 1986, pp. 74–75).

Relationships, then, are more than a pathway to a continued connection to the sacred; they are carriers of their own sacred meaning. From this perspective, relationships with family, friends, and community can be profoundly spiritual in and of themselves. Susan Sered (1989) spoke to this point in her participant observation study of elderly Jewish women in a day center in Jerusalem. Family, she discovered, was the organizing religious principle for these women. By caring for family members, the elderly women saw themselves as participating in something holy. The days of their lives were spent attempting to safeguard not only spouses, children, grandchildren, and extended kin, but also biological or mythical ancestors (e.g., biblical figures) who were remembered, watched over, and petitioned for additional help in protecting living family members. The prayers and rituals of these women were directed to ensuring the health and well-being of their kin. Mundane activities, such as cooking and cleaning for the family, also had sacred significance for them, for no act holds higher spiritual value than attending to the needs of loved ones. In this world, Sered concludes, "relationship is sacred" (p. 323).

The Pathway of Experiencing

The study of sacred scriptures (thought), the practice of religious rituals (action), and the participation in spiritual community (relationship) are all important pathways to the sacred for many people, but most would find it difficult to sustain their spirituality without what is perceived as the emotional experience of the sacred. It is the sense of an immediate encounter with the sacred, the encounter people feel deep in their bones, that provides them with the most compelling of spiritual pathways. This point may be especially true in the United States, where spirituality is generally something that people need to feel for themselves (Wuthnow, 1998).

There are many ways people seek out immediate encounters with the sacred. They range from traditional methods—scriptural study, rituals, and church attendance—to less traditional approaches: music, drugs, sex, and solitude (Hood, 1995). But of all the methods for experiencing the sacred, prayer is by far the most common in this country, where nine out of 10 people pray (Gallup & Lindsay, 1999). "Prayer" is an umbrella term that covers many forms of expression: the silent prayer, the chanted prayer, the formal prayer, the spontaneous prayer, the prayer of joy and gratitude, the prayer of pain and suffering, the conversational prayer, the pleading prayer. Although psychologists have focused on the role of prayer in facilitating physical health and mental health, from a spiritual perspective these analyses miss the point, for the most essential function of prayer is communion with the sacred. Margaret Poloma and George Gallup Jr. (1991) highlighted this notion in their study of a national sample of Americans. Many in their sample engaged in petitionary and ritual prayers. However, these expressions were less common than conversational and meditative prayers that involve simply talking with, thinking about, or listening to God. One woman described her prayers this way:

> I pray when I get up in the morning and just before I go to bed. But I don't limit myself to these two five to twenty minute prayer times. I talk to God all through the day. . . . When I am happy, I thank God for life. . . . When I feel boxed in and need direction, I ask God for his guidance. . . . Most of these prayers are silent—done in conversational style in my heart. (p. 30)

Prayer, for this woman and many others, is the vital ingredient that cements her ongoing relationship with God. Abraham Heschel (1973) tells a very different story with a similar message. Shortly after World War II, a friend of Heschel's was on his way by train from Warsaw to Paris. The train was very crowded so the friend invited a poor, emaciated Jew to share his compartment. While Heschel's friend engaged in his evening prayers, the other fellow declined, saying, "I am never going to pray any more, because of what happened to us in Auschwitz. . . . How could I pray?" (p. 302). The following morning, though, the friend noticed that his companion had started to pray. When asked why he changed his mind, the fellow said, "It suddenly dawned upon me to think how lonely God must be; look with whom He is left. I felt sorry for Him" (p. 303). At its heart, prayer is a way to experience a relationship with the divine. It expresses, in the words of Thomas Merton (1969), a "yearning for the simple presence of God" (p. 82).

Those who do not believe in a theistic God have their own ways of experiencing the sacred: they may experience what they perceive as encounters with angels or departed loved ones; they may experience a sense of transcendence through the language of music or art; or they may gain inner enlightenment through meditation. This latter practice has become particularly popular in recent years. Though meditation has a long history within western religious traditions, its upsurge in popularity has undoubtedly been shaped by the infusion of Asian disciplines in the United States in the second half of the 20th century (though many people meditate without knowledge of its deeply spiritual underpinnings). As practiced within Hinduism, Buddhism, and Taoism, meditation is not so much a way to experience an external God, as it is a way to understand the sacred in terms of inner illumination or enlightenment. Ordinary consciousness, according to Eastern thought, is limited and misleading. Meditation offers a way to cut through deceptive appearances, access deeper truths, and realize the full spectrum of human consciousness. How is that achieved?

There are many meditative practices. At a broad level, Goleman (1977) has distinguished between two types of meditation: concentration and mindfulness. Concentration forms of meditation encourage the practitioner to focus on an object, always bringing the mind back to some chosen focal point when it wanders. The object may be a mantra assigned by a trainer, as in the case of transcendental meditation (TM), or a phrase, a song, an emotion (e.g., compassion), or a movement (e.g., breathing). Mindfulness forms of meditation encourage the practitioner to engage in a detached, nonjudgmental observation of whatever the individual may be experiencing in the present moment. No event is a distraction, John Astin (1997) notes in his description of mindfulness. The challenge for the practitioner is to sustain attention, witnessing and accepting rather than avoiding or interpreting the ceaseless stream of thoughts, feelings, sensations, and perceptions that flow through his or her consciousness, including painful and distressing emotions. Some forms of meditation combine both concentration and mindfulness. For example, most popular forms of mindfulness meditation (MM) today instruct individuals to attend both to their breathing and to each moment of experience. Listen to a meditation written by Jack Kornfield (1993):

> Sit as the Buddha did on his night of enlightenment, with great dignity and centeredness, sensing your capacity to face anything that arises. Let your

eyes close and let your attention turn to your breathing. Let your breath move freely through your body. Let each breath bring a calmness and an ease. As you breathe, sense your capacity to opening body, heart, and soul.

Open your senses, your feelings, your thoughts. Become aware of what feels closed in your body, closed in your heart, closed in your mind. Breathe and make space. Let the space open so that anything may arise. Let the windows of your senses open. Be aware of whatever feelings, images, sounds, and stories show themselves. Notice with interest and ease all that presents itself to you. (p. 39)

As he or she develops increasing skill in this form of focused concentration, the meditator is said to achieve a purer awareness and a deeper spiritual connection, as we hear in the words of one Taoist sage:

> Control the mind.
> Attain one-pointedness.
> Then the harmony of heaven.
> Will come down and dwell in you.
> You will be radiant with life.
> You will rest in Tao.
> (Chuang Tzu [22:3], cited in Walsh, 1999, p. 90)

Experiences identified as encounters with the sacred are not restricted to the quiet reflection of contemplative prayer or the trance-like calm of the meditative state. For some, the experience of the sacred is less like a serene lake than it is a tidal wave that washes over the person with staggering force. In a fascinating participant observation study of the Toronto Blessing, a revivalist Pentecostal/Charismatic movement in Canada, Margaret Poloma (2003) documented a variety of manifestations of spiritual experience among group members, including deep weeping, holy laughter, dancing in the spirit, uncontrolled jerking, rolling on the floor, intense shaking, being "drunk in the spirit," and roaring like a lion. A typical participant described for Poloma how the spirit came to her:

> Almost immediately my body started rocking and shaking. I felt like something was coming from my belly. I grabbed a pillow as I felt like something was now coming out of my mouth. Then this strange language ("tongues" as I understand it) came forth with uncontrollable sobbing. I cried and talked in the strange language. I laughed and laughed. . . . I opened my eyes thinking it would go away, but it didn't. (p. 66)

Among those involved in the Toronto Blessing, Poloma points out, experiences such as this one are not isolated events. Instead, they are understood to be continuing manifestations of the Holy Spirit that reenergize and revitalize the connection to the divine.

A FEW CAUTIONS ABOUT THE
METAPHOR OF SPIRITUAL PATHWAYS

We have briefly reviewed the pathways people take to building, conserving, and enhancing their relationship with the sacred. However, the metaphor of the pathway could be misleading in a few ways. First, it may bring to mind the image of a concrete road that people never stray from throughout their lives. While some do stay on the same spiritual path, these individuals may be the exception rather than the rule. More commonly, spiritual pathways grow and evolve in different directions as people mature, their needs change, and they encounter the occasional roadblock to the sacred. Over the course of their lives, many people change congregations, try out new spiritual practices, take on different spiritual perspectives, and seek out new spiritual experiences, all in the effort to nurture and sustain their relationship with the sacred. Recall, for instance, the story of Cindy (Chapter 3) who, in her attempt to recapture and foster the sense of God's presence she had experienced as a child, shifted from Eastern mysticism to Native American religion to astrology to witchcraft to the Christian church. Cindy experienced a great deal of turmoil and relatively little assistance as she changed her spiritual path, but other people are more fortunate. They receive support and guidance in this process from many sources, such as spiritual directors, wisdom literature, spiritual exercises, and prayer. Consider, for instance, this prayer: "It would be easier, Lord, to stay with what I know, to take only well-marked paths to familiar places in my heart and soul. But if I am to come to you, then I must leave behind the comfort of what I already know and accept your invitation to journey into your infinite mystery. Take my hand, guide my steps, give courage to my heart and soul" (Kirvan, 1999, p. 131).

The metaphor of the spiritual pathway could be misleading in a second way, for it suggests that this journey may have a fixed and final destination. Yet spiritually minded people do not travel these paths as sightseers hoping to get a glimpse of the sacred and then move on in new directions. They take up the spiritual quest because they are yearning for an ongoing relationship with a spiritual presence or a sacred companion who will accompany them throughout their lives. To that end, the relationship with the sacred must be cultivated and nurtured through repetition and discipline. If the individual is to reach and remain with the sacred, he or she must persist in the spiritual journey. Thus, among the most spiritual of people, spiritual study is a task that never ends, religious rituals are enacted and reenacted on a regular basis, spiritual communities become permanent homes, and prayer and meditation are integrated into the daily rhythm of life. Why? Because the way of the sacred is a way of life, one that requires practice, determination, and discipline.

EVALUATING THE SPIRITUAL PATHWAYS

How well do these pathways work? Literally hundreds of research studies have addressed this question. The vast majority of the research on the efficacy of spiritual pathways has focused on their psychological, social, and physical effects. In perhaps the most comprehensive review of this literature, Harold Koenig, Michael McCullough, and David Larson (2001) concluded that, in the majority of studies, measures of religious and spiritual beliefs, practices, relationships, and experiences are correlated with:

- Well-being, happiness, and life satisfaction
- Hope and optimism
- Purpose and meaning in life
- Higher self-esteem
- Greater social support and less loneliness
- Lower rates of depression
- Lower rates of suicide
- Less anxiety
- Less psychosis
- Lower rates of alcohol and drug use
- Less delinquency and criminal activity
- Greater marital stability and satisfaction

In addition, they note a clear link between religious involvement, particularly frequent attendance at religious services, and longevity. Those who attend their congregations weekly or more have a 25–30% reduced risk of dying in the following 5–25 years.

Social scientists have offered a variety of psychological, social, and physiological explanations for these findings. For example, they have suggested that the beneficial effects of congregational attendance on mortality may be the result of the social support provided by the congregation, the optimism of congregation members, and better health practices among members of the congregation. And yet researchers have found that none of these variables is able to account for the relationship between congregational involvement and mortality (see McCullough, Hoyt, Larson, Koenig, & Thoresen, 2000).

There may be a simpler explanation (see Pargament, Magyar, & Murray-Swank, 2005). Perhaps there is something distinctive about spiritual pathways, something that cannot be easily reduced to other psychological, social, or physical explanations. James Baldwin (1963) captures the uniqueness of one form of spiritual expression in his description of the storefront church of his childhood:

There is no music like that music, no drama like the drama of the saints re-
joicing, the sinners moaning, the tambourines racing, and all those voices
coming together and crying holy unto the Lord. There is still, for me, no
pathos quite like the pathos of those multicolored, somehow triumphant
and transfigured faces, speaking from the depths of a visible, tangible,
continuing despair of the goodness of the Lord. I have never seen anything
to equal the fire and excitement that sometimes, without warning, fill a
church. (p. 47)

Baldwin is pointing to the power of distinctively spiritual phenomena:
the feeling of being lifted up by the music, the sense of conviction of a basic
and ultimate truth, and the merging of oneself with others in a spiritual
community of individuals who are joined by the sharing of their deepest
emotions of joy, pain, and gratitude. These may be among the most critical
ingredients in the recipe for longer life through religious involvement.

On the face of it, the findings from the empirical literature would seem
to offer clear evidence of the benefits of spiritual pathways. Yet it is important to note that these studies do not speak to the degree to which spiritual
pathways help people reach their *spiritual* goals. In fact, only a few studies
have examined the ties between spiritual pathways and explicitly spiritual
criteria. Of course, as researchers, we cannot determine whether people actually find and conserve a relationship with God or a higher power. We
have no tools to measure God. Neither can we assess the part the sacred actually plays in the human relationship. We can, however, focus on individuals' *perceptions* of a relationship with the sacred. For example, in their national survey, Gallup and Lindsay (1999) found that 97% of those who
read the Bible reported that it helped them feel "somewhat" or a "great
deal" closer to God. Similarly, 95% of those who pray reported that their
prayers had been answered. In other empirical studies, people who report
greater personal faith, attend services more often, engage in more spiritual
study, and pray more regularly also score higher on measures of closeness
to God, spiritual growth, and spiritual well-being (e.g., Ellison & Smith,
1991; Pargament et al., 1990). These studies suggest that spiritual pathways may impact people spiritually as well as psychologically, socially, and
physically.

Remember, however, that virtually any aspect of life can take on spiritual meaning. Thus, we have to be careful of drawing too fine a distinction
between the sacred and the secular, for the "biopsychosocial" dimensions
can have a spiritual significance of their own. Most religious traditions encourage the psychological, social, and physical health and well-being of
their members, but health and well-being are understood in a larger sacred
context. Thus, in the Book of Psalms, the psalmist prays for his own health
not as an end in itself, but as a means to praise God:

> Have mercy upon me, O Lord; for I am weak: O Lord, heal
> me; for my bones are vexed.
> My soul is also sore vexed: but thou, O Lord, how long?
> Return, O Lord, deliver my soul: oh save me for thy
> mercies' sake.
> For in death there is no remembrance of thee: in the grave
> who shall give thee thanks? (Psalms 6:3–6)

Finally, it is important to recognize that, even though empirical studies have linked spiritual pathways to a variety of positive outcomes, the strength of these statistical ties is only modest to moderate at best. To put it in more basic terms, the research shows that spirituality is generally beneficial, but not invariably so. Many people who follow spiritual pathways do not experience positive outcomes. Why might this be the case? Perhaps because spiritual involvement in and of itself is not necessarily constructive. In later chapters, I argue that the value of spirituality depends on the *kind* of spirituality we are talking about.

THE SPIRITUAL ORIENTING
SYSTEM AND CONCLUSIONS

In these chapters, we have seen that there is tremendous diversity in the ways in which the sacred is perceived and understood and in the paths people take to conserving their relationship with the sacred. Most people, however, are selective in the spiritual paths and destinations they choose and follow. Over time, people develop preferences for particular spiritual pathways and destinations. Based on personal, situational, and social forces, some pathways and destinations become more compelling than others. One person strives to make the world a sacred place by acts of kindness to others and efforts to bring about a more equitable society. Another seeks a personal relationship with Jesus largely through scriptural study, prayer, and devotion. One person tries to experience the sense of transcendence in daily life through meditative practices and outdoor experiences. Yet another attempts to discover ultimate truths about the origins of the universe through scientific investigation. These preferred patterns or configurations of pathways and destinations come together to form highly individualized spiritual orienting systems—frameworks of spiritual beliefs, practices, relations, experiences, and values that consistently guide and direct the search for the sacred (Pargament, 1997).

The spiritual orienting system simplifies the sacred quest and helps the person maintain stability in the process. Spiritual orienting systems are generally effective in their task. Nevertheless, there are times in life when the search for the sacred may be severely tested by trauma or transition. During these periods, the person is likely to become spiritually "disoriented" and less able to follow well-worn spiritual pathways to familiar spiritual destinations. During these times of disorientation, people embark on yet one more spiritual path, the path of spiritual coping. Spiritual coping methods are made up of the same ingredients that go into the other pathways: thoughts, practices, relationships, and experiences. But these ingredients come together to create a new pathway, one that is specifically designed to help people respond to challenges, threats, and harm to the sacred. In the next two chapters, we focus on the path of spiritual coping and the two major types of spiritual coping methods: those that attempt to protect and preserve the sacred in the face of danger, and those that attempt to transform the sacred when it can no longer be conserved.

5

In Times of Stress

Spiritual Coping to Conserve the Sacred

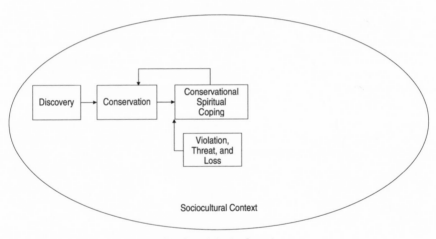

The Search for the Sacred

VIOLATION, THREAT, AND LOSS OF THE SACRED

Several years ago, I met Rachel. A bright, single, 35-year-old woman who worked with young, severely disabled children as a special education teacher, Rachel was looking for help in dealing with a long-standing depression, one she attributed to the pressures of her job and a severe case of endometriosis that left her unable to have children. Over the next months, we made little progress. Our conversations seemed to start, sputter, and stop like a car with carburetor problems. We would focus on one issue and then, without warning, she would shift to another topic. In the course of one of these herky-jerky sessions, Rachel casually mentioned that, 10 years

94

earlier, she had been gang-raped. Apart from a conversation with emergency room staff at the hospital, she had not disclosed the rapes to anyone for 10 years. It would take many more months of therapy before Rachel was able to begin talking about the horrors she had endured in any detail.

Why had Rachel kept her nightmarish experiences to herself for 10 years? Why had she chosen to live in such emotional isolation? There was no single answer. As we began to explore the last decade of her life, I learned about Rachel's mistrust of the willingness and capacity of people to grasp what had happened to her, the deep feelings of shame that accompanied her memories of the rapes, and her insistence that these rapes would not intrude into and disrupt the life she had worked so hard to construct. But I was most struck by something else. When I asked Rachel to describe how the rapes had affected her, she would sit quietly, think carefully, and finally shake her head, saying, "There are no words." I did not force the issue; Rachel had had enough of men in her life telling her what to do. But she continued to do her own thinking. One day Rachel came to a session and said she had a found a word to describe how she felt. "Contaminated," she said. "I feel as though I have been contaminated by what they did. What they did made me dirty and I can't wash it away. I feel that I am polluted to my very core, to my very being." As she spoke these words, she began to tremble.

Rachel had come upon the language of desecration. The rapes were not simply gross insults to her body and mind: she experienced them as spiritual violations, desecrations of her soul. Although Rachel had never described herself in religious or spiritual terms, the rapes had, in fact, shaken and disoriented her in a profoundly spiritual way. As we will see later in the book, addressing the spiritual character of her trauma was a key to Rachel's process of healing.

Desecrations have power. Some of the strongest words in religious language are reserved for violations of the sacred: "pollution," "profanation," "desecration," "abomination." It is important to recognize that violations of the sacred are more than traumatic events. For example, sexual abuse by the clergy is not simply an act of sexual betrayal. It is especially abhorrent because it represents a spiritual violation on several levels: a desecration of the sacred role of the clergy; a desecration of a sacred institution that may have legitimated the cleric and cloaked his acts in secrecy; a desecration of the survivor's understanding of God as a loving, protective being; a desecration of human sexuality; a violation of the rituals, symbols, and icons of a tradition that is difficult to disentangle from the offending clergy and institution, and a desecration of the survivor's soul (Pargament, Murray-Swank, & Mahoney, in press).

Well aware that people are sustained by their sanctified objects, groups bent on social destruction single out the sacred objects and spiritual pathways of their targets for desecration. During the Holocaust, for instance, the Nazis were committed to the destruction not only of Jewish lives, but of all vestiges of Jewish culture. LaMothe (1998) writes: "Sacred objects, which had held the beliefs, aspirations, expectations, hopes, and memories of a people were painstakingly destroyed by the Nazis. . . . Death camps were not only literal death camps but they were also death camps in that there were no vital-sacred objects and hence no life, only existence and necessity. This was a reality constructed with the intention of obliterating what is fundamental to human vitality . . . by means of the forced removal of sacred objects and practices" (pp. 166–167).

Many other life stressors can be perceived as violations of the sacred, from burning the American flag to pictorial caricatures of the prophet Muhammad. In a recent study of a community sample, my colleagues and I asked participants to describe a negative event they had experienced in the last 2 years (Pargament, Magyar, Benore, & Mahoney, 2005). The events they listed included a personal illness, a personal injury, illness or death of a close family member, job loss, and divorce/separation. Over 24% perceived the event as a desecration or violation of the sacred. Along similar lines, shortly after the 9/11 terrorist attack on the World Trade Center, we conducted a survey of college students in New York and Ohio about the degree to which they viewed the terrorist attacks as a desecration (Mahoney et al., 2002). Perceptions of desecration were common. For instance, approximately half of each sample agreed that "this event was both an offense against me and against God." About 30% of the two samples agreed that "something sacred that came from God was dishonored."

Empirical studies have shown that spiritual violations often shake people emotionally and physically. In one study of perceived desecration involving a sample of college students who had been recently hurt in a romantic relationship, higher levels of desecration were associated with more physical health symptoms and poorer mental health (Magyar, Pargament, & Mahoney, 2000). In the 9/11 study described above, students who perceived the terrorists attacks as a desecration also displayed higher levels of posttraumatic symptoms and depression following the attacks. In the community study above, people who appraised their negative life events as desecrations experienced stronger feelings of anger.

Perceptions of desecration can also lead to prejudice concerning the purported transgressors. My colleagues and I recently conducted a study that bears on this point (Pargament, Trevino, Mahoney, & Silberman, 2007). We tested the hypothesis that Christian anti-Semitism grows out of the perception that Jews represent a threat to Christian values. To test this hypothesis, we developed a measure to assess the degree to which Christians view Jews as desecrators of Christianity. The measure included items such as "The Jews represent a threat to the ultimate mission of Christ" and "The failure of Jews to accept Jesus Christ is an insult to the church." Our hypothesis was supported. Working with a sample of college undergraduates, we found that people who perceived Jews to be desecrators of Christianity held more anti-Semitic attitudes. Just as importantly, we found that these perceptions were greater among students who had been more exposed to messages of Jews as desecrators by the church, sacred literature, family, and media.

Not surprisingly, violations of the sacred can also impact people spiritually. Traumatic events have been associated with changes in religious beliefs, perhaps in part because these events represent spiritual violations. For example, in a study of people diagnosed with posttraumatic stress disorder (PTSD), 30% reportedly became less religious after their trauma, while 20% became more religious (Falsetti, Resick, & Davis, 2003). In a study of college students, students who reported physical and emotional abuse as children were less likely to maintain the religious beliefs they had been taught in their families (Webb & Whitmer, 2003). Other studies have shown that women with a history of childhood sexual abuse report more negative characterizations of God (e.g., Doehring, 1993; Kane, Cheston, & Greer, 1993).

Desecrations are only one way in which the search for the sacred can be disrupted. Other life events can be perceived as threats to the sacred. Heilman and Witztum (2000) describe the case of Moshe, a young ultra-Orthodox Jewish man, diagnosed with paranoid schizophrenia. Though his hallucinations were partly controlled by medications, he found that the voices and visions tended to occur on Fridays as he was preparing for the Sabbath. Moshe did not show any ambivalence about observing the Sabbath. "On the contrary, he loved the Sabbath and wanted to 'keep it holy' " (p. 118). Thus, his hallucinations were particularly distressing because they threatened his ability to experience and celebrate the sanctity of the day of rest. Indeed, Heilman and Witztum point out, "This religious disability bothered [Moshe] (and his family) as much, if not more than, the disorder itself" (p. 118).

Still other life events may be viewed as sacred losses. In our study of negative life events in a community sample, my colleagues and I found that over 38% of the participants perceived their negative event as a sacred loss (Pargament, Magyar, Benore, & Mahoney, 2005). Just as intentional violations of the sacred are likely to elicit anger and rage, the loss of the sacred is likely to lead to sadness and depression. In fact, participants in our community study who perceived their negative events as sacred losses reported higher levels of depression. We might hypothesize several other links between different types of sacred disruption and different types of emotional reactions. Perceptions of events as threats to the sacred may trigger greater anxiety. Personal violations of the sacred may result in guilt. And differences in perceptions of the sacred in a marriage may lead to marital distress. Disruptions of the search for the sacred can set the stage for a variety of strong emotions. Why? Because the deepest of all values and a way of life built on these values are at stake.

Strong emotional reactions are not necessarily problematic. Our research group found that perceptions of spiritual loss and, in some instances, spiritual violation are also associated with reports of greater spiritual growth (Magyar et al., 2000; Pargament, Magyar, Benore, & Mahoney, 2005; Pargament, Smith, Koenig, & Perez, 1998). Whether disorientation and disruption in the search for the sacred leads in positive or negative directions depends, in part, on how well individuals cope with these intrusions which (as we will see in later chapters) depends, in turn, on the degree to which the individual is spiritually well integrated. Oftentimes, the first choice in coping is to try to hold on to the sacred. We will see that conservational methods of spiritual coping are generally successful. Yet, at times, life stressors can throw the individual's world into greater spiritual turmoil. When well-worn pathways to the sacred and sacred destinations are no longer viable, the individual enters a period of spiritual struggle. In response to these struggles, the individual may engage in transformational methods of spiritual coping or disengage from the search for the sacred. In this and the following chapter, we focus on these two major spiritual methods of coping: those that are designed to conserve the sacred and those that are designed to transform the sacred.

SPIRITUAL METHODS OF COPING TO CONSERVE THE SACRED

Several months ago, a rabbi told me the following story. He had received a late-night call from a former synagogue member, a middle-aged woman who had moved to California with her family a few years earlier. Her 19-year-old son had recently returned to the local area to visit friends, and had just been arrested for driving under the influence of alcohol. Understandably, his mother was quite upset. She asked the rabbi to pick her son up from jail and bring him to his home until she could make arrangements for her son's return trip to California. The rabbi agreed. He went to the jail in the middle of the night and brought the son back to his house. Sheepish and embarrassed, the young man was reluctant to talk on the drive home. Finally, as he was about to enter the rabbi's house, he asked the rabbi, "What do I do now?" The rabbi paused for a moment and answered, "Put on a yarmulke [head covering]." The rabbi was sending an important message to the adolescent: You cope with problems by returning to your religious foundation. There you will find the spiritual roots, values, and pathways to nourish, sustain, and guide you through your tough time.

This is the kind of advice many people follow in stressful situations. They persist in their spiritual pathways. Thus, we find that 80% of a national sample in the United States indicates that they pray when faced with a problem or crisis, and 64% report that they read the Bible or other inspirational literature (Gallup & Lindsay, 1999). In a recent longitudinal study of widowed individuals and a matched control group, the widowed individuals were more likely than the controls to report that their religious and spiritual beliefs had become more important to them (Brown, Nesse, House, & Utz, 2004). Moreover, this increase was tied to declines in grief. For some groups, spirituality represents the most frequently used resource in coping. For example, in a study of African American caregivers to relatives with dementia, participants were asked to name the one special way they used to deal with caring for their confused relative (Segall & Wykle, 1988–1989). The most common response, spontaneously voiced by 65% of the group, was either prayer or faith in God. People will go to great lengths to persevere in their spiritual beliefs and practices in the face of external obstacles and barriers. In a powerful book entitled *With God in Hell*, Eliezer Berkovits (1979) presents poignant illustrations of Jews who risked their lives to persevere in the practice of Judaism during the Holocaust: one man found a place to pray in the burial pit of a concentration camp, a group of men built a makeshift sanctuary in the attic of their barracks, another man smuggled pages from the Hebrew Bible and ritual accessories into the camp under the penalty of death upon discovery, still another finished his evening prayers before he was shot to death by waiting guards.

To conserve their relationship with the sacred, people can also draw upon spiritual methods of coping designed to assist in understanding and dealing with potentially threatening or damaging situations. Spiritual methods of coping come in a variety of shapes and sizes. They involve diverse beliefs, practices, experiences, and relationships that are well suited to the task of helping people sustain themselves psychologically, socially, physically, and spiritually in the midst of crisis (see Table 5.1 for a summary). To describe the variety of conservational methods of spiritual coping in any detail would require a book of its own (actually, I have written a book on the topic; see Pargament, 1997). Here we will restrict our review to a few examples of spiritual coping: spiritual meaning making, seeking spiritual support and connection, and spiritual purification.

Spiritual Meaning Making

Life is fair. I am in control of my life. Life is good. There is a loving God who ensures that people get what they deserve. These are some of the fundamental assumptions many people live by. Crises, however, can call into question our most basic beliefs. How do we make sense of the situation of the loving mother who devoted her life to caring for her family only to suffer a progressive neurological disease that leaves her paralyzed? How do we understand a bus crash that kills a group of elementary school children going to their first day of school? How do we make sense of a society in which infertile couples desperate for children of their own are surrounded

TABLE 5.1. Conservational Methods of Spiritual Coping

- *Benevolent spiritual reappraisals:* Redefining a stressor through religion or spirituality as potentially beneficial
- *Seeking spiritual support:* Searching for love and care from the sacred
- *Seeking support from clergy/congregation members:* Seeking love and care from clergy and congregation members
- *Seeking spiritual connection:* Searching for a sense of connectedness with transcendent or immanent forces
- *Spiritual helping:* Attempting to provide spiritual support to others
- *Collaborative spiritual coping:* Seeking a partnership with the divine in problem solving
- *Spiritual purification:* Searching for spiritual cleansing through ritual

Note. Drawn from Pargament, Koenig, and Perez (2000).

by young women so desperately unhappy about their pregnancies that they seek abortions?

To these kinds of terribly profound, painful, and disorienting questions, spirituality offers the hope of an answer. From a spiritual perspective, there is a greater meaning to pain and suffering, even if we cannot understand that meaning. I like the way Clifford Geertz (1966) put it: "The effort is not to deny the undeniable—that there are unexplained events, that life hurts, or that rain falls upon the just—but to deny that there are inexplicable events, that life is unendurable, and that justice is a mirage" (pp. 23–24). Common to the religions of the world, he says, is the belief that life is ultimately comprehensible. The minimal definition of religion is not that there is a God, but that there is a God who is not mad.

In the process of spiritual meaning making, traumatic events are reappraised and often placed in a more benevolent context, a context made up of symbols, myths, and exemplary figures that offers hope for oneself and others (see Park, 2005). For example, one survivor of the September 11 attacks visited the remains of the World Trade Center and noticed a set of steel beams shaped like a cross. For her, the crucifix-like beams were a symbol of hope, reminding her of the possibilities for resurrection and rebirth in the midst of the most painful of circumstances. A man suffering from depression was able to glean a more hopeful perspective on his illness from religious readings: "I found this image was right there in scripture, you know the kind of bit in Malachi, the refiner's fire, the kind of purifying the gold and all that stuff. It kind of made me hold onto the fact that it wasn't some kind of strange twist of fate, but actually it was peculiarly and unbelievably sometimes an act of God, and therefore if that bit was an act of God, then the ultimate deliverance from it would be an act of God, and so there was hope" (Swinton, 2001, pp. 122–123). Another man facing end-stage cancer was able to draw strength and hope from his belief in God's ultimate control and the ultimate reward of heaven: "Well, I just believe that everything is written and then if it's His choice for me and it's my time, that's the way it's gonna be. And it must be a better place there [heaven], because nobody came back and complained! (laughs) So maybe I'm going to a better place and less pain that I feel I'm going to experience before I go" (True et al., 2003, p. 11).

Positive spiritual reappraisals of negative events help people conserve not only their sense of benevolence and meaning in the world, but also their relationship with the sacred. Remember that trauma can challenge basic spiritual beliefs, including the belief in a loving, all-powerful Being, but positive spiritual reappraisals protect and preserve the sacred from attack. Through a spiritual light, trauma and tragedy are not signs of an uncaring or impotent God. Instead, they are bearers of spiritual meaning and a spiritual presence. Thus, Yancey (1977) writes that "God is speaking to us through pain. . . . The symphony He is working out includes minor chords, dissonance, and tiring fugal passages. But those of us who follow His conducting through these early movements will with renewed strength, someday burst into song" (p. 77). Similarly, pain and suffering are not to be understood as pointless, but as spiritual tests and opportunities for spiritual growth. Listen to how one Hindu woman, born with a neuromuscular disorder, views her disability from a benevolent spiritual perspective:

> I was told by the swamis early in my study of Vedanta that disability was present in my life so that I could grow in new ways and progress along the path to God consciousness. I have always had rebellious tendencies, and I am sure that, had I not had a disability, I would have easily succumbed to the temptations of the '60's. . . . This life is riddled with physical frustrations but wealthy with opportunities for spiritual growth. (Nosek, 1995, pp. 174–175)

This example is not unusual. Empirical studies show that people are far more likely to view negative events from a positive spiritual perspective than attribute these events to an angry or disengaged God (Mickley et al., 1998). A woman who suffered paralysis as the result of a car accident said, "I know God doesn't screw up. He doesn't make mistakes. Something very beautiful is going to come out of this" (Baker & Gorgas, 1990, p. 5A). A husband grieving the loss of his young wife rejects critical questions about God and instead focuses on God's positive role in her life:

> Some people ask why this tragedy happened to me. . . . You know I never asked that question. . . . These are the questions to ask: Was her life rich? How many lives did she touch? Was she a blessing to her family and friends and people with whom she had contact? Will she be missed—not only by her family but by those far from her? Did she take her joys humbly and

gratefully? Did she meet her sorrows courageously? Was God present? Who can doubt it? (Krauss & Goldfischer, 1988, pp. 52–53)

Positive spiritual reappraisals do more than help people sustain hope, meaning, and comfort in stressful situations. They help people preserve their beliefs in a benevolent deity and conserve their connection with the sacred.

Seeking Spiritual Support and Connection

In difficult periods, many people seek support from the sacred. The support may come from the perception of a direct spiritual encounter, a spiritual visitation that counteracts the visitation of calamity, as Pruyser (1968) described it. A middle-aged woman, hospitalized for depression, recalled one such visitation:

> At one time I reached utter despair and went and prayed to God for mercy instinctively and without faith in reply. That night I stood with other patients in the grounds waiting to be let in to our ward. It was a very cold night with many stars. Suddenly someone stood beside me in a dusty brown robe and a voice said "Mad or sane you are one of My sheep." I never spoke to anyone of this but ever since it has been the pivot of my life. I realize that the form of the vision and the words I heard were the result of my education and cultural background but the voice, though closer than my own heartbeat, was entirely separate from me. (Hardy, 1979, p. 91)

Spiritual support can grow out of other sources as well: prayer and meditation, relationships with clergy or congregation members, ritual practice, involvement in worship services, beliefs, the study of the sacred literature, music, nature, art, and so on.

The experience of spiritual support can reduce physical discomfort. Heiligman, Lee, and Kramer (1983) described the case of a 68-year-old woman who underwent a surgical procedure to remove a carcinoma of the colon. Following this kind of surgery, most patients experience a painful process of recovery. But this woman was an exception; she required no analgesic medication. Puzzled, the physicians asked her why she had not requested any analgesia. The patient answered that she did not need any medication because angels were watching over and caring for her. Though they did not say anything to her, the angels had a human-like appearance, gave off a bright glow, and offered a comforting presence.

Spiritual support can serve a host of psychological and social purposes as well. Karolynn Siegel and Eric Schrimshaw (2002) illustrated this point in their interview study of older adults living with HIV/AIDS. In coping with their illness, many of their participants sought out spiritual support that provided them with a number of different benefits. To some, it was a source of emotional comfort. One man said, "I think the main support that I receive is my Buddhist practice. That is what has sustained me for the last 25 years. No matter how deep in despair I have become, I've found refuge in Buddhism. . . . It helps me find my center. And it helps me find peace and tranquility and love" (p. 94). Others described the strength and empowerment they gained from spiritual support. "I'm speaking to my higher power, my God," said one man. "And I give thanks to that power. It has been a source of strength. You know, it's like tapping in to some sort of power source that I can recharge my batteries" (p. 95). Others spoke about the sense of community and connectedness they derived from the support of their religious congregations. One Roman Catholic man said, "Religion to me is not mass from 7 to 8, it's the gathering of everybody from 6 to 9, with mass in the middle. Because I always go there for the interaction, and I always stay for the social and other business afterwards. It's not just—the liturgy is fine, and I'm getting more into that, but I'm not as liturgy centered as I am community centered" (p. 96).

Though spiritual support serves key physical, psychological, and social functions that may have a spiritual meaning of their own, it is important to emphasize that many people seek spiritual support first and foremost to conserve their relationship with the sacred. For theists, an ongoing personal relationship with God in the midst of crisis has tremendous value in and of itself. As one man with HIV put it, "I talk to God and I feel good, feel supported. Like there is someone who is always there for me. I talk to Him, and I ask Him for things. I talk to Him at night, in the morning, and I go to church. Knowing that He is there for me, and that I can talk to Him personally has been very good for me" (Siegel & Schrimshaw, 2002, p. 97). In life crises, people can also draw closer to the inspirational models of their faith tradition. Christian theologian Thomas Oden (1983) writes: "When we are being washed helplessly by a nurse, we may recall our radical dependence upon God, and the cleansing of baptism. When we have to spend hours in isolated silence we are in a position like that of Jesus who endured suffering silently. When we feel the buffering of thorns, Christians recall that God's own Son wore a crown of thorns" (p. 254).

Spiritual support is a vehicle for sustaining many sacred aspects of life, not only the divine. For example, beliefs in the afterlife provide a way to continue to hold on to sacred ties with loved ones even after they have died. This point was illustrated for me recently, following the death of my Uncle Sammy. The last 10 years of my uncle's life were terribly painful for him as he struggled with cancer, heart disease, Parkinson's disease, and diabetes. The years were equally painful for his wife. My aunt and uncle had been devoted to each other through almost 60 years of marriage (family members would pronounce "Aunt Mitzi and Uncle Sammy" as if they were one word), and my aunt had taken on the burden of caring for my uncle over the many years of his illness. My wife and I were concerned about how my aunt was coping with her loss after the funeral and shiva (a 1-week mourning ritual within Judaism), so we called her to see how she was doing. My aunt said she was doing well. Between calls from family and friends and invitations to go out, she had little time to herself. She admitted, though, that she enjoyed just being in her apartment by herself. She didn't feel alone there. On the contrary, she said, that's where she felt her husband's presence most strongly. Surrounded by the objects, photographs, and memories of their years together, she sensed Sammy was still there for her.

My aunt's experience is not atypical. In the United States, about 80% of the population believes in some form of afterlife (Harley & Firebaugh, 1993). And many people who have lost a loved one experience a continued attachment with the deceased person. For example, in a study of bereaved parents of pediatric cancer patients, 88% reported that they felt a continued connection with their deceased child (Sormanti & August, 1997). The sense of continued attachment can express itself in many ways: hearing a voice, experiencing a dream, smelling an aroma, feeling a touch, catching a glimpse of the deceased, having flashbacks, or simply sensing a presence (Benore & Park, 2004). One bereaved mother said, "I talk to him all the time. I 'keep him up on' what's going on at home and with all of us. I feel the strongest connection at the cemetery. I imagine his spirit in the trees behind his grave. When I begin to talk to him the wind almost always rustles the leaves, which tells me he's there" (Sormanti & August, 1997, p. 464). Visits to the grave, conversations with the deceased, holding on to cherished objects, rituals that venerate the memory of the loved one, and asking the departed for guidance are all ways to sustain a sacred connection with the person who died and integrate his or her memory into the core of the self. One man who had lost his partner to AIDS put it this way: "For a while after he was gone, I felt very empty. But then I started realizing that everything I saw in him I really did experience and that is part of me. So now, it makes me feel very full rather than empty" (Richards, Acree, & Folkman, 1999, p. 117).

Beliefs in the afterlife can also help people hold on to the sense that at least a part of who they are will continue after they die. Most people in the United States believe they will go to heaven where they will enjoy immortality (Spilka et al., 2003). Immortality may be defined in a spiritual or mystical sense (living on in some physical or spiritual form), in a biological sense (living on through children), in a creative sense (living on through achievements and accomplishments), or in a natural sense (living on as part of nature) (Lifton, 1973). Kushner (1989) speaks to these different manifestations of immortality:

> The words I have written and spoken, the hearts I have touched, the hands
> I have reached out to, the child I leave behind, will gain me all the immor-

tality I need. More than that, I am assured that even when the last person who ever knew me dies, and the last copy of my book has been removed from the library shelf, the essential me, the nonphysical me, will still live on in the mind of God, where no act of goodness or kindness is ever forgotten. (p. 173)

Though they may take different forms, beliefs in immortality help people sustain the conviction that they contain an indestructible sacred core, one that will transcend death itself.

Spiritual Purification

Threats to the sacred can come from within as well as outside the person. The religions of the world articulate a wide range of personal acts that represent offenses against God, from gluttony, greed, pride, lust, and sloth to jealousy, slander, hate, adultery, theft, and murder. Though the specific transgressions may vary to some degree from tradition to tradition, they share a common feature: each is said to create a breach between the individual and the sacred.

To repair the breach, many people engage in rituals of purification. Ritual sacrifice, repentance, punishment, cleansing, liturgies of atonement are among the many methods of purification (see Paden, 1988, for a review). In Western culture, spiritual confession is perhaps the most common purification ritual. Rites of confession are practiced by most religious groups in the United States, and are also prominent in 12-step programs, support groups, and counseling. Spiritual confessions may be public or private, but every confession has two important components: an acknowledgment that the person has committed a spiritual violation and a request for forgiveness (Swank, 1992). Acts of penance and restitution are also commonly part of spiritual confessions within many traditions.

The act of catharsis involved in admissions of wrongdoing is certainly helpful in and of itself, as research by James Pennebaker (1997) has shown. Pennebaker has studied the effects of the "confession" of traumas, secrets, and mistakes. One example involved a woman who recalled an incident as a 10-year-old when she failed to pick up her toys one evening before her grandmother came for a visit. Her grandmother slipped on one of the toys, broke her hip, and died a week later during hip surgery. Confession through letters or conversation, Pennebaker has found, is tied to a number of physical and mental health benefits. Although Pennebaker uses the term "confession," he has not explored the spiritual dimension of this practice. Spiritual confessions, though, may be distinctive, for confessions of this kind are designed to help people reestablish themselves in proper relationship to the sacred.

In an experimental investigation, Aaron Murray-Swank (1992) assigned college students to one of three groups: a secular confession group, in which participants wrote an essay about something they had done wrong; a spiritual confession group, in which the participants wrote a letter to God about something they had done wrong and asked for His forgiveness; and a control group, in which the participants wrote an essay about the contents of their apartment, dorm, or house. The results were interesting and complex, but one finding stood out. Both immediately after the experiment and 2 weeks later, participants in the spiritual confession condition reported significantly more closeness to God than students in the secular confession and control groups.

This finding suggests that there is something distinctive about a spiritual confession. Perhaps it has to do with the individual's sense that the divine is uniquely approachable and willing to forgive even the greatest of mistakes. One student in Murray-Swank's study began her letter to God this way: "Dear God, I am writing this letter to get some things off my chest that I can't talk to anyone but you about. I hope that you can find forgiveness in your eyes and help me along in my journey as you always have" (p. 58). Of course, people who see God as a less compassionate being may have different reactions to spiritual confession. In this vein, Murray-Swank found that, among students who made a spiritual confession, those who held more loving images of God experienced increases in their positive affect over the 2-week period of the study, while those who held less loving God images reported decreases in their positive emotions.

The Many Methods of Spiritual Coping

This discussion has merely sampled from the rich variety of spiritual methods of coping. Before I move on, two additional points are worth noting. First, many of the spiritual coping methods assume that the individual perceives him- or herself in a relationship with an active personal God. Certainly that assumption holds true for most people in the United States, but it does not apply to everyone in this country, nor does it apply to everyone in other parts of the world. For instance, in Scandinavian countries where people generally view God in less personal terms, researchers have identified other forms of spiritual coping. Van Uden, Pieper, and Alma (2004) articulated and assessed "receptivity," a method of spiritual coping that reflects an openness to and trust in the eventual discovery of meaning and solutions to life's problems without specifying the agent that makes it possible. One item from their scale read: "When I find myself in times of trouble, I have faith in the eventual revelation of their meaning and purpose." In a sample of students from the Netherlands, they found that higher levels of receptive coping were associated with lower levels of anxiety and higher levels of basic trust. In contrast, the researchers found that scores on several of the spiritual coping scales developed in the United States that assume a personal relationship with an active God were unrelated to anxiety and trust in the Dutch sample. As the psychology of religion and spirituality advances, we are likely to identify still additional forms of spiritual coping among Buddhist, Hindus, and spiritual groups that perceive the sacred in different terms (see also Tarakeshwar, Pargament, & Mahoney, 2003a).

Second, although we have focused on the ways individuals engage in spiritual coping, it is important to note that spiritual coping methods can also be interactive. Following the Oklahoma City bombing and the September 11 terrorist attacks, communities all across the United States joined together and coped with these terrible traumas by means of shared prayers and rituals. On a more regular basis, many couples, families, and congregations engage in spiritual dialogue, joint practices, and shared spiritual experiences as forms of coping. The communal nature of these practices may add a distinctive dimension to the coping process.

In one of the first studies of shared spiritual coping, Gina Yanni (2003) examined the ways parents and their college-age children coped with religious disagreements that arose between them. Drawing on the work of family systems theorists, Yanni defined a relational form of spiritual coping in which God is "detriangled" from the conflicts and becomes instead an advocate for love and harmony between parent and child. Her measure of "Positive Religious Detriangulation" consisted of ways of coping in response to conflict such as "I suggest that God loves us both even if we disagree about certain issues" and "I suggest that we turn to God or our faith to be patient with each other." Parent–child dyads that scored higher on this measure appeared to have healthier parent–child relationships, including greater parent–child satisfaction, more intimacy and perceived family support, and more constructive conflict resolution methods. Generally, dyads who talked about religious and spiritual matters more frequently, including their views on God, religious beliefs, spiritual struggles and doubts, and differences of opinion, experienced a variety of personal benefits and benefits in their relationship: more happiness, greater parent–child satisfaction, less verbal hostility and negative communication patterns, and greater intimacy. The findings from Yanni's pioneering study of spirituality and the family underscore the importance of moving beyond an exclusively individualistic focus in our efforts to understand the search for the sacred. It is important to attend to the expressions of spirituality at multiple levels—couples, family, and community, as well as individual. Yanni's findings also raise another central question.

DO THEY WORK?

As we have seen, testaments to the value of spiritual coping are plentiful, but what do the data show? As I noted in the first chapter, studies of diverse groups, from combat veterans and medically ill patients to victims of physical abuse and people with serious mental illness, indicate that 50–85% of individuals in these groups felt that religion and spirituality was helpful to them in coping (Pargament, 1997). Spiritual coping has also been significantly associated with measures of health and well-being in cross-sectional and longitudinal studies with various populations, such as women coping with breast cancer (Gall, 2000), informal caregivers (Pearce, 2005), Latinos dealing with arthritis (Abraído-Lanza, Vasquez, & Echeverria, 2004), older adults living in deteriorating neighborhoods (Krause, 1998), church members (Bjorck & Thurman, in press), and adults in the community under stress (Loewenthal, Macleod, Goldblatt, Lubitsh, & Valentine, 2000). In a meta-analysis of 49 studies, Gene Ano and Erin Vasconcelles (2005) found that measures of positive religious coping (e.g., benevolent spiritual reappraisals, seeking spiritual support and connection) were consistently tied to better psychological adjustment. For example, in a study of patients and their loved ones dealing with the stress of kidney transplant surgery, spiritual coping was associated with better adjustment among both patients and their significant loved ones concurrently and at 3 and 12 months after surgery (Tix & Frazier, 1998). These findings remained significant even after controlling for the effects of other general coping factors, such as internal control, cognitive restructuring, and social support. Tix and Frazier concluded that spiritual coping represented a distinctive resource for people coping with this major medical challenge. Other studies have also pointed to the distinctive role spirituality plays in the coping process (see Pargament, Magyar, & Murray-Swank, 2005).

It is important to add that spiritual coping appears to be particularly helpful to people with fewer personal and social resources facing more trying situations. Greater benefits of spiritual coping have been reported by members of minority groups, the elderly, less educated and poorer people, individuals who are more personally insecure, and those dealing with more stressful situations (see Smith, McCullough, & Poll, 2003; Pargament, 2002, for a review). Confronted with their own limitations, many people find spiritual methods of coping especially compelling.

Some might argue that findings such as these are reflections of the "sugarcoating" power of spiritual coping. Within psychology, there is a long history of stereotyping religion and spirituality as merely a defense against reality, a form of denial or passivity in the face of events that call for action (see Pargament & Park, 1995). Admittedly, we can find examples of spiritually based passivity and denial, but empirical studies suggest that these examples are exceptions to the rule. For the most part, spiritual methods of coping have been linked more to an active than to a passive coping style. For example, people in the United States are more likely to agree with the item "When it comes to deciding how to solve a problem, God and I work together as partners" than with the item "God solves problems for me without my doing anything" (Pargament et al., 1988). Thus, people generally see themselves more as active partners with God than as individuals who simply defer to God the responsibility for solving their problems while they themselves sit passively by. Furthermore, in the process of spiritual meaning making, denial is relatively unusual. More commonly, people face the reality of traumatic events, but place them into a larger, more meaningful context. As one caregiver to parents with Alzheimer's disease said, "It is the most rewarding and devastating experience of my life; I would not have given up this period to care for my parents for anything. There has been combativeness, wandering—lots of frustrations. But I'm learning for the first time to take each day at a time. This illness is teaching me to gain strength from the Lord" (Wright, Pratt, & Schmall, 1985, p. 34).

The evidence indicates that spiritual methods of coping are effective in helping people sustain and enhance their mental health in times of crisis. But how effective are they in helping people conserve the sacred? To the spiritually minded, this is the most important question. Here the evidence is even more compelling. Spirituality is exceptionally resilient to life stressors, including the most extreme situations. Empirical studies show that most people maintain their levels of spiritual and religious involvement through periods of crisis (see Pargament, 1997). For instance, in his survey study of Jewish Holocaust survivors, Reeve Brenner (1980) found that 61% reported no change in their religious behavior before the Holocaust, immediately after the Holocaust, and at the time of the study. Stability over time in religious beliefs and practices was also the hallmark for heart attack patients recovering from their illness (Croog & Levine, 1972). This stability seems to be attributable, at least in part, to the conservational power of spiritual methods of coping. A number of studies have also uncovered strong relationships between spiritual coping and indices of spiritual growth and well-being. For example, in a 2-year longitudinal study of medically ill, elderly, hospitalized patients, my colleagues and I found that those patients who made more use of conservational spiritual methods of coping (e.g., benevolent religious reappraisals, seeking spiritual support and connection, spiritual helping, collaborative spiritual coping, spiritual purification) reported strong increases in their feelings of closeness to God, their sense of spirituality, and their closeness to their church over the 2-year period (Pargament, Koenig, Tarakeshwar, & Hahn, 2004).

CONCLUSIONS

Overall, studies show that people are not left empty-handed when they encounter situations that violate, threaten or damage the most sacred aspects of their lives. They can draw on spiritual methods of coping, a powerful set of resources to help reorient and sustain themselves psychologically, socially, physically, and spiritually.

There are times, though, when the sacred cannot be fully protected. External life events or internal developmental changes have a way of insisting on change. Try as we might to hold on to the sacred, not even the conservational methods of spiritual coping may be sufficient to preserve the status quo. During these times, we may experience greater spiritual confusion and disorientation, struggle to find our way in the search for the sacred, and ultimately transform our relationship with the sacred. In the next chapter, we shift our focus to the topics of spiritual struggles and transformation.

6

In Times of Stress

Spiritual Coping to Transform the Sacred

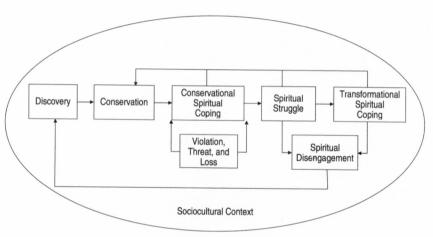

The Search for the Sacred

PRELUDE TO TRANSFORMATION:
SPIRITUAL STRUGGLES

Joe came to my office in crisis. After many years of marital conflict, he had left his wife and was now living with a friend. His 20-year marriage had been marked by frequent arguments, physical abuse by his wife, and failed attempts to work through their problems. The crisis for Joe, though, was not the separation per se; if anything, he felt tremendous relief being on his own. The crisis was instead spiritual. Joe had been a member of the Jehovah's Witnesses for much of his life. The church had been central to his being. There Joe met with other family members and friends. There he derived a great deal of support and satisfaction through his role as a leader of the church. And there he knew who he was. Joe's church, however, frowned on his decision to end his marriage. Siding with his wife, his clergyman, family members, and friends had cut off contact with Joe. He was no longer welcome in the church. Joe struggled with a number of spiritual questions: How could the church that he had loved abandon him at the low point of his life? How could he remain part of a religion that seemed to blame the victim of a failed marriage? How could the God he worshipped and trusted permit such a terrible injustice? Addressing these spiritual struggles became the focus of therapy.

Spiritual struggles are signs of spiritual disorientation, tension, and strain. Old roads to the sacred and old understandings of the sacred itself are no longer compelling. In their place, people struggle to reorient themselves and find a new way to the sacred or a new understanding of the sacred. We can distinguish among three types of spiritual struggles: interpersonal, intrapersonal, and divine (see Pargament, Murray-Swank, Magyar, & Ano, 2005, for review). Interpersonal spiritual struggles involve spiritual conflicts and tensions with families, friends, and congregations, such as the conflicts Joe experienced with the members of his church. Neal Krause and his colleagues (Krause, Chatters, Metzer, & Morgan, 2000) conducted focus groups with older church members and identified a number of types of negative spiritual interactions, such as gossiping, cliquishness, hypocrisy on the part of clergy and members, and disagreements with church doctrine. These negative behaviors were especially upsetting to the churchgoers because they violated members' expectations about how people in a religious community should express their spiritual values with each other. One woman complained, "They get off in a corner and talk about you and you're the one that's there on Saturday working with their children and ironing the priest's vestments and doing all that kind of thing and washing the dishes on Sunday afternoon after church. But they don't have the Christian spirit" (p. 519). Spiritual struggles among family members may carry additional meaning, for they undermine not only the unity of the family but also the spiritual bond between the family and the sacred (Mahoney, 2005).

Spiritual struggles can take intrapersonal as well as interpersonal forms. Many people experience uncertainty and doubt about spiritual matters. They may question their own ultimate value, efficacy, or spiritual purpose in life (Hill, 2001). Or they may have serious doubts about their religious traditions, as we hear in the words of one adolescent: "Is Christianity a big sham, a cult? If an organization were to evolve in society, it would have to excite people emotionally, it would have to be self-perpetuating, it would need to be a source of income, etc. Christianity fits all of these. How do I know that I haven't been sucked into a giant perpetual motion machine?" (Kooistra, 1990, p. 95). Julie Exline (2002) describes another type of intrapersonal struggle, the tension between the pursuit of virtues as en-

couraged by many religious traditions and the desire to gratify human appetites. These tensions may be hard to resolve, Exline notes, given the
temptations offered by the environment and the limited human capacity for
self-control.

A third form of spiritual struggles involves tension between the individual and the divine. Within monotheistic traditions, most people view
God as a loving, all-powerful Being who works directly in our lives to ensure that good things will happen to good people. Critical life events, however, can throw this set of beliefs into question, as we hear in the painful
doubts voiced by a 14-year-old Nicaraguan girl:

> Many times I wonder how there can be a God—a loving God and where
> He is. . . . I don't understand why He lets little children in Third World
> countries die of starvation or diseases that could have been cured if they
> would have had the right medicines or doctors. I believe in God and I love
> Him, but sometimes I just don't see the connection between a loving God
> and a suffering hurting world. Why doesn't He help us—if He truly loves
> us? It seems like He just doesn't care. Does He? (Kooistra, 1990, pp. 91–
> 92)

Like this adolescent, many people struggle to redefine their relationship
with the divine in response to pain and suffering. For example, in a study
of homeless men, 50% reported that their social condition elicited negative feelings toward God (Smith & Exline, 2002). Similarly, in a survey of
diabetic, congestive heart failure, and oncology patients, George Fitchett
and his colleagues (2004) found that approximately 20% described moderate to high levels of religious struggle, defined by feelings of alienation,
abandonment, anger, or punishment in relationship to God. A minority
of the survey participants went further, indicating that they felt they were
engaged in a battle with malevolent forces from the spiritual or demonic
realm.

Spiritual struggles can also involve various combinations of these types
of interpersonal, intrapersonal, and divine conflicts. For example, the divine can be brought into interpersonal conflicts as an ally or as a referee
who is said to side with one person or the other. Mark Butler and James
Harper (1994) illustrate this process of "divine triangling" in their work
with religious couples:

> In a middle session of therapy, the wife in such a couple told the therapist
> that her husband needed to pray more. Looking through her purse, she
> claimed she could produce a list on which she had recorded the daily time
> she spent praying. Of course, the husband countered that if his wife were
> free of sin, she could cast the first stone. He then made a long speech about
> God's unconditional love for him and God's disgust for vain and repeti-
> tious prayers. (p. 282)

In the process of divine triangling, the tension between the couple is displaced onto God, but the end result is typically an escalation of the conflict rather than a successful resolution, for the stakes are raised considerably when the couple competes for God's favor.

Spiritual struggles can grow out of many critical events. In a study of more than 5,000 university students, 25% of the sample reported that they had experienced considerable distress related to religious or spiritual concerns (Johnson & Hayes, 2003). Their concerns were tied to a number of the stresses and strains associated with young adulthood and the transition to college: breakup of a relationship, homesickness, suicidal thoughts and feelings, and sexual assault. Other researchers have linked spiritual struggles to major traumas and PTSD (Ai, Peterson, & Huang, 2003; Ali, Liu, & Humedian, 2004). For example, Ali et al. (2004) interviewed British Muslims after 9/11 and found that many participants reported feelings of loss and confusion about their faith. Developmental changes and the process of searching for the sacred itself can also lead to spiritual struggles. Theologian Abraham Heschel (1973) spoke to this point when he wrote that "knowing God is not consoling but demanding, offering challenge rather than pleasure . . . in a deep sense, the more knowledge we acquire, the more uncomfortable we become" (p. 189).

This is not to say that spiritual struggles are a sign of pathology or weak faith. Consider the spiritual struggle contained in these words: "I am told that God lives in me—and yet the reality of darkness and coldness and emptiness is so great that nothing touches my soul. . . . I want God with all the power of my soul—and yet between us there is terrible separation. . . . Heaven from every side is closed" ("God's Silence," 2003, p. 6A). Readers might be surprised to know that this is the voice of Mother Teresa who experienced profound feelings of divine abandonment as she began her work with homeless children and dying people in the slums of Calcutta. Yet Mother Teresa's example is not unusual. From Moses to Jesus to Buddha, the heroic figures of the world's great religious traditions also faced spiritual turmoil of their own, only to be strengthened and steeled through the process.

Not all spiritual struggles are so momentous. Spiritual struggles may be temporary, consisting of a fleeting feeling of anger toward God or a passing question of whether the person is being punished for his or her sins. Christian apologist C. S. Lewis (1961) described some of these feelings one night soon after the death of his wife: "Step by step we were 'led up the garden path.' Time after time, when He seemed most gracious He was really preparing the next torture" (p. 27). But the next morning he recanted: "I wrote that last night. It was a yell rather than a thought. Let me try it over again" (p. 27). Similarly, Exline and Martin (2005) found that 80% of college students who experienced negative feelings toward God reported that their feelings decreased over time. Thus, spiritual struggles may be short-lived expressions of spiritual pain that are quickly followed by a return to established conservational spiritual pathways.

For many people, though, struggles represent a major turning point in life, a spiritual fork in the road that can lead to renewal, growth, and positive transformation in one direction, or despair, hopelessness, and meaninglessness in the other. A few empirical studies have shown a link between spiritual struggles and higher levels of growth. For example, in a sample of adults who belonged to churches close to the site of the Oklahoma City bombing, people who experienced more spiritual struggles also reported higher levels of personal growth as a result of their traumatic experience (Pargament et al., 1998). Findings such as these are consistent with the sentiments of psychologists of religion, from William James (1902/1936) to Daniel Batson (Batson, Schoenrade, & Ventis, 1993), who argue that the deepest faith is fashioned in the workshop of question and doubt.

Though spiritual struggles may lead to growth, they are not always a prelude to greater well-being, for struggles may also presage pain and decline. The portrait painted by the research in this area is quite clear. Interpersonal, intrapersonal, and divine spiritual struggles have been consistently tied to higher levels of anxiety and depression, lower levels of physical functioning and quality of life, and relational distress (see Exline & Rose, 2005; Fitchett et al., 2004; Pargament, Murray-Swank, et al., 2005; and Yanni, 2003, for reviews). These struggles appear to add a distinctive element to psychological functioning. For example, Burker, Evon, Sedway, and Egan (2005) found that spiritual struggles, particularly reports of feeling punished by God, were predictive of greater depression and anxiety among patients with end-stage lung disease, even after controlling for a standard measure of nonreligious coping.

Adding further to the pain are the feelings of spiritual emptiness that can accompany spiritual struggles. Listen, for example, to the following words about survivors of childhood sexual abuse:

> The death of our God-images causes us pain because we enter a period which is void of any image. Before a new one emerges, we reside in darkness and emptiness. We find it very difficult to pray, and we sense little comfort. We struggle intellectually and emotionally; we yearn for some felt experience of God, yet God is silent. Finally, we begin to wonder if there even is a God because our felt experience seems to be part of the past. (Flaherty, 1992, p. 126)

Spiritual struggles may also signal a temporary or lasting disengagement from the sacred quest. In their study of undergraduates, Exline and Martin (2005) found that 9% resolved their negative feelings toward the divine by deciding not to believe in God.

Spiritual struggles may even increase the risk of dying. In the 2-year longitudinal study of medically ill elderly hospitalized patients mentioned earlier, my colleagues and I found that patients who voiced more spiritual struggles showed greater declines on measures of psychological, physical, and spiritual functioning (Pargament et al., 2001, 2004). Strikingly, higher levels of spiritual struggle (particularly struggles with the divine) at the beginning of the study were also associated with a 22–33% greater risk of dying over the 2-year period, even after controlling for other variables including demographic, physical health, and mental health variables. This was, as far as we know, the first study to demonstrate that certain forms of spirituality may *increase* the risk of dying.

Empirical studies thus suggest that spiritual struggles may lead to growth or decline. What determines which direction the spiritual struggler follows? I believe it depends in part on the individual's ability to engage in a successful spiritual transformation. (Later in the book, I consider other determinants of whether spiritual struggles and the search for the sacred, more generally, lead to growth or decline.)

SPIRITUAL METHODS OF COPING
TO TRANSFORM THE SACRED

Although people may seek out new values and purposes for the simple excitement and energy they spark in their lives, these cases may be the exception rather than the rule. Not until tried-and-true methods for understanding and dealing with the world have failed again and again do most people contemplate basic change. Ebeneezer Scrooge, of *Christmas Carol* fame, remained stuck in his miserly ways for much of his life, seemingly immune to the pain and suffering that surrounded him. Only when the ghosts of the past, present, and future dragged him into merciless self-confrontation did he undergo his famous transformation.

By "spiritual transformation," I refer primarily to fundamental changes in the place of the sacred or the character of the sacred in the person's life, and secondarily to a fundamental change in the pathways the individual takes to the sacred (Pargament, 2006). Spiritual transformation can be difficult and painful. Furthermore, it is not always successful; some transformations lead to failure and decline. Nevertheless, transformation is another natural and normal part of the search for the sacred. Rupp (1997) writes:

> A cup is a container for holding something. Whatever it holds has to eventually be emptied out so that something more can be put into it. I have learned that I cannot always expect my life to be full. There has to be some emptying, some pouring out, if I am to make room for the new. The spiritual journey is like that—a constant process of emptying and filling, of giving and receiving, of accepting and letting go. (p. 11)

Many people construct their own distinctive methods of spiritual transformation. In addition, the major religious traditions have developed a variety of methods that are specifically designed to facilitate the process of transformation to a more authentic spiritual existence. It is also important to recognize that, although the spiritual pathways (knowledge, practice, relationship, experience) reviewed in Chapter 4 are generally conservational in nature—helping people to sustain and solidify their relationship with the sacred—they can also lead to profound change at times. A complete review of the methods of spiritual transformation would take us beyond the scope of this book (see Pargament, 1997, for a review). Here I will illustrate a few of the most significant forms of spiritual transformation: sacred transitions, revisioning the sacred, and centering the sacred.

Sacred Transitions

Several years ago a colleague of mine died suddenly at work. He was a dedicated psychologist who had made lasting contributions to the community. His death was deeply felt and his funeral was attended by many people. My colleague was Jewish and, although he had married a Roman Catholic woman and raised his children in that tradition, he had requested a Jewish funeral. Within Judaism, it is traditional that family and friends participate in the graveside internment by shoveling dirt onto the coffin. Oftentimes, this is the emotional culmination of the funeral service, a time when many loved ones share their deepest feelings of grief and loss. This funeral was no exception. Afterward, a few people came up to me and voiced their displeasure with the seeming heartlessness of this ritual. Funeral services, they said, should be comforting, not distressing. They were only partly correct.

Providing comfort is one function of a religious funeral service, but not the only one. Funerals are also designed to facilitate transformations in sacred status. They mark the fact that a momentous event has occurred: a living member of the community is now deceased and those who loved him or her have now become mourners. Prayers and rituals are offered to help speed and secure the transition of the departed to the hereafter. Roman Catholics pray to God to release the deceased from their sins so that they can enjoy a better place in the afterlife. Muslims whisper into the ear of the departed the answers to questions that the angels may pose to determine whether they will go to paradise or hell. Similarly, the new status of the bereaved is marked by distinctive attire (e.g., dark clothes) and visits from family and friends. And the funeral service itself can dispel any tendency on the part of mourners to deny the reality of their loss. Viewing the body, listening to memorial talks, and accompanying the casket to the grave all underscore the significance of this transition. The graveside ritual in which family and friends shovel dirt on the casket of the deceased in front of a witnessing community also forces a confrontation with the reality of change, both the changed status of the person who has died and the changed status of those who mourn his or her death.

Rites of passage can facilitate other critical life transitions. Particularly noteworthy are the transition rituals that have been developed by Native Americans to help veterans of war redefine their role in life and reintegrate themselves into family and community after the trauma of combat. Steven Silver and John Wilson (1988) describe a number of these rituals. For example, upon their return from war, Native Americans may participate in a sweat lodge ritual developed by the Sioux Indians. The sweat lodge is a domed tent constructed out of three tree branches. The tent contains a pit filled with rocks that have been heated to a very hot temperature, a variety of ceremonial instruments, and religious symbols signifying the power of the universe. Participants who enter the sweat lodge experience darkness, extreme heat, and feelings of claustrophobia. Seated around the pit, they chant prayers led by a medicine man who explains that life is filled with pain and suffering, but, by sharing these hardships together and praying to the "Grandfathers" for healing, pain and suffering can be overcome. Water is repeatedly poured on the rocks to make steam and prayers and rituals continue. After an hour or more in the sweat lodge, participants reenter the outside world.

Silver and Wilson (1988) liken the sweat lodge ritual to a process of rebirth. As they crawl naked into the tent, participants are reminded of their own smallness, helplessness, and dependency. The interior of the tent itself is womb-like; members are packed tightly together, surrounded by heat and darkness, suspended in time, with no way to escape. There, they accept the reality of their histories, reexperience their pain and suffering, and release their destructive thoughts. Throughout this process, members are "carried" by the wisdom of the medicine man, prayers to the Grandfathers, and spiritual connection with others. These spiritual resources help participants view their life experiences from a new perspective, gain greater mastery over their emotions, and define themselves and their place in the community in a new light. At the conclusion of the sweat lodge ceremony, participants are propelled from "the interior or the womb" back into the world "with a profound sense of release, rebirth, and a personal renewal of spirit" (p. 352).

Without the benefit of rituals, combat veterans who have returned to the posttrauma civilian world run the risk of becoming frozen into a "warrior-like" identity, one marked by numbness, terror, hyperarousal, and rage. Native American transition rituals are designed to prevent that from happening. Those who participate in transition rituals do not return to their old stations in life. Instead, they assume new roles in the tribe that signify their accumulated wisdom and experience. As Silver and Wilson stress, "The warrior is not asked to give up his experiences; they are the basis for assuming new responsibility, rank, and prestige" (p. 345). In this sense, Native American rituals of transition provide warriors with an opportunity

to emerge from the experience of combat as valued members of their com- .
munities who have achieved a new sacred status.

Our movement through the lifespan is far from linear. It is punctuated by
dramatic changes—birth, coming of age, marriage, shifts in roles, death—
that represent "hinges of time" (Friedman, 1985, p. 164) in which a door
swings open, the finite character of life is revealed, and we capture a glimpse
of larger forces at play in the universe. From baptisms to funerals, rites of passage announce the fact that ordinary time has been suspended and a process
of transformation is underway in which an individual will be shepherded
from one sacred place in life to another. Sacred transitions may be linked to
yet another form of spiritual transformation: revisioning the sacred.

Revisioning the Sacred

Understandings of God, Maria Rizzuto (1979) wrote, are "infinitely plastic" (p. 45). Images of the sacred rooted in the earliest of childhood experiences may not stand up well to the full range of challenges and demands
people face over the course of their lifespan. These images must be re-
created in response to the crises and transitions of life if they are to remain
relevant and sensitive to human needs. For example, over time, the God
who is initially viewed as a father may take on the character of mother, sister, brother, friend, foe, distant relative, or lover.

Beliefs in a loving, all-powerful God are especially vulnerable to
challenge when people encounter injustice and suffering. In his classic
book *When Bad Things Happen to Good People* Harold Kushner (1981)
recounted his own painful process of spiritual soul-searching triggered by
the death of his 14-year-old son. Kushner was unable to reconcile his understanding of God with his tragic loss. How could an all-powerful God
permit such a tragedy? How could a loving God cause such pain? Spiritual methods of coping that conserved the essential character of God
were simply inadequate from Kushner's vantage point. He refused to ex-
onerate God from blame, even if there were any long-term value to the
death of his son: "If a human artist or employer made children suffer so
that something immensely impressive could come to pass, we would put
him in prison. Why then should we excuse God for causing such unde-
served pain, no matter how wonderful the ultimate result may be?"
(p. 19). Neither could he reinterpret his son's death as a blessing: "We try
to persuade ourselves that what we call evil is not real, does not really
exist, but is only a condition of not enough goodness, even as 'cold'
means 'not enough heat,' or darkness is a name we give to the absence of
light . . . but people do stumble and hurt themselves because of the dark
and people do die of exposure to cold" (pp. 27–28). Ultimately, Kushner
transformed his understanding of the divine from a loving, all-powerful
Being to a loving, but limited God.

I do not believe the same things about Him that I did years ago, when I was growing up or when I was a theological student. I recognize his limitations. He is limited in what He can do by laws of nature and by the evolution of human nature and human moral freedom. . . . I can worship a God who hates suffering but cannot eliminate it, more easily than I can worship a God who chooses to make children suffer and die, for whatever exalted reason. . . . Because the tragedy is not God's will, we need not feel hurt or betrayed by God when tragedy strikes. We can turn to Him for help in overcoming it, precisely because we can tell ourselves that God is as outraged by it as we are. (p. 134)

Other people who see God as a distant, even punitive, being may revision the divine as a compassionate figure who is present in times of greatest pain. Recall the story of Cindy who had been unable to rediscover the God of her childhood until the death of her mother, when she realized that God had, in fact, been carrying her throughout her life. Some religious groups encourage this type of transformation. Thomas Csordas (1983) describes a ritual among Catholic Pentecostals called the "Healing of Memories." In this ritual, Jesus is visualized walking alongside the individual throughout his or her entire lifetime to demonstrate that, even though he was not perceived, "He was always really there" (p. 356). This transformation is reinforced by "holy hugs" and embraces from members of the religious community that symbolize being touched by the hand of God. Similarly, many Jewish survivors of the Holocaust and their children have shifted in their representations of God from an external being to an immanent force present within the individual, even in the midst of evil. For example, one child of a Holocaust survivor writes:

Think of the divine power, the spiritual strength, of a mother comforting a child on the way to the gas chamber. If God was present at Auschwitz, it was in the mother, in her words, in her emotions, in the instinct that kept her from abandoning her child. . . . God was within every Jew who told a story or a joke or sang a melody in a death camp barracks to alleviate a friend's agony. God permeated every Jew who held a dying parent, or a brother or sister, or a friend, or even a stranger. (Rosensaft, 2001, pp. 190–191)

Among Christians, visions of the sacred can shift from one aspect of the Trinity to another. For example, Melissa Smith (2004), a survivor of clergy sexual abuse, has written a poignant account of her determined effort to transform her vision of the sacred. As a young girl, Melissa had felt a strong connection to God. "I remember loving God and feeling loved by him," she recalls. "God was with me as a constant companion, a friend. I felt a warmth that was God's presence inside of me. I loved God; I loved life and because of these truths, I loved people" (p. 5). At the age of 14, however, Melissa's life changed. Her family priest began to molest her and Melissa descended into a private hell of anorexia, alcohol, migraines, and self-destructiveness. Even more painful to Melissa were her spiritual struggles. "What caused me the most unspeakable agony," she says, "was the loss of trust in a loving and forgiving God" (p. 8). Over the next 10 years, Melissa tried to find a new way to envision the sacred in her life. Her old image of God the Father was no longer viable, for it elicited memories of "Father the Molester." But she was able to experience a sense of divine love through her relationships with people, through conversations with a caring priest, and through participation in the sacraments. Ultimately, Melissa changed her sacred vision from an exclusive focus on God to a focus on Jesus as the bridge to God. "I came to realize that Jesus was my way back to the Father," she says. "God let himself be known through the compassion, understanding, forgiveness and love of the Son. Suddenly I had the bridge I needed to approach God again. . . . Through Jesus there was finally a connection with God. No longer was God an intellectual exercise. God was living deep within me, and my ability to love God and feel God's love was alive. There is no way to express adequately the joy I felt and still feel" (p. 10).

Understandings of the sacred can also change from narrow conceptualizations of a God concerned only with one's personal well-being to broader perspectives regarding the sacred. This is just the kind of transformation that Martin Luther King Jr. fostered by framing the fight against segregation in spiritual terms:

> How does one determine when a law is just or unjust? A just law is a man-made code that squares with the moral law or the law of God. An unjust law is a code that is out of harmony with the moral law. To put it in the terms of Saint Thomas Aquinas, an unjust law is a human law that is not rooted in eternal and natural law. . . . All segregation statutes are unjust because segregation distorts the soul and damages the personality. . . . So I can urge men to disobey segregation ordinances because they are morally wrong. (King, 1973, p. 200)

Centering the Sacred

New visions of the sacred represent more than cognitive changes. They are often accompanied by other spiritual transformations in which the sacred is realigned within the individual's hierarchy of significant values and strivings. The shift may be from self-centered pursuits to a desire to make the world a better place. It may involve a change from a focus on anger, bitterness, and injustice to a focus on forgiveness and peace of mind. It may entail a process of detachment from intensely pleasurable but ultimately destructive pursuits, such as drugs or alcohol. Or it may involve a spiritual conversion from a life devoid of divinity to one in which God becomes the focal point of existence. In any case, the sacred moves from a marginal position to the very center of the individual's life and definition of him- or herself. There are three important steps in the process of centering the sacred. First, the individual recognizes the limitations of current strivings. Second, he or she decides it is time to let go of old values. Third, the individual replaces old sources of significance with the sacred.

Recognizing the Limitations of Current Strivings

In this book, I have stressed the idea that people are goal-directed beings. We seek significance. And yet there is no guarantee that people will attach themselves to life-enhancing values. The bonds that individuals form with alcohol, drugs, materialism, promiscuity, hatred, and self-aggrandizement can be every bit as tenacious as the connections they form with more virtuous strivings. And people may cling as forcefully to destructive values that are being threatened as they cling to constructive ones. Singular powerful experiences, such as the confrontation with death, may be enough to force a challenge to existing priorities (e.g., Edmonds & Hooker, 1992). But only with repeated frustration and failure do some people recognize that they have been living misdirected lives. Tragically, some never reach the realization that they have been, in the words of Starbuck (1899), "striving at a wrong angle" (p. 115). Those who do, however, may experience an epiphany, a critical moment when they face the limitations of their dreams. For example, Brenda was a 29-year-old woman who had married at an early age to escape her abusive father. When her husband left her, she began to drink heavily and to drift from one relationship to another. Over the next 10 years, violent relationships with men and heavy drinking became the defining features of her life. One night, hospitalized after a particularly brutal beating, Brenda reached an epiphany: "I'm sitting there on the table, and they were taking pictures of all the marks and bruises, and I was waiting to hear whether or not my skull was fractured. They had just told me that my eardrum was broken. . . . I felt like I was going to faint, and I knew, sitting there on that table, that there had to be something different, there had to be a better way, there had to be more than this" (Pargament, 1997, p. 246). At this critical juncture, Brenda came face to face with the fact that she was heading down a road leading to a dead end. She decided she needed to make a change.

Letting Go

Letting go of old values is very hard to do. Why? Because even though the old values have proven themselves to be no longer viable, they have served as an organizing force that has given at least some semblance of meaning, purpose, and direction to life. Giving up old sources of significance often leaves people feeling totally disoriented. Better to lose an arm or a leg than suffer the loss of a dream, some would say. But letting go of old dreams is a necessary part of life, as necessary as letting go of an old breath is to taking in a new one (Brenner, 1985).

The religions of the world recognize the importance of letting go. Muslims are told "Whosoever surrenders himself to Allah, doing good meanwhile, has taken hold of the surest hand-grip" (Koran 31:21). Hindus are instructed "Seek refuge in Him, making a total surrender of your being—body, mind and soul" (Bhagavad-Gita 18:62). Buddhists are told "Throw your life into the abode of the Buddha, living by being moved and led by the Buddha" (Zenji, cited in Beck, 1989, p. 149).

Spiritual resources can play an important role in helping people let go of old values. For example, the practice of meditation is designed to help individuals detach themselves from destructive longings. One expert in mindfulness meditation suggests the following: "When you become aware of an attachment, stop whatever you are doing and try to identify the underlying emotions, body sensations, thoughts, feelings, and tensions. Bringing careful awareness to the experience of craving, rather than mindlessly acting it out, gives insight into it and even more importantly, can reduce it" (Walsh, 1999, p. 95). Prayer can also serve as a resource in letting go of crippling emotions and yearnings. A member of Narcotics Anonymous put it this way: "It's a big change in my life you know. . . . I always pray and I ask God to please take that [the craving for drugs] away from me. . . . I could get angry inside or upset inside and that stupid thinking will come back to me and say 'yeah, I need a hit now' then I have to pray and I say the serenity prayer, 'Lord grant me the serenity.' . . . I have to let that go. I can't always have that with me" (Green, Fullilove, & Fullilove, 1998, p. 327).

Among clinicians who have been trained to help clients take control of their lives, the idea of "letting go" may sound an alarm. But letting go should not be equated with passivity or avoidance (Cole & Pargament, 1999). Instead, it implies a recognition of a hard reality: old objects have lost their former significance. The act of surrendering untenable goals can enhance the individual's ability to define new goals and act to achieve them. Of course, it may make a great deal of difference who or what the individual is surrendering to. Surrender to the sacred may have very different implications than surrendering fatalistically to chance or to an uncaring universe. In this vein, as part of our larger interest in religious coping, my colleagues and I explored the value of spiritual surrender (Koenig, Pargament, & Nielsen, 1998). We created a spiritual surrender scale made up of items such as "Did my best and then turned the situation over to God" and "Did what I could and put the rest in God's hands" and administered the measure to hospitalized patients coping with medical illnesses. We found that higher scores on spiritual surrender were associated with less depression, better quality of life, and more stress-related growth.

The act of letting go creates a value and meaning vacuum. To fill that void, the individual looks to other sources of significance. When a spiritual transformation takes place, the shift is profound and may represent a change from "playing God" to "seeking God" (Cole & Pargament, 1999, p. 185).

Placing the Sacred at the Center

William James (1902/1936) wrote that "to say that a man is 'converted' means . . . that religious ideas, previously peripheral in his consciousness, now take a central place, and that religious aims form the habitual centre of his energy" (p. 165). To frame it in the language of this book, the sacred becomes a vital part of the individual's identity and, as a result, the individual may feel an expanded and empowered sense of self. Listen to the way one man described this change: "When I let our Higher Power become part of me, I become infinitely larger, wiser, calmer, strong—and more importantly: caring, loving, and kinder. . . . On my own, I am like a blind man in a dark room" (Peradotto, 2006, p. 43).

The movement of the sacred from the periphery to the center of life may occur gradually through a process of introspection and self-discipline or more rapidly as the result of a dramatic sacred experience or encounter. Many people report feelings of being "swept up" or "carried away" by a force that is in some ways both transcendent and immanent, as we hear in an account cited by James (1902/1936): "The Holy Spirit descended upon me in a manner that seemed to go through me, body and soul. I could feel the impression, like a wave of electricity, going through and through me. Indeed, it seemed to come in waves and waves of liquid love; for I could not express it in any other way. It seemed like the very breath of God. I can recollect distinctly that it seemed to fan me, like immense wings" (p. 250). Even though this report is over a hundred years old, many like it can be found today. In their study of people who had experienced "quantum change," defined as "vivid, surprising, benevolent, and enduring personal transformation," William Miller and Janet C'de Baca (2001) found that the majority experienced the feeling that they were in a holy presence that some defined as God, others defined in terms of other sacred entities, and still others could not put it into words.

Most often, it is a divine entity that becomes the sacred nucleus of the individual's life and identity, but other sacred objects can also become central. For instance, Hayes, Strosahl, and Kelly (1999) describe a potentially critical shift in the way the individual understands him- or herself. This shift involves a transformation from a self defined by fusion with actions (e.g., I am a drug addict), emotions (e.g., I am miserable), or other labels (e.g., I am fat), to an understanding of the self-as-transcendent, an observ-ing self, stable and immutable, that is capable of accepting whatever thoughts or feelings the individual encounters without being defined by them. The individual can also shift from a life preoccupied by self-centered interests to a life that focuses on caring for other people or humanity as a whole. People who experience a "universal conversion" report a sense of deep transcendent connection with others and a desire to devote themselves to their well-being. Other people move a religious group or leader to the center of their lives. In this case, the individual attributes divine qualities to the group and looks to its leaders, members, beliefs, and practices for iden-tity, power, and spiritual support. Marc Galanter (1989) illustrates this point with the story of a drug-addicted woman who converted to the Di-vine Light Mission:

> Once I got to know them, I realized they loved me. They took me up, and it was as if they were holding me in their arms. I was like a baby whose mother guides its moves and cares for it. When I wanted to take heroin, or even to smoke [marijuana], I knew they were with me to help me stay away from it, even if I was alone. And their strength was there for me, even be-fore I could hardly meditate at all, I could rely on their invisible hand, moved by Maharaj Ji's wisdom, to help me gain control. (p. 30)

Whatever its form, the movement of the sacred from the edge to the center of the individual's life and identity marks a radical transformation in values and significance. Empirical studies bear this out. In their study of people who experienced quantum change, Miller and C'de Baca (2001) found that the five most highly valued personal characteristics for men shifted from "wealth, adventure, achievement, pleasure and be respected" before the change to "spirituality, personal peace, family, God's will, and honesty" after the change. For women, the top five values changed from "family, independence, career, fitting in, and attractiveness" to "growth, self-esteem, spirituality, happiness, and generosity" (p. 131). One person described the change in core values this way:

> My motivations and my whole sense of direction have changed. My values changed. What I thought was important changed. I just completely shifted gears. It's given me a sense of purpose and direction I never had before, and I've been searching different avenues but never found exactly what I was supposed to be doing. I've tried a lot of different things, a lot of different jobs, traveled a lot, had lots of experiences in my life. Yet always there was that kind of restless searching, searching. Now I feel like I know exactly what I'm supposed to do. (Miller & C'de Baca, 2001, p. 130)

With a new sense of motivation and purpose, many people also feel newly empowered to reach their goals. Illustrative of this point, Brian

Zinnbauer and I (1998) compared three groups of college students: students who had experienced a conversion to God, Jesus, or a Higher Power in the last 2 years, nonconverts who had become more religious or spiritual over the same time, and students who had not changed in their religiousness or religious denomination. In comparison to the students who had not changed religiously, both converts and nonconverts who had become more religious reported greater perceived stress 2 years earlier, and increased closeness to God over the past 2 years. Furthermore, the groups of converts and more religious students indicated significant improvements in self-esteem, self-confidence, and personal identity, unlike the religiously unchanged students who reported no alterations in their sense of themselves. It seems that the students who were frustrated with the limits of their personal goals and powers were able to find a resolution by recentering their lives around the sacred, and this new focus appeared to strengthen and empower the students in the pursuit of their strivings.

CONCLUSIONS

In response to spiritual struggles, many people engage in transformations. But spiritual transformation is not easy. For instance, to center the sacred, people have to confront the limits of a way of life. They must then undergo the painful process of letting go of old sources of significance. And then they face the task of rebuilding their lives and reorienting themselves around a new core of values. Hard as this kind of change is, it is not impossible. Research on spiritual transformation is just getting underway, yet empirical studies from different domains (e.g., 12-step programs, conversion, forgiveness) suggest that many people are, in fact, able to make profound spiritual transformations (e.g., Emrick, 1987; Freedman & Enright, 1996; Nicholi, 1974). Many clinicians can tell their own inspirational stories about remarkable clients whose existences appeared to be hopeless, yet who found the wherewithal to turn their lives around.

The search for the sacred does not end, even when successful transformation has occurred, for the individual is faced once again with the task of sustaining and enhancing his or her relationship with what has been transformed. And so the process continues.

It is important to reiterate that spiritual transformations can end in failure as well as success. Rites of passage may feel empty and meaningless to some people who are then left unable to move from one sacred phase of life to another. In the effort to build a more spiritual life, some people commit themselves to following destructive religious leaders or narrowly conceived gods that cannot hold the sacred. In attempting to make spiritual sense of their suffering, some people are unable to arrive at any vision of a God who tolerates such pain in the world. Listen, for example, to the way one victim of incest addresses God:

How could you in all your greatness have abandoned me, a little girl, to the merciless hands of my father? How could you let this happen to me? I demand to know why this happened? Why didn't you protect me? I have been faithful, and for what, to be raped and abused by my own father? I hate and despise you. I regret the first time I ever laid eyes on you; your name is like salt on my tongue. I vomit it from my being. I wish death upon you. You are no more. You are dead. (Flaherty, 1992, p. 101)

Ultimately, spiritual transformation can result in spiritual disengagement: disconnection from God, detachment from a religious community, or distance from any sense of transcendence, ultimacy, and timelessness in the world. Like a divorce, spiritual disengagement can occur angrily, but anger may only signify a continued spiritual struggle. Spiritual disengagement is best defined by a loss of interest in things sacred. The search for the sacred no longer matters, and furthermore it no longer matters that it no longer matters.

Although spiritual disengagement could be the final word when spiritual transformation fails, the spiritual spark may not be fully extinguished. Yearnings for the sacred can smolder for a while beneath the ashes of disappointment and pain only to be rekindled once again at some point later in life when the sacred is rediscovered and the individual ventures again onto the spiritual pathway. Thus, while the "You are dead" letter from the incest victim to God could indeed signal the beginning of spiritual disengagement, the passion in the letter suggests that it might also mark the beginning of an important new conversation with God.

People are active beings striving for significance. Spirituality, the search for the sacred is one critical element of that striving. In the last chapters, we have described spirituality as a process, a cycle of discovery, conservation, and transformation that evolves over the lifespan. Individual spiritual journeys unfold in remarkably diverse ways, depending on many individual, social, and situational factors as well as the response people perceive from the sacred. Some experience the journey as relatively "smooth sailing," but many encounter rough waters at times. The sense of sacred presence seems to come and go, as if God is engaged with the person in a game of cosmic peek-a-boo (Bakan, cited in Havens, 1968). Gaps and inconsistencies in spirituality can be discovered. Like an onion, new layers of spiritual experience and practice grow over old ones which, though hidden, can reveal themselves at the oddest of times. Thus, the man who has long proclaimed his atheism may be stunned to find himself feeling betrayed by

God when he is diagnosed with a terminal illness. The devout churchgoer may find herself equally surprised that she can no longer pray when she loses a loved one.

That spirituality ebbs and flows over the lifespan, that it can take many shapes and forms, that it can evolve and affect people in a variety of ways, and that it can be downright puzzling does not make spirituality anything other than one more normal dimension of human experience. The processes of discovery, conservation, and transformation of the sacred are not signs of psychopathology; neither should they be mistaken for indicators of extraordinary health and well-being. They are simply part and parcel of what it means to be human.

Yet any understanding of spirituality cannot stop here, for spirituality is more than a normal and natural part of life; it is also linked to life at its best and to life at its worst. The search for the sacred can lead to expressions of the greatest of human potential, but it can break down too, turning what was a potentially valuable aspect of human experience into a destructive force that wreaks havoc. How do we distinguish the spirituality that leads to growth from the spirituality that leads to decline? How do we distinguish the spirituality that is a part-of-the-solution from the spirituality that is a part-of-the-problem? To understand spirituality and address it in psychotherapy, we must be able to answer these questions.

7

Problems of
Spiritual Destinations

At its best, spirituality can be an integral part of life, one that fills the most ordinary of experiences with color, depth, and meaning. But if spirituality can be a part of the highest of human expressions, it can also be a part of the lowest. "Spirituality" is not a synonym for "goodness." Throughout history, people have justified forced conversions, suicide, torture, and genocide in the name of whatever they hold sacred. And the ties between spirituality and ugliness are not a thing of the past, as a quick review of any newspaper will show.

There are many types of spiritual problems. We are familiar with the sensational stories of parents who deny medical treatment to their children for religious reasons, cult members who commit mass suicide, clergy who sexually abuse their most vulnerable parishioners, and violent confrontations between people with conflicting visions of the sacred. Less sensational but far more common are the individual cases of people whose search for the sacred has broken down. A gay man cannot find a place for himself in his church. A college student is plagued by feelings of sinfulness that are made only worse by his scrupulous attention to ritual. An elderly woman suffering from a progressive illness cannot reconcile her disease with her belief that God would never allow her to suffer. And we should be alert to less obvious spiritual problems: the husband traumatized by the discovery that the wife he has worshipped has been unfaithful; the physically abused adolescent who develops an addiction to drugs; the successful businessman who feels emptiness rather than satisfaction in his life.

What makes a problem a spiritual problem? What criteria do we use to decide whether spirituality is a part of the problem, a part of the solution, or simply irrelevant to the problem at hand? How can we make sense of spiritual problems? These are not theoretical questions. They are questions that have very practical implications, for if we are to address spirituality successfully in psychotherapy we have to understand not only the normal process of spirituality, but also the ways in which spirituality goes awry. In this chapter and the next, we turn our attention to spiritual problems.

CRITERIA FOR EVALUATING SPIRITUALITY

There are three criteria for evaluating spirituality: truth-based criteria, pragmatic criteria, and process criteria.

Truth-Based Criteria

A number of years ago, Elizabeth, a 28-year-old woman, came in to see me at the request of her parents. A year and a half earlier, Elizabeth had lost her 5-month-old daughter in a car accident. Elizabeth described her deep conviction that her daughter was in heaven with the angels, looking down on those she loved, and protecting her family on earth. Elizabeth would often talk to her daughter, sharing day-to-day events and letting her know she was still in her mother's thoughts. On the anniversary of her daughter's birthday, Elizabeth asked her parents to come to a remembrance party and say a few words about their granddaughter and what her short life had meant to them. At this point, truly alarmed about the sanity of their daughter, Elizabeth's parents asked her to seek psychotherapy for her "religious delusions."

Was Elizabeth's daughter in heaven? Did Elizabeth, in fact, have a relationship with a spiritual presence? My PhD in psychology offered little help with these questions. They were, after all, unanswerable from a scientific point of view. We have no way to measure heaven, spiritual presences, or the divine. Scientific study cannot authenticate the truth of God's existence, divine revelation, biblical miracles, or life after death. And yet, to the spiritually minded, the value of spirituality has everything to do with its truth. Elizabeth did not feel she was in any sense delusional. Quite the contrary, her experience of an ongoing spiritual connection with her daughter in heaven was utterly convincing, as real to her as any of her relationships with loved ones on earth. As discussed earlier, this sense of being in touch with the "really, real" (Geertz, 1966) is a hallmark of spiritual experience. It is also a hallmark of organized religions that grow out of the sharing of divinely revealed truths. The major traditions of the world provide their adherents with a vision of ultimate reality: how the world was created, how people came to be, what is sacred, and what happens when we die. According to most traditions, to recognize and live by spiritual truths is the key to the good life. The failure to see and live out these spiritual truths is, on the other hand, the road to trouble.

Of course, the spiritual truths of one person may not be the spiritual truths of another. Elizabeth's parents were as convinced that their daughter was out of contact with reality as Elizabeth was that she was experiencing the "really, real." And I was being asked to arbitrate. There was a spiritual problem here, I concluded, but it was not one that could be resolved by any scientific evidence I could marshal regarding the truth of life after death, heaven, and angels. From a psychological point of view, the criterion of truth cannot be easily applied to evaluations of spirituality.

This is not to say that therapists do not live and work according to deep-seated values, beliefs, morals, ethics, indeed truths, of their own. However, the therapist has no special divine authority. This is one of the ways psychotherapy differs from religiously based forms of help, such as pastoral counseling, which is guided by the truths and authority of a particular religious tradition. For the therapist, morality, ethics, and truth are personally, professionally, and culturally based, but they are no more privileged than those of anyone else. In fact, it is the right of clients to define truths as they see them that is perhaps the most basic of all truths that therapists live by (though there are exceptions to even this truth). Truth-based criteria, then, are simply insufficient as guides for evaluating spirituality. To evaluate spirituality, we have to look to additional criteria for guidance.

Pragmatic Criteria

William James (1907/1975) offered a different way to understand the merits of spirituality. Rather than focus on the roots of religion, he proposed, consider its fruits. The right religion, the "true" religion, he believed, is the one that works best. James's approach was unabashedly pragmatic: "[Pragmatism] will count mystical experiences if they have practical consequences. She will take a God who lives in the very dirt of private fact—if that should seem a likely place to find him. Her only test of probable truth is what works best in the way of leading us" (p. 44).

From a pragmatic point of view, Elizabeth's spiritual beliefs were not problematic. She derived a great deal of comfort and reassurance from the knowledge that her daughter was in heaven. She was not preoccupied by her beliefs and they were not interfering with her ability to engage herself in the world. Elizabeth continued to be a productive worker, a loving wife, and a mother who was devoted to her surviving child.

Applying pragmatic criteria to the evaluation of spirituality is not always so easy, however. In many instances, the clinician may not know whether a particular approach to spirituality is likely to be helpful or harmful to a client. After all, clients come to treatment in the midst of problems;

they are in the process of a journey and it can be difficult to predict where their journey may take them.

Empirical studies could help clarify matters. In fact, hundreds of studies have been conducted on spirituality. In the tradition of William James, social scientists have taken a pragmatic approach to the evaluation of spirituality over the past century, focusing their attention on the question "How well does spirituality work?" through studies of the correlates and consequences of various spiritual beliefs and practices. This body of research has revealed important links between spirituality and health and well-being. Unfortunately, though, the findings as a whole have not been particularly helpful to clinicians, perhaps because the research has been too far removed from the clinical context. For instance, a modest correlation between frequency of prayer and life satisfaction in the general population may be statistically significant, but it may not be clinically significant to the psychologist who needs more individualized and contextualized information, such as information about the kinds of prayer that are likely to be most helpful to an elderly Hispanic man who is unsure whether to pursue chemotherapy for advanced cancer. Similarly, the finding that fundamentalist religious beliefs are associated with greater optimism, while interesting, may be of limited value to the clinician who wants to know about the potential costs as well as the benefits of these beliefs. And findings of ties between spirituality and measures of health and well-being, though noteworthy, may miss the mark for spiritually minded clinicians who are most interested in the impact of various spiritual beliefs and practices on *spiritual* criteria of well-being.

This picture has begun to change. As we have seen in earlier chapters, researchers have begun to identify more clinically relevant questions, to measure spirituality in richer ways, to focus on spirituality among discrete groups of people in times of trouble, and to pinpoint both the costs and the benefits of various forms of spirituality (Pargament, 2002b). The knowledge that is emerging from this body of research should be of greater value to clinicians as they grapple with the difficult task of evaluating spirituality.

I doubt, though, that pragmatism will ever prove to be wholly sufficient as a way of evaluating spirituality, for there are important limits to this approach. One grows out of the fact that people can achieve positive results in spite of themselves. Several months ago, I came across a newspaper account of a man who withdrew his life savings from the bank, went to Las Vegas, and wagered all of his money on one spin of the roulette wheel. He won. In essence, he lucked out; his foolish strategy led to a fabulous result. On the other side of the coin (to mix a metaphor), there are all too many examples of people who do the right thing only to suffer terrible consequences: the good Samaritan who is robbed by the person she stops to help, the loving parents whose child becomes incorrigible, the fitness devotee who dies of a heart attack at an early age. "Just plain surviving is fatal in the end," a writer once put it (Estleman, 2004, p. 56). To judge the quality of an effort purely by its results would lead us to applaud the man who treated the roulette wheel as a sound investment strategy and to deride the good behavior of those who suffered negative outcomes. A fairer evaluation of spirituality requires attention not only to spiritual *outcomes*, but also to the spiritual *process*.

Process Criteria

Although a beautiful work of art can give the appearance of seamlessness and simplicity, the impression is misleading; hundreds of bits and pieces have to come together "just so" to create something beautiful. Consider, for example, what it takes to produce a memorable symphonic performance: every instrument must be properly tuned, each of the musicians must be highly skilled, the entire ensemble must blend and coordinate its sounds, no musician can ignore the overarching direction of the conductor, and so on. When all of these elements cohere, an orchestra can produce extraordinary sounds, sounds capable of transporting the listener from his or her preoccupation with daily worries to a place of transcendent beauty. There are only so many ways for a work of art, such as a symphonic performance, to come together. Beauty is beauty. Only highly trained musicians can tell the difference between a Beethoven symphony played by the New York Philharmonic and the same piece played by the Philadelphia Orchestra. But there are thousands of ways a performance can go wrong. One out-of-tune instrument, a single mistimed entrance, the squeak of a sole clarinet can spoil the entire piece.

At its best, spirituality, like a work of art, reflects the harmonious interplay among dozens of bits and pieces. It is not easy to put this process into words, but a few social scientists and theologians have tried. They describe the highest levels of spirituality in terms of balance, dynamism, comprehensiveness, flexibility, and interconnectedness. For example, Gordon Allport (1950) likened mature religion to "a rich pudding, smooth and simple in its blend, but intricate in its ingredients" (p. 9). Orlo Strunk (1965) described mature religion as "a dynamic organization of cognitive–affective–conative factors possessing . . . depth and height" (p. 144). This is the language of process. When judged by the standards of process, the value of spirituality rests on its quality rather than its truth or its outcomes.[1]

---

[1]Of course, evaluations of spirituality according to process, pragmatic, and truth-based criteria are not necessarily inconsistent with each other. In general, a well-integrated spirituality is likely to have good results. And a higher truth can be attributed to the value of integration, as in the case of religious traditions that sanctify the values of balance, harmony, and the Golden Mean.

How do we define an efficacious spiritual process? The answer to this critical question does not lie exclusively within or outside of any particular religious tradition. Nor does it lie in a single belief, practice, or experience. Nor does it lie solely within the individual, for spirituality is more than a quality of a person; it is a quality of a person in interaction with situations and their larger context. I would say that the most effective spirituality is a *well-integrated spirituality*, one whose component parts work together in synchrony with each other. Conversely, spiritual problems are reflections of a *dis-integrated spirituality*, one whose parts are out of balance and working against each other. Elizabeth provides a case in point. She had a spiritual problem, but it could not be detected by pragmatic criteria. Her belief that her daughter was in heaven with the angels was a source of comfort rather than distress to her. Neither were her family's more secularized beliefs dysfunctional. The problem, instead, involved a lack of fit, a collision between their two disparate spiritual views of the world. The ultimate solution did not call for individual therapy that focused on Elizabeth's problem, but instead on family therapy in which Elizabeth and her family could share their different spiritual points of view more openly and more respectfully.

Evaluating spirituality as a process may seem complex and confusing, but I believe clinicians engage in just this kind of evaluation regularly in treatment. My colleague Eric Butter and I (2003) conducted a study that speaks to this point. We developed several vignettes that described people engaged in well-integrated and poorly integrated spirituality. Poorly integrated vignettes presented portraits of individuals who were facing spiritual conflicts with their larger social system, using spiritual methods of coping that were ill suited to the problem at hand, and seeking sacred and secular goals that were out of balance. Well-integrated vignettes described people who were spiritually supported by the social system, made use of spiritual coping methods that fit their problems, and sought a balanced set of goals. For example, in one well-integrated vignette, a young man faced with a terminal illness decides it is time to discontinue active treatment and surrender "everything to God's will" (see Table 7.1). In a comparable poorly-integrated vignette, a young man diagnosed with a treatable illness also decides to discontinue active treatment and surrender control to God. We asked 83 mental health professionals and 83 clergy to evaluate the level of adjustment of the person in each vignette and to rate the degree to which religion was helpful or harmful in that scenario. It is important to underscore the fact that none of the vignettes presented an outcome. The only difference between the vignettes was their degree of spiritual integration. Would mental health professionals and clergy be able to evaluate these vignettes purely on the basis of these process criteria? Would mental health professionals and clergy agree in their evaluations, or would they apply different standards to these vignettes? The results were clear. Despite the lack of informa-

TABLE 7.1. Well-Integrated versus Poorly Integrated Spiritual Vignettes

Well integrated

Mark started complaining of headaches, nausea, and dizziness recently. After seeing a doctor, Mark was diagnosed with an aggressive form of cancer, with a rapidly growing tumor in his brain, and cancer throughout 70% of his body. The doctor didn't have to tell Mark how long he has to live; he knows that his time is very, very limited.

Mark feels there is nothing he can do now to improve his health. He believes this situation is in God's hands. He believes that nothing he could do would make any difference in how things are going to turn out. He believes that he can do nothing to help himself and if he puts things in God's hands, it will all be ok. He is waiting for God to take control of his life and comfort him. Mark has surrendered everything to God's will.

Poorly integrated

Ben was alarmed when he started having pains in his chest and was having trouble breathing. After seeing a doctor and going through a battery of stress tests, Ben was told that his blood pressure was high and that he was at risk for a heart attack. The doctor prescribed a medication and encouraged him to eat a more balanced diet and to exercise regularly. The doctor tried to reassure Ben that as long as he starts taking care of his heart, he has no reason to be concerned. The doctor stressed to Ben how important this early intervention will be, and that he was lucky for catching it before anything serious occurred.

Ben feels there is nothing he can do now to improve his health. He believes this situation is in God's hands. He believes that nothing he could do would make any difference in how things are going to turn out. He believes that he can do nothing to help himself and if he puts things in God's hands, it will all be ok. He is waiting for God to take control of his life and comfort him. Ben has surrendered everything to God's will.

Note. From Butter and Pargament (2003). Reprinted by permission.

tion about outcomes, both mental health professionals and clergy judged religion to be more helpful in the well-integrated than in the poorly integrated vignettes, and both groups assessed the participants in the well-integrated scenarios as better adjusted than those in the poorly integrated vignettes. Furthermore, clergy and mental health professionals did not differ from each other in their ratings. In short, both groups demonstrated a sensitivity to the *process* of spirituality in their evaluations.

In the remainder of this chapter and in the next one, I will evaluate spirituality as a process, supplementing this discussion with empirical research and pragmatic evaluative criteria when possible and truth-based criteria at times. We will see that people can follow many spiritual trajectories in their lives: some smooth, some bumpy, some leading toward growth, some leading toward decline. Whether these trajectories lead in the general direction of growth or decline, I will argue, depends on the degree to which spirituality is well integrated (see Figure 7.1).

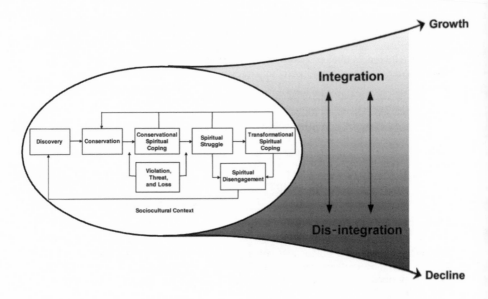

FIGURE 7.1. Spiritual trajectories.

What do I mean by "spiritual integration"? A well-integrated spirituality is defined not by a specific belief, practice, emotion, or relationship, but by the degree to which the individual's spiritual pathways and destinations work together in synchrony with each other. At its best, spirituality is defined by pathways that are broad and deep, responsive to life's situations, nurtured by the larger social context, capable of flexibility and continuity, and oriented toward a sacred destination that is large enough to encompass the full range of human potential and luminous enough to provide the individual with a powerful guiding vision. At its worst, spirituality is dis-integrated, defined by pathways that lack scope and depth, fail to meet the challenges and demands of life events, clash and collide with the surrounding social system, change and shift too easily or not at all, and misdirect the individual in the pursuit of spiritual value.

In this and the chapter that follows, I elaborate on this definition and the meaning of spiritual integration. As with a symphonic performance, there are far more ways for spirituality to go wrong than to go right. Thus, I will focus more on spirituality at its worst than spirituality at its best. We will see that dis-integration can occur among members of every religious tradition, as well as among those who do not identify with any religious tradition. To lend some order to this discussion, I consider two types of spiritual dis-integration: problems of spiritual destinations (this chapter) and problems of spiritual pathways (the next chapter).

PROBLEMS OF SPIRITUAL DESTINATIONS

Not all gods are alike. Earlier, I described the variety of ways in which people perceive the sacred in their lives. I reviewed a host of viable sacred forms. Certain representations, however, are not "up to the job" of the sacred. In the words of James Jones (1991), they are unable to "bear the full weight" of the divine, contain the "range of the experience of the holy," or fulfill all of the functions of the sacred (p. 123). Who are these inadequate gods? There are "small gods" that fail to capture the sacred in its range and depth, "false gods" that serve as poor substitutes for the sacred, "demons" that spare people from acknowledging the darkness within others or themselves, and "gods at war" that create intractable conflicts within the person. Sacred objects that are not up to the task do not have the power associated with stronger objects. They fall short in generating the sacred qualities of transcendence, boundlessness, and ultimacy. They are less capable of eliciting spiritual emotions, providing organization and coherence, and serving as a resource to the individual. As a result, the person who pursues a less-than-adequate form of the sacred is likely to be crippled from the start, no matter how proficient he or she may be in spiritual study, spiritual practice, or any of the other spiritual pathways. Without a strong and compelling destination, the search for the sacred can fall apart, with dangerous consequences for the individual and those around him or her. Below I consider three types of problems associated with spiritual destinations (see Table 7.2).

"Small Gods": The Problem of Insufficiency

One of the oddest things about religious education is that it often ends just when it should be beginning. For many adolescents, religious confirmation signals the culmination of formal religious education. And yet adolescence is the time when young adults are able to replace child-like conceptions of divinity and the sacred with more sophisticated spiritual understandings

TABLE 7.2. Spiritual Dis-integration: Problems of Spiritual Destinations

- Problems of small gods
- Problems of false gods
- Problems of sacred clashes within
  - Ambivalence toward the sacred
  - Self-degradation in relation to the sacred
  - Demonization of self and others
  - Internal sacred wars

that are better suited to the complexities of adult life. This premature closure leaves many people with "small gods." Of course, it could be said that all representations of God are too small because the human is incapable of fully grasping the character of the divine. Even so, some spiritual understandings are more encompassing than others. Smaller gods represent a problem because they fail to shed light on the profound dilemmas of life.

J. B. Phillips (1997) presents some apt illustrations in his book *Your God Is Too Small*. He describes the Grand Old Man "who was a great power in His day, but who could not possibly be expected to keep pace with modern progress" (p. 24); the god of Absolute Perfection who insists on complete and total loyalty and flawless performance; the Heavenly Bosom who provides limitless solace and comfort without ever asking for anything in return; and the Resident Policeman who serves as the "nagging internal voice that at worst spoils our pleasure and at best keeps us rather negatively on the path of virtue" (p. 15). To this list, I might add the Distant Star god who observes life from a great distance but fails to warm the world with the qualities of sacredness.

These limited representations of the sacred are ill-equipped to deal with the full spectrum of human potential and the full range of life challenges. For instance, clients with an overly strict conscience often view God as a "Resident Policeman" who frowns upon enjoyable experiences in life and spoils moments of pleasure with the threat of ultimate punishment. But small gods are not limited to punitive beings. People who see the sacred as purely loving and protective are equally vulnerable to disappointment and disillusion, for they may be unable to reconcile their narrow, albeit positive, representation of the sacred with their experiences of pain, suffering, and evil in the world. As William James (1902/1936) observed, a religion based on this "healthy-minded" but narrow perspective is also incomplete: "There is no doubt that healthy-mindedness is inadequate as a philosophical doctrine, because the evil facts which it refuses positively to account for are a genuine portion of reality; and they may after all be the best key to life's significance, and possibly the only openers of our eyes to the deepest levels of truth" (p. 160).

Small gods can also create problems for whoever lies outside of the sacred sphere. Within every religious tradition we find people convinced that God is theirs and theirs alone, committed to the belief that they hold exclusive claim to ultimate truth or divine revelation. Pity those who do not fall within this sacred umbrella! For example, in a study of over 11,000 people from 11 European countries, researchers found that people who believed that "there is only one true religion" were significantly more prejudiced against ethnic minorities (Scheepers, Gijsberts, & Hello, 2002). The consequences for outsiders can go beyond prejudice because small gods are likely to be perceived as vulnerable gods that require protection from external dangers. Over the centuries, slavery, religious bigotry, terrorism, and geno-cide have all been justified as legitimate responses to the threats that outsid-ers pose to the sacred. As such, these acts of violence come with a sacred seal of approval. Take, for example, this description of Ratko Mladic, com-mander of the Serbian military forces that committed atrocities and geno-cide in Srebenica: "To him the Bosnian Muslims were not fellow members of a once-shared nation. They were the worst kind of foreigners. They were Turks, blood enemies of his nation. His, then, was the holiest of missions: to capture sacred soil for his own people" (Halberstam, 2001, p. 296).

Small gods can leave even purported insiders open to injury. In an inci-sive analysis of why the Roman Catholic Church refused to acknowledge the prevalence of clergy sexual abuse for so long, canon lawyer and U. S. Air Force Chaplain Thomas Doyle (2003) suggested that the problem was partly tied to the narrow view of the sacred held by many priests who had been educated prior to Vatican II. Before Vatican II, Doyle wrote, the Ro-man Catholic Church defined itself as the "Perfect Society," one that had been established and favored by God and could do no wrong. From this perspective, "the 'good' of the Church equaled the 'good' of the clergy, es-pecially the hierarchy" (p. 206). While Vatican II redefined the Catholic Church more broadly as "the People of God," the more constricted per-spective continued to exert itself through the leadership of clerics who had come of age before Vatican II. "In many ways," Doyle writes, "the bishops defined the Church as themselves. Consequently when faced with threats to institutional stability such as the sex abuse phenomenon, the bishops' in-stinctive response was to protect the Church as they knew it" (p. 208). Thus, for many years, the accusations of parishioners who had been victim-ized by their pastors were met with denial, silence, or quiet transfers of offending clergy to other parishes. The victims of the abuse were left feeling abandoned and betrayed by their spiritual communities. Doyle concluded that the confusion of the Roman Catholic Church hierarchy with the total-ity of the sacred was the root cause of the clergy sexual abuse crisis. And the problem will not be solved until there is a clear commitment to the larger view of the sacred, one that encompasses the people as well as the in-stitution of the Catholic Church.

"False Gods": The Problem of Idolatry

Because they fail to contain the range of human needs and potentials, small gods often become even smaller, shrinking in size and power until they are nothing more than hollow entities. What remains of God, as Douglas Porpora (2001) put it, is "the smile of a Cheshire cat, stripped of surround-ing features. Such a God is a cipher, a 'floating signifier' without referent" (p. 18). And such a God leaves people with a spiritual vacuum at their core.

Remember, though, that the loss of the sacred is not necessarily final, for the spiritual impulse is not easily eliminated from the human psyche. Optimally, the spiritual vacuum will be filled by a more encompassing God. Unfortunately, however, inadequate substitutes for the sacred can also rush in to fill this spiritual void. Take, for example, the story of Julie Yau (2003). As a child, she was exquisitely sensitive to God and the spiritual dimension of nature: "I was about six when I began praying and talking to God. I was always aware of the Omnipresence as someone I could talk to. . . . I was connected to the mysterious. . . . Butterflies and bees, mountains and grass, starfish and sand were all enchanting parts of a magical world that I watched with innocent eyes" (pp. xiv, 18). Yet she was inordinately sensitive to the pain in the world as well as its beauty, and her experience of the sacred did not provide her with a way to affirm and contain her emotions. As she moved into adolescence, Julie was overwhelmed by the intensity of her feelings and intuitions. Believing that something was wrong with her, she cut herself off from her sense of sacredness. In its place, she developed a "merciless hunger" and food became the center of her life. It took several years of struggle with an eating disorder for Julie to realize that she was trying to satisfy her "spiritual rumblings" with food. "Underneath," she wrote, "I was emotionally and spiritually famished, unable to find a way to fulfill my spiritual yearning" (p. 90). With that realization, Julie began to recover from her disorder. Central to her healing, she believed, was the rediscovery of the sacred, but a sacred now large enough to affirm and contain her own personal gifts and strengths: "Reaching out to God inwardly, outwardly and through nature, the complexity of my disorder began to smooth out, and I recognized my own inner resources for healing" (p. 92).

Food is only one of many possible substitutes for people in search of something to satisfy their spiritual hunger. Others turn to alcohol, drugs, or sex to fill a spiritual vacuum (e.g., Coleman, Kaplan, & Downing, 1986). Listen to this example:

> As my alcoholism progressed, my thirst for God increasingly became transmuted into a thirst for the seemingly godlike experiences that alcohol induced. Alcohol gave me a sense of well-being and connectedness—and wasn't that an experience of God? Alcohol released me from the nagging sense that I was never good or competent enough—and wasn't that God's grace? Alcohol dissolved my worries about the future, allowing me to live in the present—and wasn't that a divine gift? At my core there was a thirst, a thirst for whatever would fill the emptiness. (Nelson, 2004, p. 31)

Self-worship is another common substitute for God in Western culture. To become totally self-contained, exclusively devoted to the satisfaction of one's own needs and desires, is the ultimate ideal for many people. Many others idolize celebrities who distract them from the emptiness within themselves (McCutcheon, Lange, & Houran, 2002). Still others devote themselves even more passionately to money, material gain, and consumption. On a recent trip to New York City, my wife and I decided to visit the home of Franklin Roosevelt. I was delighted to see a long line of fellow history buffs waiting to board the bus. But, as it turned out, Aileen and I were in the wrong line. Those in the long line were heading off to a retail shopping outlet. (Aileen and I were the only ones taking the bus to visit Roosevelt's home.) Group shopping trips are a sign of the times. "The visit to the shopping mall has taken on the character of a regular religious ritual," Dell deChant (2003, p. 2) has noted. Here "consumption has become the place of final truth, of absolute seriousness," and the economy has become the "ground of the sacred" (p. 4). One man illustrated the point succinctly: "Some people are Catholics, some are Protestants. Me, I'm an Oldsmobile man." The list goes on; in search of the sacred people can turn to everything from baseball and politics to nationalism and racial pride.

The choice of sacred objects is not trivial. "There are real dangers involved when the sacred gets attached to the wrong things," Parker Palmer (1998, p. 25) notes. Those who worship false gods can pose a threat to themselves. Witness the terrible consequences faced by people who center their lives around drugs, alcohol, or food. Or consider the price paid by people who devote themselves to an abusive spouse or a despotic authority figure. People who worship false gods can threaten others as well as themselves. "Ask anyone whose family or history was touched by the Nazis' murderous attachment of the sacred to blood, soil, and race," says Palmer (p. 25).

The sanctification of other seemingly more innocent objects can also lead to trouble when it becomes idolatrous. Earlier I described how people naturally attempt to extend the reach of the divine into their day-to-day lives. Through the process of sanctifying relationships, themselves, and time and place, they try to illuminate life with radiance from the sacred core. In this process, people seek a symbolic form for what is so difficult to represent: their own sense of the sacred. As Paul Tillich (1957) pointed out, only symbolic language can express the ultimate. Problems arise, though, when the sacred object that symbolizes the divine is perceived to be divine in and of itself rather than as a manifestation of the divine or a container of sacred qualities. Essentially, the symbol is confused with what it represents. In Tillich's (1957) terms, a "preliminary concern" is elevated over an "ultimate concern" and the result is idolatry. Similarly, theologian Robert Neville (1996) points out that, although religious symbols offer a "window" from which to view the divine, they should not be confused with the divine itself: "When the symbols of a particular religious tradition are fresh and living, people see through them to the divine. They do not notice the symbols as such any more than they notice the glass in a window or think about columns of mercury when hearing the temperature from the TV weather announcer" (p. 29). Paradoxically, Neville notes, "only religious symbols that are broken are true" (p. 243), for only a broken symbol conveys its own limitations and points beyond itself toward the ultimate source of holiness.

Confusing their sacred objects with divinity itself, people become vulnerable to trouble. They may overestimate the powers of other people and find themselves devastated when those they have deified prove to be human. As Schreurs (2002) wrote: "Putting their hope for infinite love in one lover, friend, parent, or leader after another, they heap disappointment upon disappointment and end up in bitterness because the love they are actually receiving never meets the standard of being 100 per cent unconditional and infinite" (p. 121). For instance, a few years ago, I worked with Barbara, an attractive 45-year-old who had been emotionally neglected by her parents as a child and later abandoned by her husband. The immediate problem she presented, however, involved her pastor. He was a kind and attentive man. Even so, there were times when he forgot to return her phone calls, failed to ask her how she was doing after a worship service, and seemed more concerned about other members in the church than her. While exploring her feelings regarding the pastor, I first thought that Barbara was seeking someone who could fill the emotional holes that had been left by her parents and spouse. And yet she had passed up numerous promising opportunities to form new romantic relationships. "They're just not there for me in the way I need them," she said. What were her expectations of men, and her pastor in particular, I asked? Barbara responded, "I expect him to always be there for me to love me and care about me." But what about his responsibilities to other people in the church? I wondered. "Well, I know he has those," Barbara said, "but I need to know that I come first." It struck me that Barbara was yearning for something that no person could satisfy. Perhaps, I suggested, she might look more directly to God for the enduring and unconditional love she was seeking from the pastor. "Oh no," she replied. "God cares about everyone. You know, he loves everyone and all that. I need someone who can make me feel that I'm special." I realized that God, for Barbara, had taken on the guise of the perfunctory parents she had experienced as a child. And, like her parents, this God could not meet her deepest needs. Barbara had largely given up on God and instead developed an idolatrous attachment to her pastor, an attachment that could only fail because the pastor was only human.

People can also define themselves as their own gods, taking themselves and others down an even more deadly path. Jim Jones, leader of the People's Temple at Jonestown, Guyana, exhorted his followers to replace the "sky-God" of the Bible with himself, the "socialist worker God": "You prayed to the sky-God and he never heard your prayers. You asked and begged and pleaded for help with your suffering, and he never gave you any food. He never provided a bed. He never gave you a home. But I, the social-ist worker God, have given you all those things" (Kimball, 2002, p. 77). For those who accepted Jim Jones as their God, the results were deadly.

Commenting on the dangers of self-worship after World War II, Carl Jung (1945/1967) said, " 'God-almightiness' does not make man divine, it merely fills him with arrogance and arouses everything evil in him. It pro-duces a diabolical caricature of man, and this inhuman mask is so unendur-able, such a torture to wear, that he tortures others. He is split in himself, a prey to inexplicable contradictions" (p. 215). Whatever form idolatry takes, it generally breaks down because the worshipper fails to see beyond the object to what it represents. Inevitably, the object proves itself to be fragile, unable to bear the full weight of the divine, and when it cannot, the individual is left without sacred symbol or sacred core.

Sacred Clashes Within: The Problem of Internal Conflict

I have noted that a person can hold very different images of the sacred simultaneously. The same individual can view God as loving at one level, punitive at another, and detached at still another. This shouldn't be alto-gether surprising, given the fact that the portrait of the sacred is drawn from such different materials: representations of parents, culture, organized religion, personal needs, temperament, sacred experiences, and spiritual longings. Of course, people can live with a lack of internal consistency in their spiritual perspectives, but, at times, divergent understandings of the sacred collide with each other or with the way people understand them-selves.

Psychodynamic and object relations theorists, such as Fairbairn and Kohut, have written most extensively about these internal spiritual con-flicts. James Jones (2002) provides an exceptionally clear and cogent sum-mary of this literature and goes on to make his own valuable contribution. According to this body of work, the child's understanding of the sacred de-velops, first and foremost, out of relations with his or her parents. When these relations are troubled, conflicts with the sacred can follow. If the child lacks the kind of parenting that results in a strong sense of self, he or she is unable to develop a cohesive "self-structure." What remains instead is an "object hunger," a powerful desire for an object that can be idealized, one that can offer self-affirmation and self-cohesion in return. Seeking to satisfy this hunger, the child develops representations of the sacred that unfortu-nately contain the seeds of the same tension and conflict that defined the child's relations with his or her parents. Below I consider four examples: the problem of ambivalence toward the sacred, the problem of self-degradation, the problem of demonization, and the problem of sacred wars.

Ambivalence toward the Sacred

Jones (2002) presents the case of Stanley, a successful musician who had suffered from disappointment and depression for much of his life. Stanley grew up with a hypercritical father, a high school teacher who was merciless and sarcastic in his evaluations of his students and equally disparaging of his son, whom he treated like just another student. Stanley's mother, a concentration camp survivor, was so anxious and fearful for her children that she kept them at home for much of high school. Music represented a shelter for Stanley. Here he could excel and avoid his father's criticism, since his father was uninterested in this form of art. In his 20s, Stanley began to explore religion. He lived in a Tibetan Buddhist center for 2 years, but was devastated when he discovered that the leader was struggling with alcoholism and having affairs with several of the female initiates. He became deeply involved in a Pentecostal Christian group only to reject it after he learned that they did not believe in evolution. Eventually, he married a woman who showed an interest in his music, but he left her when he found her to be pretentious. Her final words to him were "You could rain on anybody's parade" (p. 36). The pattern in Stanley's life was clear. Over many years, he had seesawed from uncritical devotion to various sacred objects to deep disillusion with them. At the root of Stanley's terrible ambivalence, Jones believes, was the damage he had suffered as a child in his ability to idealize or denote things as sacred. Jones writes:

> If the need for idealization is not met, if a child is not allowed to idealize, or if idealized objects fail too early, the child may block the capacity to idealize. Such a person cannot idealize . . . [and] must disparage and debunk everything. But the need for objects of idealization does not disappear . . . it propels the individual into a frantic search for objects of idealization that are sooner or later bound to fail and so further reinforce his/her cynical attitudes. (p. 33)

Self-Degradation

Conflict with parents can also manifest itself through self-degradation in relationship to the sacred. When disappointed, frustrated, or hurt by their fathers or mothers, children may split the "badness" off from their parents and take it on themselves to preserve the sense that their parents are good. Toward the same end, children can also project their own good qualities on to their parents. This pattern of "incorporating the bad and projecting the good" often becomes the model for subsequent relationships, including relationships with the sacred. According to Erich Fromm (1950), this pattern is the essence of "authoritarian religion" in which

> [the person] projects the best he has onto God and thus impoverishes himself. Now God has all love, all wisdom, all justice—and man is deprived of these qualities, he is empty and poor. . . . He is [then] caught in a painful dilemma. The more he praises God, the emptier he becomes. The emptier he becomes, the more sinful he feels. The more sinful he feels, the more he praises God—and less able is he to regain himself." (pp. 50–51)

Certainly, the recognition of human finitude and limitations is central to wisdom and growth, Fromm noted, but authoritarian religion takes this understanding to another, ultimately destructive level.

> It is one thing to recognize one's dependence and limitations, and it is something entirely different to indulge in this dependence, to worship the forces on which one depends. To understand realistically and soberly how limited our power is an essential part of wisdom and of maturity; to worship it is masochistic and self-destructive. The one is humility, the other self-humiliation. (p. 53)

Demonization of Self and Others

In its most extreme form, self-degradation can express itself as demonization of the self. The self is perceived as more than sinful, it is seen as demonic. Recently, I saw Crystal, a 30-year-old mother of three young children, in psychotherapy. Crystal had suffered from obsessions and compulsions for much of her life. While in her early 20s, she had worked with a cognitive-behavioral psychologist who had helped her to eliminate many of her disturbing thoughts and behaviors. However, Crystal admitted that she continued to be plagued by a few obsessions and compulsions, thoughts and actions that she had been too ashamed to admit to her first therapist. As a young child, she had watched the movie *The Exorcist*, and since that time she had had fears that she too could become possessed by the devil. To ward off that possibility, she had developed a personal ritual of clenching her hands, arms, and shoulders. At an intellectual level, Crystal recognized that her feelings and behaviors were absurd. After all, she did not believe in the devil or possession. Nevertheless, she continued to worry about the demonic and to "clench" her arms and shoulders. Moreover, the problem was getting worse. Clenching was leading to tingling feelings in her upper body, which only fueled her fears of possession.

In my conversations with Crystal, I learned that she had grown up as the oldest of three sisters. Her father had left the family after the youngest sister was born. Her mother, tormented by chronic back pain, was an unpredictable force in the family, at times screaming uncontrollably at the children, at times isolating herself in her room for days on end, and at times reminding the children how much she loved and cared about them. In spite of the treatment she had received from her mother, Crystal insisted that her mother was a good woman who had done the best she could raising the children.

At one point in therapy, I asked Crystal to imagine what she would be like if she became possessed. She had never considered this question before and her response was quite interesting. What she feared most, Crystal said, was not being able to be there for her children. She did not imagine grotesque changes in her bodily form, spitting foam, or committing brutal murders. Possession instead meant mistreating her children or simply leaving them without a mother. I sat without comment. After a long pause, Crystal said, "That sounds like my mother."

Crystal's deepest fear was not possession by the devil, but possession by her mother. However, by attributing the problem to demonic forces within herself, Crystal was able to preserve the sacred image of her mother who was, after all, "a good woman who had done the best she could." Of course, Crystal's effort to protect her mother's image came at a terrible cost to herself. Rather than confront the darker side of her mother, Crystal worried that her own soul was at risk. I will have more to say about the treatment of Crystal later in the book.

The dialectical tension between self and sacred can lead in a different direction, from demonization of the self to demonization of the other. Jones (2002) points out that some individuals, unable to tolerate the badness they have internalized, deal with their pain by projecting it onto another "despised group" (p. 60). In fact, the splitting of the good and the bad can result in a reversal of the "bad me—good God" model of authoritarian religion into a "good me—demonic other" model. Children who are raised by parents with unrealistically high expectations may respond by developing a sense of themselves as "all good" and others unlike themselves as "all bad." This type of splitting can have terrible consequences. Many psychologists have maintained that the failure to acknowledge the dark side within oneself sets the stage for acts of hatred and violence. Allport (1950), for example, wrote: "Hate behaves like jaundice; the sufferer overlooks the state of his own liver; to him it is the world out there that appears maliciously yellow" (p. 156).

Religious groups can support this type of splitting and intensify it even further through the language of the demonic. From this perspective, those who fall outside of the individual's sacred sphere are not only bad, they are allied with the powers of darkness against the sacred. To root out the demonic and protect the sacred, religious groups may be willing to take extreme steps with potentially disastrous results. For example, Bowman (2000) describes the case of a woman with a dissociative disorder who confided her guilt about masturbating to members of her church. Fellow congregants told her that masturbation was displeasing to God and demanded that she wear mittens as a form of penance, which in turn only reinforced her feelings of guilt and self-hatred. When the woman turned to acts of self-mutilation, the congregation labeled her as "demon-possessed," attempted to exorcise her self-mutilating alter egos, and, when that proved unsuccessful, shunned her. Bowman reports that the spiritual damage this woman suffered was profound and long lasting.

The demonization of others can have larger social impact as well. Consider Osama bin Laden's (1998) prophetic warning of a jihad against the United States prior to 9/11:

> The ruling to kill the Americans and their allies—civilians and military—is an individual duty for every Muslim who can do it in any country in which it is possible to do it, in order to liberate the al-Aqsa Mosque and the holy mosque [Mecca] from their grip, and in order for their armies to move out of all the lands of Islam, defeated and unable to threaten any Muslim. This is in accordance with the words of Almighty Allah, "and fight the pagans all together as they fight you all together." . . . We also call on Muslim ulema, leaders, youths, and soldiers to launch the raid on Satan's U.S. troops and the devil's supporters allying with them.

Demonic language can be used by any religious group and both sides of a conflict. Muslim extremists have labeled the United States "the Great Satan"; Christian crusaders in the Middle Ages depicted Muslims as less than human; Ian Paisley, a Protestant leader in the conflict between Northern Irish Protestants and Catholics called the pope "a black coated bachelor from hell" (Juergensmeyer, 2000, p. 183); and Christian white supremacists have called Jews "children of Satan" (Silberman, Higgins, & Dweck, 2005).

These dehumanizing appraisals are not as uncommon as one might expect. For example, in our study of college students from Ohio and New York City following the 9/11 terrorist attack on the World Trade Center, we found that a significant proportion of the students demonized the terrorists (Mahoney et al., 2002). Fifty-five percent of Ohioans and 42% of New Yorkers agreed that "these people are on the devil's side" and 64% of Ohioans and 49% of New Yorkers agreed that "the devil is at work in these people's actions." Students who were more likely to demonize the terrorists were also more likely to agree that "no punishment is too extreme for these people" and that "these people should suffer for all of eternity." Furthermore, they were more likely to support extremist reactions, such as the use of nuclear and biological weapons. Similarly, beliefs in Satan have been tied to higher levels of prejudice toward gays, lesbians, and ethnic minorities (Wilson & Huff, 2001).

It is important to stress that the danger here lies not in the language of the demonic per se, be it the demonization of self or others. Only powerful language can give adequate voice to the intense fear, anger, and pain people feel when their deepest values have been threatened or when they have suffered. Further, the notion of Satan or an evil force at large in the universe may offer a particularly compelling way to make sense of what seems incomprehensible, including one's own acts or the acts of others. The language of the demonic serves other important purposes: it preserves the individual's sense of God and the sacred; it contributes to the individual's identity by defining what the person stands against; and it is often accompanied by the comfort and hope that the demonic can be controlled and contained. Many viable religious traditions have found an important place for the demonic in their theologies (Parkin, 1985).

Problems arise, however, when people are unable to integrate their understanding of evil with the way they come to terms with themselves, other people, and the world. Dis-integration may occur when people experience themselves as being on the losing side of the battle with the demonic, when they identify themselves exclusively with evil, or when they deny the darker side of themselves and project it on to others. This latter danger is especially salient today when, to paraphrase Carl Jung (1945/1964), terrorists "dissociate and jump over their own shadow to see dark in others" (p. 203). And the step between projecting evil onto others and then attempting to eliminate those others has proven to be all too small. What is truly diabolical, psychologist David Bakan (1966) concludes, is not the denied part of oneself but the separation of the denied part *from* oneself. Similarly, the greatest challenge is not how to eliminate the unacceptable parts of oneself but how to live with them, how to accept the fact that both we and others "contain the capacity for both good and evil" (Bowman, 2000, p. 134).

Internal Sacred Wars

Even though various representations of the sacred can exist side by side within the person without apparent conflict, they can also clash, at times with devastating results. Carrie Doehring (2004) brought a movie to my attention that depicts just such a conflict. *Breaking the Waves* tells the story of Bess, a simple young woman who lives by the sea in a Scottish village. Bess looks deeply at life around her and seems to be transported to another dimension by the rough beauty of the Scottish highlands and the physical sensuality of her relationship with her husband. Bess's native spirituality, however, collides with the stern God of her family and her Calvinist Presbyterian church. This God views pleasure and joy as sinful distractions, insisting instead upon self-denial as the pathway to grace. Bess has no way to reconcile these different ways of experiencing and understanding the sacred. Her experiences of pleasure in life are followed by conversations in which she takes on God's voice and chastises herself for her joy. Bess cannot purge herself of the spiritual pleasure she takes from life, but neither can she turn her back on her God. She is left with two warring representations of the sacred: a God who cannot support her mystically sensual experiences, and a physical spirituality that cannot accommodate an austere God.

The conflict must come to a head. After her husband leaves Bess to return to his job on an oil rig in the North Sea, she experiences excruciating loneliness. Unable to sustain herself because of the harshness of her God and the coldness of her religious community, she begs God to return her husband to her. Shortly after, her husband is crippled by an accident and comes home paralyzed from the waist down. Bess is herself crippled with guilt for the divine punishment she feels she has brought down upon her husband. When her husband asks her to engage in sex with strangers and share her stories with him, Bess is caught between the deep love she feels for her spouse and her religious prohibitions. Her solution to this sacred conflict is shocking: she becomes a prostitute. This is a terrible sacrifice, for sex with strangers is reprehensible to Bess. Yet her willingness to desecrate the act of sexual intimacy in response to her husband's request, she believes, represents the greatest gift of love. At the same time, the violation of her body represents a form of atonement for her sins, a repayment to God that will bring her back into his good graces. Her sacrifice seems to be supported by a God who (speaking in Bess's voice) compares her to Mary Magdalene. Bess is never able to find a more successful resolution to her conflict, one that might soften and enlarge her understanding of God or one that might legitimize the sacredness of her experiences in the physical world. Ultimately, Bess makes the supreme sacrifice, consistent with her sacrificial understanding of Christ's crucifixion. She knowingly places herself in the hands of a sexual sadist who murders her. This is by no means your typical movie ending, but it does illustrate the destructive potential of internal sacred wars.

CONCLUSIONS

In the search for the sacred, people strive toward many spiritual destinations. At best, people seek a relationship with a sacred large enough to encompass life as a whole, a sacred that is not confused with those symbolic forms that attempt to give it expression, a sacred that accepts the full range of human possibilities including the darker side, and a sacred that provides an overarching and coherent vision to orient and guide peoples' lives. But not all sacred ends are worthwhile; some are dead ends. Small gods, false gods, demons, and gods at war are signs of spiritual dis-integration, signs of a lack of depth and unity in ultimate purpose and direction that have powerful implications for the health and well-being of individuals and their larger communities. The problem of spiritual ends can also have spiritual "ripple" effects that leave even greater spiritual dis-integration in the wake of the misdirected pursuit of spiritual value. In the next chapter, we turn our attention to forms of spiritual dis-integration that involve the pathways people take to their destinations.

8

Problems of
Spiritual Pathways

Several years ago, I came across a disturbing account of a man who
had murdered his wife, three children, and mother for ostensibly religious
reasons.

> With [my daughter] being so determined to get into acting I was also fear-
> ful as to what that might do to her continuing to be a Christian. . . .
>   Also, with [my wife] not going to church I knew that this would
> harm the children eventually. . . .
>   At least I'm certain that all have gone to heaven now. If things had
> gone on who knows if this would be the case. . . .
>   It may seem cowardly to have always shot them from behind, but I
> didn't want any of them to know even at the last second that I had to do
> this. . . .
>   I'm only concerned with making my peace with God and of this I
> am assured because of Christ dying even for me. ("Memorandum . . . , "
> 1990, p. 25)

Obviously, there was something very wrong with the spiritual life of this
man, but what was the problem? On the face of it, he was pursuing a legitimate spiritual goal, one shared by many fellow believers: he was trying to
ensure the spiritual salvation of his loved ones. Yet the pathway he took toward this seemingly reasonable sacred goal was horribly flawed. Unable to
tolerate spiritual differences among the members of his family and frozen in
his spiritual perspective, he could not imagine other ways to resolve his
conflicts. Ultimately, he selected a "solution" that was totally dispropor-

tionate to his goals: murdering his loved ones to save their souls. Certainly, problems in this man's understanding of the sacred may have set the stage for the tragedy that followed. For example, his was a small god who could not encompass more than the narrowest of spiritual expressions. Perhaps even more to the point, this man had no qualms about engaging in idolatry, setting himself up as his own god who served as judge and jury of his family. But the problems with this man went well beyond his understanding of the sacred and his choice of sacred goals. Spiritual dis-integration manifested itself dramatically in the path he took toward his destination. This is merely one example. There are many others.

At times, people become spiritually disoriented, and their ways of thinking, acting, feeling, relating, and coping fail to form traversable pathways to the sacred. As a result, the individual engaged in the spiritual quest gets stuck, lost, collides with others, reaches a dead end, or falls over a cliff. In this chapter, we take a closer look at several different forms of dis-integration associated with spiritual pathways: problems of breadth and depth, problems of fit, and problems of continuity and change (see Table 8.1).

PROBLEMS OF BREADTH AND DEPTH

At its best, spirituality is more than a loose set of beliefs, practices, relationships, and experiences. It is, instead, a way of being that is broad and deep, touching on virtually every dimension of life. Not everyone integrates spirituality so fully. In Western culture, which values the freedom to choose one's beliefs and practices, people are encouraged to construct their own customized spiritual pathways. Of course, people do not have to "go it alone" in their search for the sacred. To assist them in the process, our culture provides a variety of spiritual options from which people can pick and choose. One rapidly growing, nondenominational, evangelical church provides a vivid illustration. Inspired by the U.S. shopping mall, the church offers its 6,000 members a "boutique" approach to worship: "Here simultaneous services, all with their own mood, music, and prayer leaders, range from rock and roll cool for Generation X and the baby-boomer crowd to old fashioned and hymn-filled traditionalists to coffee-shop casual for people wanting informality and a cup of java with their prayers" (Cineplex Church, 2002). This smorgasbord approach to spirituality may satisfy the appetites of some, but it may leave others spiritually malnourished.

Ultimately, go-it-alone or cafeteria-style spirituality can create holes in the spiritual lives of people. In our culture, we can find a variety of forms of spirituality that lack breadth: the self-contained spirituality focused solely on personal gratification without concern for others; the spirituality of hollow practice cut off from sacred feelings of awe and uplift; the spirituality of pure experience ungrounded in the wisdom of great spiritual teachers,

TABLE 8.1. Problems of Spiritual Pathways

- Problems of breadth and depth
- Problems of fit
  - Problems of fit between spiritual pathways and destinations
    - Spiritual extremism
    - Spiritual hypocrisy
  - Problems of fit between spiritual pathways and situations
  - Problems of fit between the individual and social context
- Problems of continuity and change

---

past and present; the spirituality of mind alone devoid of rituals that symbolize and enact life's deepest truths.

Perhaps even greater than the problem of spiritual breadth in our culture is the lack of height and depth in spirituality (Strunk, 1965). Summarizing the findings from a national survey on the topic of spirituality, pollsters George Gallup Jr. and D. Michael Lindsay (1999) concluded that "spirituality in the United States may be three thousand miles wide, but it remains only three inches deep" (p. 45). To illustrate their point, they note that even though nine out of 10 adults have a copy of the Bible in their homes, only 35% of this largely Christian population knows who delivered the Sermon on the Mount and only 40% know what the Trinity is.

Without spiritual breadth and depth, people are likely to experience spiritual dis-integration in their search for the sacred. A few years ago, I worked with a 50-year-old man in psychotherapy who was recovering from serious injuries he had suffered in a car accident that had also killed his wife. Until recently, Charles felt he had been coping well with the tragedy. A mechanic by trade and a problem solver by nature, he had dealt with his accident by focusing on the most visible of his problems: his physical injuries and rehabilitation. Lately, though, he had been experiencing waves of sadness that seemed to sweep over him for no apparent reason. He was also troubled by obsessive thoughts over trifling matters, such as where he had put his spare car keys. Like the waves of sadness, his thoughts seemed to come out of nowhere, keeping him awake at night and leaving him with the feeling that his life was out of control. In the course of our conversations, it became clear that Charles had never really grieved over the death of his wife and his own physical losses. I told Charles that he had been making a wonderful physical recovery from his accident and then suggested to him that perhaps his depression and anxiety were signs that he was ready to begin his emotional recovery. He agreed. But Charles' emotional recovery was, in some respects, more difficult than his physical recovery, for spiritual reasons.

As we talked about the accident, Charles repeatedly returned to some troubling spiritual questions. Why had God chosen to take his wife's life and his own health? Why was God inflicting him with such great sadness and disturbing thoughts? The fact that he was even asking these questions came as a surprise to Charles, who had never seen himself as a particularly religious or spiritual person. His parents, nominal Methodists, had sent him to Sunday school for a few years as a child, but he remembered only bits and pieces of what he had been taught. Neither was his family much for religious ritual, with the exception of Christmas, a day more for eating and gift giving rather than one filled with religious meaning. Though Charles and his wife had sent their children to Sunday school, they rarely attended religious services. Indeed, religion played little part in the life of the family. Because of his injuries, Charles had been unable to attend the funeral of his wife. Here was a man with the thinnest of spiritual backgrounds, struggling with the deepest of spiritual questions, as we hear in the following exchange from a session:

CHARLES: I was doing so well and then all of these thoughts and feelings just happened.

K.I.P.: You talk about your thoughts and feelings as if they descended on you from above.

CHARLES: Above or below.

K.I.P.: What do you mean?

CHARLES: That's just the way it feels (*pause and hesitation*). Sometimes I wonder whether they're the work of the devil.

K.I.P.: I haven't heard you talk about the devil before. Could you say more about how you see the devil involved in your life?

CHARLES: I don't know. I remember something I heard about or read about years ago in the Bible. This Job fellow had suffered a lot. He had lost his wife, his kids, everything. And it turns out the devil had made a bet with God that Job wouldn't keep his faith if he lost everything.

K.I.P.: So how do you make sense of that?

CHARLES: I don't know. Maybe the devil was trying to test Job.

K.I.P.: Is that how you're feeling too?

CHARLES: I guess. Maybe the devil is causing all of this trouble to try to turn me away from God or Jesus.

K.I.P.: How do you think God or Jesus feels about this?

CHARLES: I'm not sure where I stand on that. I have a hard time imagining how they think and feel about things.

K.I.P.: Do you remember how the story turned out for Job?

CHARLES: Not really.

Though Charles was wrestling with weighty spiritual questions, he was not well equipped to resolve them. His spiritual knowledge was fragmentary at best and what he knew was the source of more anxiety than comfort. His beliefs were unexamined and had only the loosest of connections with the way he understood himself and the world around him. Missing was any relationship with a religious community or pastor that could have supported him and guided him through his struggle. The rituals he had practiced in his life were hollow, empty of meaning and substance. Largely absent from his coping repertoire were spiritual methods of understanding and dealing with the tragedy, including rituals to signify the sacred losses he had suffered and help him through the process of transformation. Finally, his relationship with God was marked by ambivalence and uncertainty. He felt a sense of loyalty to a God who, he feared, may have been responsible for the misfortunes of his life.

Yet beneath the surface of his pain and confusion, Charles was expressing a profound spiritual yearning. He was seeking answers to ultimate questions about suffering, meaning, responsibility, and God. But he was crippled in his search for the sacred by his lack of spiritual breadth and depth. His was a "spirituality in exile" (Schreurs, 2002). Charles's psychological distress, in turn, was at least partly linked to his ongoing spiritual struggle. It would have been difficult, if not impossible, to help Charles in psychotherapy without attending to the spiritual dimension in his life. I will consider how spiritually integrated psychotherapy addresses problems of spiritual breadth and depth in a later chapter. For now, let me note that spiritual progress and therapeutic progress were inseparable in my work with Charles. Charles needed help broadening and deepening his spiritual pathways before he could grieve more fully for his losses and finally experience emotional relief.

Charles's case isn't unusual. Empirical studies have linked the spirituality that lacks breadth and depth to other problems. Consider some examples from a few streams of research. The findings from one set of studies suggest that people with a less extensive history of religious and spiritual involvement are less likely to find their spirituality helpful to them in stressful times. For example, among individuals diagnosed with a serious mental illness, those who had reported a shorter history of religious coping showed higher levels of symptomatology, including depression, hostility, obsessive–compulsiveness, anxiety, paranoid ideation, and psychoticism (Tepper et al., 2001). After finding similar results from their own longitudinal study of religion and life satisfaction, another group of researchers likened religious involvement to a sound investment strategy: "Long-term investment in religious capital yields dividends that can compensate for subsequent declines in other human stock" (Wink & Dillon, 2001, p. 102). Another set of studies indicates that people who compartmentalize spirituality from other aspects of their lives are more vulnerable to psychological problems. For instance, as part of a larger study of religious integration, Michael Wein-born (1999) asked members of liberal and conservative churches about the extent to which they agreed with statements such as "Religion is only one part of my life" and "There's a time and place for religion, and a time and a place for other things in life." Greater religious compartmentalization, Weinborn found, was associated with reports of less life satisfaction, poorer problem-solving skills, and lower religious well-being. Yet another line of research has shown that people who feel that their relationship with God is shaky also experience higher levels of psychological distress. For ex-ample, Lee Kirkpatrick and Philip Shaver (1992) asked a sample of adults to read a set of three statements that describe three varieties of attachment to God—secure, avoidant, and anxious/ambivalent—and then to select the attachment that best reflected their relationship to the divine (see Table 8.2). In comparison to those who described a secure relationship with God, adults with an insecure attachment to God (i.e., avoidant or anxious/am-bivalent) reported more loneliness, depression, and anxiety; poorer physical health; and lower overall life satisfaction.

All in all, these studies suggest that, without scope and depth, spiritu-ality loses power. It may be unable to serve important psychological func-tions, and it may actually contribute to more psychological trouble. Not only that, a thin, fragmented spirituality can lead to still other spiritual problems, for the disparate bits and pieces of spiritual life may clash and collide, resulting in further dis-integration.

PROBLEMS OF FIT

Few of us achieve the perfectly integrated life. In the pursuit of those things that matter most to us, we have to deal simultaneously with the obstacles life puts in our way; our own ever-changing needs and preferences; pres-sures from family, friends, and community; and massive amounts of infor-mation from the external world. Small wonder, then, that we live with some conflicts and inconsistencies. As one person put it, "Today, if you are not confused, you are just not thinking clearly." Spiritual conflicts and inconsistencies are also commonplace. For instance, surveys show that ap-proximately one in four Evangelical Christians uses alcohol or holds non-Christian beliefs, including beliefs in astrology and ghosts (Gallup & Lindsay, 1999). Among secular and some Orthodox Jews in Israel, interest in the occult has risen dramatically over the past 30 years. There, the use of graphology, palm reading, numerology, and even foot reading has found its way, not only into popular culture, but into politics, the media, and psy-chotherapy (Beit-Hallahmi, 1992). Despite the popularity of Pope John Paul II, significant numbers of Roman Catholics in the United States dis-sented from his teachings: 44% disagreed that homosexual behavior is

TABLE 8.2. Three Styles of Attachment to God

Anxious/Ambivalent

God seems to be inconsistent in His reactions to me. He sometimes seems very warm and responsive to my needs, but sometimes not. I'm sure that He loves me and cares about me, but sometimes He seems to show it in ways I don't really understand.

Avoidant

God is generally impersonal, distant, and often seems to have little or no interest in my personal affairs and problems. I frequently have the feeling that He doesn't care very much about me, or that He might not like me.

Secure

God is generally warm and responsive to me. He always seems to know when to be supportive and protective of me, and when to let me make my own mistakes. My relationship with God is always comfortable, and I am very happy and satisfied with it.

Note. Drawn from Kirkpatrick and Shaver (1992, p. 270).

always wrong, 58% believed that the Catholic Church should relax its standards on forbidding abortions, and 89% believed that people who use birth control are still good Catholics (Gallup & Lindsay, 1999).

Fortunately, most of us can live just fine with some degree of spiritual inconsistency. At times, though, the inconsistencies become more problematic. The elements that make up an individual's spirituality may grate and grind against each other, like fingernails on a chalkboard, or they may collide with each other with explosive force. In any case, spirituality fails to cohere and the individual encounters problems of spiritual "fit." Below I consider a few examples.

The Fit between Spiritual Pathways and Destinations

Spiritual Extremism

There is no shortage of clichés in U.S. culture. In fact, I recently discovered a website devoted to clichés (clichesite.com for those of you interested in extending your mastery of trite phrases). Many of our clichés speak to the primary value of success. "All's well that ends well," we are told. In stronger terms, we hear "The ends justify the means" and "Nice guys finish last." In the spiritual realm, however, the success-at-all-costs mentality can be particularly troubling. As I noted earlier, people will go to great lengths to preserve and protect what they hold sacred. But any length? Is it acceptable, after all, to engage in immoral acts to attain spiritual goals? Precious as these goals are, most people would likely say "No." They would reject criminal acts that serve elevated purposes, unlike the man who murdered his family to save their souls. Why? Because the pathways people take to their destinations have a value of their own. To draw on a different cliché, it matters a great deal how "you play the game." In his philosophy of non-violence, Mahatma Gandhi repeatedly stressed the importance of means: "They say 'means are after all means.' I would say 'means are after all everything.' As the means so are the ends. There is no wall of separation between means and ends" (Prabhu & Rao, 1967, p. 484). Higher ends cannot be achieved through unprincipled actions, he argued. Or, in the example above, murder cannot be justified on spiritual grounds because the act itself represents a violation of the sacred.

From a spiritual perspective, acts of spiritual extremism are problematic because they undermine the goals they are intended to achieve. Religious scrupulosity provides another case in point. Greenberg, Witztum, and Pisante (1987) draw on the thoughts of St. Ignatius of Loyola when they define scrupulosity as a form of religious overconcern, "an inclination in devout people to go too far in the right direction [because they are] too anxious to be certain they have not sinned" (p. 29). Fears and doubts about whether a sin has occurred lead the scrupulous individual into compulsive rituals that only partially allay those fears, resulting in yet further acts of penance. In spite of the religious meticulousness of scrupulous people, their careful attention to the minutiae of religious life subverts their ultimate spiritual goals. For example, Greenberg et al. (1987) describe the case of one Orthodox Jewish man who was so fearful of transgressing the religious injunction to be "clean at all orifices" before prayer services that he spent 20 minutes after each visit to the toilet and prior to his three daily prayers cleaning and checking his anal area. As a result, he was often late to prayer and unable to fulfill a religious obligation more critical than the cleanliness of orifices. Similarly, Greenberg and Witztum (2001) describe an Orthodox Jewish woman so concerned about violating the prohibition against menstrual impurity that she continually checked herself for signs of menstruation, immersed herself repeatedly in the ritual bath, and avoided intercourse with her husband. In the process, however, she broke the higher commandment in the Torah to procreate.[1]

Whether they are directed toward others or oneself, acts of spiritual extremism are not hard to understand. To preserve and protect the sacred, people often feel compelled to take extraordinary measures. However, ex-

---

[1]As an interesting side note, additional studies suggest that Jews as a group may be more prone to scrupulosity in religious practice than Protestants as a group (Abramowitz, Huppert, Cohen, Tolin, & Cahill, 2002). Conversely, Protestants may be more vulnerable to scrupulosity about immoral thoughts than Jews. These findings may reflect more basic theological differences in emphasis that Judaism and Christianity place on moral thoughts and moral actions (see Cohen & Rozin, 2001). While Judaism places greater emphasis on avoiding immoral actions than avoiding immoral thoughts, Christianity tends to give equal emphasis to both.

traordinary measures can turn into extreme measures. And extremism, particularly extremism of the spiritual variety, can become self-perpetuating, for it contains its own rewards, both spiritual and secular. Commenting on the violent religious fanatics of the world (e.g., David Koresh, Jim Jones, Shoko Asahara, bin Laden, Dan Lafferty), Krakeur (2004) speaks to this point:

> As a result of his (or her) infatuation, existence overflows with purpose. Ambiguity vanishes from the fanatic's worldview; a narcissistic sense of self-assurance displaces all doubt. A delicious rage quickens his pulse, fueled by the sins and shortcomings of lesser mortals, who are soiling the world wherever he looks. His perspective narrows until the last remnants of proportion are shed from his life. Through immoderation, he experiences something akin to rapture. (pp. xxii–xxiii)

Thus, what developed out of a natural yearning for the loftiest of goals becomes a self-sustaining, fanatical pursuit in which the most extreme of methods, including cruelties to others and oneself, are legitimated in the name of the sacred. Missing from this pursuit are the balancing virtues of humility, forgiveness, mercy, and compassion. Ultimately, however, spiritual extremism fails in many instances because it leads people away from rather than toward their spiritual destinations.

Spiritual Hypocrisy

Here's a great way to put some life into a party. Bring up the topic of spiritual hypocrisy. Perhaps no subject is guaranteed to raise the hackles of more people than this one. Most everyone, religious or nonreligious, has a sharp comment about people they know who wear their religion on their sleeves, yet fail to put their faith into practice. Harry Truman, a U.S. president who was never one to mince words, had this to say about hypocrisy: "Who is to blame for present conditions but sniveling church members who weep on Sunday, play with whores on Monday, drink on Tuesday, sellout to the Boss on Wednesday, repent about Friday, and start over on Sunday" (Keyes, 1995, p. 66). Many people base their discomfort with religious institutions on sentiments similar to Truman's (though Truman was himself a lifelong Baptist). But the world's religions offer harsh words of their own for those who make a show of their faith without living it out. In their sacred text, Muslims read: "Woe to those who pray and are heedless of their prayers, to those who make display and refuse charity" (Koran 107:4–7). Christians are told: "Beware of practicing your piety before men in order to be seen by them; for then you have no reward from your Father who is in Heaven" (Matthew 6:1). Jews are taught: "He who exploits the crown [of Torah for personal benefit] shall fade away" (Mishnah 4/7).

Some examples of spiritual hypocrisy are relatively mild: the insurance salesman who attends church regularly primarily to make new business connections, the woman who sits on the board of various religious charities because it makes her look good in the eyes of the community. Examples such as these can be understood as a poor fit between motivation and practice. Certainly, there is nothing wrong with selling insurance or seeking approval and status in the eyes of family and friends. But to attend church solely to sell insurance or to participate in charitable activity solely to create the appearance of spiritual devotion is problematic, for religious institutions are designed primarily to serve spiritual needs. Of course, religious institutions might welcome the involvement of people such as these, with the hope that their psychological and social needs will eventually take on a larger spiritual character. Nevertheless, there is a basic incongruity for those who remain on a spiritual path for nonspiritual reasons.

A few empirical studies suggest that this kind of incongruity may be linked to greater distress and poorer psychological functioning. Several years ago, my colleagues and I (Pargament, Steele, & Tyler, 1979) examined the relationships between religious participation, religious motivation, and measures of psychosocial competence in a sample of Jewish, Protestant, and Roman Catholic congregation members. We subdivided the church/synagogue members into four groups: frequent attenders with strong religious motivation, infrequent attenders with strong religious motivation, frequent attenders with low religious motivation, and infrequent attenders with low religious motivation. Of the four groups, the frequent attenders without strong religious motivation showed the poorest psychosocial functioning, including the greatest sense of control by powerful others and chance, and the lowest sense of efficacy, personal control, trust in others, and active coping skills. Ryan, Rigby, and King (1993) reported comparable findings in a more recent study of several Christian samples. They distinguished between religious motivation based on personal choice (which they called "identification") from religious motivation based on guilt, anxiety, and external pressures (which they called "introjection"). While religious identification was tied to better mental health and higher self-esteem, religious introjection was associated with poorer mental health. These studies suggest that religious participation without a basic amount of internalized religious conviction may be a source of conflict and distress for people.

In more extreme instances, the problem of spiritual hypocrisy represents a deliberate misuse of spiritual pathways to reach not simply nonspiritual but antispiritual destinations. From priests who sexually molest the children under their care to televangelists who bilk unsuspecting elders of their savings, leaders of congregations from every tradition can cloak their behavior in the prestige of their positions and the authority of their institutions. Lay members and nonmembers of religious institutions can engage in spiritual misuses of their own, concealing prejudice and bigotry to outsiders with the appearance of spiritual tolerance, participating in spiritual practices only to allay the guilt that accompanies immoral behavior, appealing to religious doctrine to justify the authority and power of an elite few. Offensive as these behaviors are, they become even more reprehensible when they are surrounded with an aura of sanctimony.

Before concluding this section, I need to briefly mention another form of spiritual dis-integration closely related to spiritual hypocrisy: spiritual inauthenticity. This involves the pursuit of non- or antispiritual ends in spite of spiritual yearnings that are a more authentic reflection of the individual's aspirations. I recall my client Larry, a 55-year-old man who had been struggling with alcoholism for decades. Over the years, Larry had made many attempts to change—via 12-step groups, inpatient and intensive outpatient programs, and psychotherapy—but none had been successful. And yet even though he continued to drink heavily, he also continued to seek help for himself. Why, I wondered? Was he, in fact, sincere in his efforts to stop drinking? Or was he simply using his occasional forays into treatment to reduce the anxiety and guilt he felt about a behavior that he had no real intention of changing?

I asked Larry why he persisted in his efforts to change in spite of his repeated failures. Larry paused for a moment and then said that even during the worst of his drinking binges, he felt something gnawing at him. It was like a little voice in the back of his mind telling him, "It doesn't have to be this way. You're bigger and better than this." This was new ground for us in therapy. I wanted to help Larry learn more about this part of himself, so I asked him to describe the tone of this voice. He said, "It's kind, but it has an edge too. Like it's telling me that I'm not a total bastard, but it's not letting me off the hook either. 'There's something to you,' it's saying. 'Don't throw it down the toilet.' "

Over time, Larry decided that he was hearing the voice of his own soul, the deepest and truest part of himself. This was a revelation for Larry. Until this point, he had believed that he was, at his deepest level, nothing more than an alcoholic—and therefore dishonest, self-serving, and worthless. The notion that there was a more profound dimension to himself, one that was challenging him to live more authentically, represented a powerful new understanding. The focus of therapy shifted to discussions of how Larry could live in a more spiritually authentic way. Through this process, Larry began to experience extended periods of sobriety for the first time in his adult life. Later in this book, I will discuss other interventions that are designed to help clients access their spiritual strivings and achieve greater spiritual authenticity.

The Fit between Spiritual Pathways and Situations

Part of the power of spirituality lies in its richness and diversity. As we have seen in earlier chapters, many different spiritual pathways are available to people who encounter critical life events. People can pick and choose among these varied pathways for the best route to their destination. But this requires "situation wisdom" (see Oden, 1983), the ability to know when to do what. This is just the type of wisdom members of 12-step programs seek through the Serenity Prayer: "God grant me the serenity to accept the things I cannot change; courage to change the things I can; and wisdom to know the difference." At times, though, people misread their situation and select a spiritual path poorly suited to the demands of the events they are facing. They may err in their explanations about the causes of events or they may err in the steps they take to resolve their problems.

Several years ago, I consulted on a project to promote prostate cancer screening through outreach to church ministers. The members of the advisory board of the project included a number of religious leaders. We spent a long time talking about the psychological, social, and religious barriers to participating in prostate cancer screening as well as steps churches might take to lower these barriers. As our work was winding down, Reverend Thomas, a man in his 60s who had been silent for much of our discussion, admitted that he had been diagnosed with prostate cancer a few years earlier. He also confessed that he had told no one about his condition. Why? Rev. Thomas told us that he believed his illness was a sign that somehow he had fallen out of favor with God. Although he could not identify what he had done to displease the Lord, he felt that his suffering, like that of Adam and Eve, was the result of his own spiritual disobedience. And how could he, a leader of the church and a model to its members, reveal to others his illness, the naked sign of his own sinfulness?

Certainly, many forces, psychological and social, contributed to Rev. Thomas's spiritual response to his illness. But regardless of its roots, he was making an error of explanation. Prostate cancer, he believed, was the result of his moral failings. In explaining his disease, he was overlooking naturalistic causes of prostate cancer that have been well established through scientific studies as well as more compassionate spiritual explanations (e.g., cancer as a spiritual test or opportunity for spiritual growth). His narrow spiritual explanation left him ill-equipped to sustain himself or to assist others in his role as a leader of his church. It also led to an error of control—a misjudgment about appropriate solutions to the problem.

Convinced that his illness was purely the result of a spiritual failing, Rev. Thomas sought out purely spiritual solutions. Nonspiritual options, including medical treatment and support from family and friends, were rejected. Instead, Rev. Thomas believed that prayer, self-reflection, and attempts to live a spotless spiritual life were the correct responses to his illness. The problem in this case was not with these spiritual coping strategies per se. After all, prayer, soul-searching, and spiritual purification have been proven to be valuable to many people faced with many different situations. Had he been facing an untreatable disease, Rev. Thomas's spiritual approach to problem solving would have made more sense in his case as well. But in the context of a situation that demanded some level of active human agency and control, his narrow spiritual coping methods were insufficient and put him at greater risk.

This story is not unique. Baider and De-Nour (1987) interviewed 10 Arab Muslim women who had had a mastectomy and found that none of the women had discovered the lump in their breasts by touching it and only three of the 10 discovered the lump by seeing it. Most had not realized that they had a problem until the disease was advanced and most had not told others about their symptoms until several months had passed. Even after their surgery, the women were generally unaware of their disease and treatment. How do we explain this remarkably passive and dangerous approach to coping? Interviews with these women suggested that their passivity grew out of their deferral of responsibility and control to God. One woman put it this way: "It is God's will what happens to me, and I am here just to obey God. God is with me and my fate is his." Another said, "It is not in our power to decide our destiny. You, or doctors, cannot help me because it is beyond human decisions. Illnesses are part of our destiny" (p. 9).

The deferral of responsibility for problem solving to God is not, for the most part, an effective coping method because most problems call for a certain degree of direct human action. In a study that speaks to this point, my colleagues and I developed a measure of three styles of religious coping that varied according to where people place the responsibility and control for problem solving (Pargament et al., 1988). In the deferring approach, the responsibility for problem solving is perceived to be God's and God's alone (sample item: "Rather than trying to come up with the right solution to a problem myself, I let God decide how to deal with it"). In the self-directing approach, the responsibility for problem solving belongs solely to the individual (sample item: "I act to solve my problems without God's help"). In the collaborative approach, the responsibility for problem solving is shared between the individual and God, that is, the individual and God work together to solve problems (sample item: "When I feel nervous or anxious about a problem, I work together with God to find a way to relieve my worries"). Working with a sample of church members, we found that a more deferring religious problem-solving style was tied to less self-efficacy, lower self-esteem, poorer problem-solving skills, and greater intolerance for differences between people. In contrast, the self-directing and collaborative styles were associated with higher levels of self-efficacy and problem-solving skills. The deferring approach was not generally effective in coping with problems.

But wait a minute, you might say. Isn't this too sweeping a conclusion? Aren't some problems, in fact, largely uncontrollable? What about a terminal illness, unemployment as a result of downsizing, an accident, or a betrayal in a romantic relationship? Wouldn't deferral to God or collaboration with God make more sense in these situations? On the other hand, wouldn't a self-directing approach to uncontrollable problems and their solution be as helpful as hitting your head against a brick wall? One research study showed that the value of the religious coping styles may indeed vary from situation to situation. Carl Bickel and his colleagues (1988) found that more self-directing religious problem solving was associated with *more* depression among church members dealing with uncontrollable events. In contrast, faced with the same situations, members who made use of more collaborative religious problem solving experienced *less* depression.

Exclusively secular forms of coping that fail to attend to the demands of the situation make as little sense as exclusively spiritual forms of coping that are equally disconnected from the realities of life. Situational wisdom requires the judicious application and integration of resources, both spiritual and nonspiritual, in the effort to understand and deal with life's greatest problems. Paul Johnson (1959) conveys this kind of wisdom in his description of prayer:

> Prayer does not work as a substitute for a steel chisel or the wing of an airplane. It does not replace muscular action in walking or faithful study in meeting an examination. These are not the proper uses of prayer. But prayer may help to calm the nerves when one is using a chisel in bone surgery or bringing an airplane to a landing. Prayer may guide one in choosing a destination to walk toward, and strengthen one's purpose to prepare thoroughly for an examination. (pp. 142–143)

The Fit between Individual and Social Context

In spite of the fact that the search for the sacred unfolds in a larger social and cultural context, the influence of family, organization, institution, community, and culture on spirituality is easy to overlook. Just as we rarely notice the air that nourishes us in our daily lives, we can neglect the power of the larger context that supports our spiritual journeys. Not until it becomes less supportive does the social context seem to emerge out of the background and become more visible. Members of religious minority groups, gays, lesbians, and others who have engaged in acts discouraged by religious traditions (e.g., abortion, divorce) are well aware of the larger religious institutional context in the United States and their marginal place within it. For example, Kelly Schuck and Becky Liddle (2001) surveyed 66 lesbian, gay, and bisexual people and found that almost two-thirds of them reported conflicts between their sexual orientation and their religion, including its teachings, scriptural passages, and prejudice from members and clergy in the congregation. Participants in the study also described several emotional consequences of this conflict: guilt and shame, depression, self-loathing, suicidal ideation, feelings of rejection by the congregation, and fears of being rejected by God and going to hell.

These findings aren't uncommon. Oftentimes, the lack of fit between the individual and his or her social context sets the stage for problems. Marital partners from different religious traditions have lower marital satisfaction, greater marital conflict, and higher divorce rates than religiously homogenous couples (Mahoney, Pargament, Tarakeshwar, & Swank, 2001). Similarly, children who are raised in neighborhoods in which they are in the religious minority suffer more depression, psychosomatic symptoms, and lower self-esteem than children raised in neighborhoods in which they are a part of the religious majority (Rosenberg, 1962).

People who encounter periods of spiritual struggle may also have difficulty locating a context that will be accepting and nurturing. Illustrative of this point, Wick (1985) presented the case of a man who served in the Vietnam War and thereafter was unable to find a place for himself in his religious community. John, a Roman Catholic, went off to Vietnam with the blessings of his family and parish priest. He was involved in heavy combat, lost a few close friends, and began to lose faith in the conflict. John sought solace and advice from his military chaplain, who responded, "Kill as many as you can" (p. 15). John was unable to resolve his moral qualms about the war and the part he was playing in it. When he returned home, he developed PTSD and sought help from his own pastor. The pastor told him, "You are a mass murderer. I cannot help you" (p. 16). John's condition deteriorated. He could find no resolution to his own moral confusion and the conflicting religious voices in his head: "As he walked he heard the chaplain say, 'Kill as many as you can'; then the pastor, 'You are a mass murderer'; then the chaplain again, 'kill'; the pastor, 'mass murderer.' And on it went: 'Kill, mass murderer, kill, kill as many as you can. . . . Right then John felt, he could do it. He could kill them all . . . all, all, all, including himself" (p. 16). Instead of hurting others or himself, however, John vowed never to see a priest (or a psychiatrist) again.

Why is spiritual discord so problematic? Perhaps because the discord *is* spiritual. Remember that we are talking about sacred matters here—beliefs, practices, emotions, and aspirations of the most vital importance. Differences in the sacred sphere can threaten or challenge the deepest of values. Some, like John, leave unsupportive religious settings. Other people, unwilling to face spiritual conflicts directly, create unworkable spiritual compromises or gloss over their differences. In his book on interfaith marriage, Reeve Brenner (2007) warns of the problems that arise when Jewish and Christian couples try to resolve their differences by creating a mixed "Chewish" faith for their children:

> The first year or two you'll try to celebrate both sets of holidays and it will be fun. Chanukah comes, you spin the dreidl. Christmas comes, you decorate the tree. You do Passover, then Easter. By the third or fourth year, either stress takes over or imbalance takes over. You are trying to do it all: both synagogue and church and all the holidays and soccer, piano, and Tae Kwon Do and everything else a child requires—and you're going out of your mind. (p. 8)

The attempt to practice both faiths, Brenner argues, leads to competition, shallowness, and a lack of commitment. "The only way you can have a dual religion," he maintains, "is to cut the heart out of both" (p. 16).

Spiritual intolerance is another even more damaging way to defend faith from threat or challenge. Intolerance is not hard to recognize in its barest forms—shunning, religiously based prejudice, fanaticism, and wars all represent attempts to deal with spiritual differences by derogating or destroying the spiritual outsider. But spiritual intolerance can also manifest itself more subtly, as Agneta Schreurs (2002) demonstrates when she reports her experiences while leading a psychotherapy group of religious sisters. One of the Roman Catholic sisters, a charming woman in her 70s, admitted to the group that she was afraid of death. The group responded with stories of others who had died peacefully, suggestions to meditate on Jesus' fear the night before he was executed, and reassurances that she had no reason to be afraid. None of these responses, however, was helpful to the fearful sister. Schreurs pointed out to the group that they appeared to be having difficulty tolerating the sister's fears. Why was this the case? Over the course of the session, it became clear that the fears of the older sister represented a challenge to their own deep-seated belief that "nuns have an exemplary faith and lead exemplary Christian lives, and therefore have no reason to fear death" (p. 79). The group, rather than accepting the elderly sister's spiritual struggles as very real and difficult, had tried to talk the sister out of her turmoil in an effort to secure their own shaken spiritual beliefs.

The lack of integration of the individual within his or her social context does not inevitably lead to trouble. Poor fit can stimulate important personal and social change. In their study of lesbian, gay, and bisexual people, Schuck and Liddle (2001) found that a significant percentage of the participants had made positive spiritual transformations. Some reinterpreted the teachings of their tradition and achieved a different understanding of themselves and God. As one person put it, "Once I realized that God was a loving God, and not the vindictive, vengeful God organized religions make him [out] to be, all my experiences have been positive. This has been especially helpful to me as I continue to live through the AIDS crisis" (p. 74). Other participants tried to create fundamental changes in their churches and synagogues or switched their affiliations to gay-affirmative congregations. One member who had made a successful transition commented, "I feel completely free to be myself . . . and express my gifts and have them appreciated" (p. 73).

Finally, though it seems all too rare in the world today, spiritual differences among people could lead to enriching dialogue rather than to destructive diatribes, and to shared experience rather than to alienation. After all, as Paul Tillich (1957) wrote, "Man is integrated only in part and there are also elements of disintegration in all dimensions of his being" (p. 108). Through dialogue and sharing, people could achieve a greater appreciation for the strengths and limitations of their own spiritual world and the spiritual worlds of others.

Yossi Klein Halevi (2001) provides a powerful illustration. A rabbi and journalist in Israel, Halevi set out on his own spiritual adventure in search of peace and understanding among the faiths. Rational dialogue alone, he found, could not produce a solution to interfaith conflicts. However, by participating in the celebrations of Christian monastics and the prayers of Muslim mystics, not as a Christian or as a Muslim but as a committed Jew, Halevi was able to break through age-old barriers and build a deep connection with unlikely Christian and Muslim partners based on the sharing of sacred experience. But it takes tremendous courage to experience unfamiliar religious worlds, worlds that seem alien and forbidding. In fact, it may require a spiritual transformation, not to a new God or a new faith, but to a recognition of the universality and richness of the spiritual impulse. Fittingly, Halevi concludes his book by describing just this kind of personal transformation: "The one enduring transformation that I carry with me from my journey is that I learned to venerate—to love—Christianity and Islam. I learned to feel at home in a church, even on Good Friday, and in a mosque, even in Nuseirat. The cross and the minaret have become for me cherished symbols of God's presence, reminders that He speaks to us in multiple languages—that He speaks to us at all" (p. 314).

This kind of transformation can take root only in a certain kind of soil, one in which differences become opportunities for learning and growth rather than threats to the sacred. Gandhi (1962), for one, was able to give voice to this attitude: "For me, the different religions are beautiful flowers from the same garden, or they are branches of the same majestic tree. Therefore, they are equally true, though being received and interpreted through human instruments equally imperfect" (p. 407). Difficult as it may be, it is only through an openness to spiritual differences, a willingness to engage in spiritual dialogue, and a sincere desire to share spiritual experience that people may be able to reach the most profound understanding of themselves and each other. As we will see, this sentiment lies at the heart of spiritually integrated psychotherapy.

PROBLEMS OF CONTINUITY AND CHANGE

Continuity and change are part and parcel of spiritual life. Long periods of stability, when people are focused on sustaining their relationship with the sacred, can be followed by periods of sharp or gradual change, when people seek out new ways to understand and approach the sacred. As I noted earlier, conservation and transformation are two of the key components of the search for the sacred. Regulating these two processes, though, is not always easy. Should I stay the course? For how long? Is it time to make a change? People regularly struggle with these questions. A popular country singer likens the dilemma to a game of poker: "You got to know when to hold 'em, know when to fold 'em, Know when to walk away and know when to run."

The failure to transform when change is called for can result in serious problems, and spirituality can be implicated in this process. Several years ago, a 35-year-old woman named Kathy came to my office for help. It wasn't hard to tell that she was depressed: Kathy walked hunched over as if she were weighted down by a terrible burden, she had the look of a wounded animal in her eyes, and she spoke in the halting, tentative voice of a frightened child. I soon learned that Kathy had suffered a long history of physical and verbal abuse by her parents. They had nicknamed her "BUD," which stood for big, ugly, and dumb, and still called her by that name. Kathy continued to visit her parents weekly, although they persisted in their verbal abuse, even in front of Kathy's children. I asked Kathy why she maintained her relationship with her parents and she responded by saying that she had learned from the Bible to "honor thy father and mother." Though Kathy had grown up chronologically, she had not matured in her view of herself and of her parents, nor in her understanding of Scripture or of the sacred. And, as a result, the pattern of abuse continued.

Like Kathy, many people lock themselves into a set of spiritual beliefs and practices. To them, spirituality is a crystalline object, set in fixed and final form, and the idea of spiritual change can be quite threatening. To reconsider and question spiritual matters may feel like an act of betrayal against the sacred itself. By simplifying life into a few key rules, good and bad, in-group and out-group, truth and falsehood, the individual can replace questions, confusion, and doubt with meaning, clarity, and conviction.

There is a steep price to pay for this kind of spiritual rigidity, however. From at least some theological perspectives, those who cling too tightly to their beliefs, practices, and concepts of the sacred are engaging in a form of idolatry. Recall from the last chapter that theologians have warned against confusing symbols of the sacred with what the symbols represent. As finite beings, Tillich (1957) and Neville (1996) wrote, we cannot fully grasp the infinite. Instead, we must rely on symbols to express our ultimate concerns, for only symbols are able to point to something beyond themselves. And yet symbols can never fully contain the infinite and for that reason they should not be viewed literally. "Literalism," Tillich (1957) wrote, "deprives God of his ultimacy and, religiously speaking, of his majesty. It draws him closer to the level of that which is not ultimate, the finite and condi- tional. . . . Faith, if it takes symbols literally, becomes idolatrous" (p. 52). Instead, symbols are to be held with an appreciation for their limitations, their "brokenness," and an openness to deeper and richer forms of sacred representation. Tillich (1957) went on to write, "Faith, conscious of the symbolic character of its symbols, gives God the honor which is due him" (p. 52).

On a more pragmatic note, a spirituality that lacks flexibility is likely to become woefully inadequate as time and circumstances change. Earlier, I described a 2-year longitudinal study of medically ill elderly hospitalized patients in which we found that people who reported spiritual struggles showed greater declines on measures of psychological, physical, and spiri- tual functioning (Pargament et al., 2001, 2004). Not only that, but higher levels of spiritual struggle, especially struggles with the divine, were tied to a greater risk of dying over the next 2 years. My colleagues and I were sur- prised by these findings. After all, as I noted before, there are many exam- ples of remarkable religious figures—Moses, Buddha, Muhammad, Jesus— who experienced their own periods of storm and struggle yet came through them strengthened and transformed. And a few studies have tied greater spiritual struggles to reports of personal growth (Pargament et al., 1998). But the spiritual struggles in our study of medically ill elders were linked to decline, even death.

Perhaps, we wondered, the problem had less to do with spiritual strug- gles per se than with an inability to resolve these struggles. Many people might work through their conflicts. Recall the findings from one survey that indicated that 80% of college students who reported negative feelings toward God said that their feelings decreased over time (Exline & Martin, 2005). Those who were unable to resolve their struggles, however, might be at greater risk for problems. To test this possibility, we conducted some ad- ditional analyses on the survivors in the patient sample. We compared survivors who reported spiritual struggles over the 2-year period (chronic spiritual strugglers) with those who reported spiritual struggles at only one point in time (acute spiritual strugglers) and those who reported no spiri- tual struggles (nonstrugglers). As you might have guessed, it was the group of chronic spiritual strugglers who experienced significant declines in qual- ity of life, mood, and independent functioning over time. In some sense, the chronic spiritual strugglers appeared to "get stuck" in their struggles. These findings need to be replicated but they suggest that the failure to work through or resolve spiritual struggles may have been the factor that placed these elderly patients at greatest risk for dying. The inability to change when spiritual change is called for seems to set the stage for trouble.

Equally problematic is the inability to sustain a spiritual approach to life. Without commitment and continuity, the search for the sacred can take the form of faddish jumps from one spiritual trend to another or frenetic but superficial samplings from various spiritual pathways. Virtually every spiritual group, traditional and nontraditional, espouses the importance of practice, determination, and perseverance in whatever spiritual pathways the individual follows.

Continuity and change—how does the individual integrate these two processes? "Knowing when to hold 'em and when to fold 'em" makes a nice lyric but it's tough to put into practice. Some do, though, and with good results. Using a variety of measures, Daniel McIntosh and his colleagues identified groups of people who were both strongly committed to their faith and religiously flexible and found that highly committed/flexible people showed fewer symptoms of physical illness (McIntosh & Spilka, 1990), better adjustment to a negative life event, and greater well-being (McIntosh, Inglehart, & Pacini, 1990). Thus, both continuity and change are essential parts of a search for the sacred. How we integrate continuity and change, how we know when to "hold 'em" or "fold 'em," may be one of the features that distinguishes spirituality at its best from spirituality at its worst.

CONCLUSIONS

In this part of the book, I have presented a way to make sense of spirituality, not as a theoretical exercise but as a necessary foundation for clinical practice. Understanding spirituality, I believe, is an essential prerequisite for working with spirituality in psychotherapy. Thus, in preceding chapters we have considered what spirituality is and how it develops and changes over time and circumstance.

The last two chapters have focused on a particularly important issue: how to evaluate spirituality. Readers looking for easy answers may have been disappointed, for I have assumed that evaluations of spirituality cannot be boiled down to one, two, or three factors. No single quality holds the key to an effective or an ineffective spirituality. Certainly, some individual beliefs and practices are generally more helpful than others, but researchers and practitioners have to be careful not to oversimplify their evaluations of spirituality—oversimplifications can only distort what is a rich and complex process. Recall the definition of spiritual integration I presented in Chapter 7: the effectiveness of the search for the sacred lies not in a specific belief, practice, emotion, or relationship, but in the degree to which the individual's spiritual pathways and destinations work together in synchrony with each other. At its best, spirituality is defined by pathways that are broad and deep, responsive to life's situations, nurtured by the larger social context, capable of flexibility and continuity, and oriented toward a sacred destination that is large enough to encompass the full range of human potential and luminous enough to provide the individual with a powerful guiding vision. At its worst, spirituality is defined by pathways that lack scope and depth, fail to meet the challenges and demands of life events, clash and collide with the surrounding social system, change and shift too easily or not at all, and misdirect the individual in the pursuit of spiritual value. Thinking about spirituality as a process that can be, to varying degrees, well integrated or poorly integrated does add complexity to the task of the clinician, but this is just the kind of thinking that is often required of clinicians—sifting, weighing, and balancing dozens of factors as they develop a picture of their clients' lives and move toward treatment.

It is important to stress that an individual's level of spiritual integration is neither fixed nor final. Like the other ingredients that make up the search for the sacred, spiritual integration is a dynamic construct. Over the course of life, a person may move toward or away from greater spiritual integration depending on a host of personal, social, and situational factors. A high level of integration does not mean that the search for the sacred is complete. Neither is dis-integration necessarily the last word in the search for the sacred. No matter how inconsistent, fragmented, shallow, or disorganized an individual's spirituality may be, transformation remains a possibility. Even so, making fundamental change is often difficult to do without help. Spiritually integrated therapy represents one resource that could facilitate the individual's efforts to achieve not only greater personal well-being but also a more coherent and compelling spirituality. With this perspective on spirituality in mind, we now turn to the practical task of addressing spirituality in psychotherapy.

Part III

ADDRESSING
THE SACRED

9

An Orientation to Spiritually Integrated Psychotherapy

My new client is in the waiting room. Other than her name, I know nothing about her personally, and yet the fact that she has chosen to seek help from a psychologist says a great deal about her already. She is frustrated about her life, or she wouldn't be here. Her problems, she feels, have exceeded her ability to cope. She is hopeful that somehow things can get better, or she wouldn't be seeking out help. She is courageous enough to share very personal problems with a stranger. And she is open enough to allow this stranger to learn something about her world and her place in it. As I open the door to meet her, I feel a sense of appreciation for what she is doing, and I try to convey my respect for her courage and willingness to take this risk, this leap of faith. More than that, even after almost 30 years of practice, I still feel a bit nervous about the responsibility that has been given me. Who am I to believe I might be able to help her? What is it that I have to offer someone who has most likely exhausted many solutions before coming to therapy?

What grounds me in my work with this and every client I see is my therapeutic orientation—my perspective on people, problems, myself, and the process of change. This perspective is the product of theory, research, practical experience, personality, and social context. It is my road map for working with clients, helping me to identify problems, solutions, directions for change, and the role I should play in this process. Without this map, I would be lost in the therapy room; oriented by this map, I can feel reasonably confident in the work to come.

In this chapter, I introduce one particular therapeutic orientation, the orientation of spiritually integrated psychotherapy. Spiritually integrated psychotherapy is an approach to treatment that acknowledges and addresses the spirituality of the client, the spirituality of the therapist, and the process of change. This chapter presents the orientation of spiritually integrated psychotherapy to each of these three critical therapeutic ingredients. The essential features of this orientation are summarized in Table 9.1.

THE ORIENTATION OF SPIRITUALLY INTEGRATED PSYCHOTHERAPY TO THE CLIENT

Spiritually integrated psychotherapy rests on the assumption that spirituality is a vital dimension in the lives of many clients. It is not to be dismissed as a static or compartmentalized set of beliefs, practices, or emotions used occasionally to improve mood or health. It is, instead, a set of pathways that people follow in search of the sacred. The sacred is key here. As Schreurs (2002) wrote, "[The] whole point of spiritual life is that there is a transcendent reality you can know, albeit partially, albeit permanently in need of connection and albeit at various levels of intensity" (p. 162). Spiritually integrated psychotherapy is grounded in the therapist's appreciation of the client's spiritual dimension and its far-reaching potential.

When people come to psychotherapy, they do not check their spirituality at the door. Spiritually integrated psychotherapy assumes that spirituality is often interwoven with the problems that clients bring to psychotherapy, the solutions to those problems, and the client's larger social and cultural context.

The Spiritual Dimension of Problems

Most clients do not present religious or spiritual problems when they come to psychotherapy, at least not according to the diagnoses of mental health professionals. In a survey of a random sample of more than 300 psychologists who were members of the American Psychological Association, most (94%) indicated that they had never given their clients a religious/spiritual problem V code in their diagnoses (Hathaway, Scott, & Garver, 2004). The V code signifies distress associated with loss of faith, questions about spiritual values, and problems associated with conversion. There are good reasons, however, to question these apparently low levels of religious and spiritual concerns in diagnoses. First, on a pragmatic note, V codes are not billable to most third-party insurers, so therapists may underuse this category for economic reasons. Second, therapists as a group often overlook the spiritual dimension in their work with clients. For example, in the Hathaway et al. study (2004) over half of the psychologists indicated that they rarely or never examined how a psychological disorder might impact

TABLE 9.1. The Orientation of Spiritually Integrated Psychotherapy

Orientation of spiritually integrated psychotherapy to the client

- Clients do not leave their spirituality outside the therapy office.
- Spiritual problems can be a cause of psychological problems.
- Psychological problems can be a cause of spiritual problems.
- Spirituality can be a source of solutions to problems.
- Spirituality can be a source of resistance to solutions.
- The client brings a larger social, cultural, and religious context to psychotherapy.

Orientation of spiritually integrated psychotherapy to the therapist

- Therapists do not leave their spirituality outside the therapy office.
- Therapists vary in their degree of professional spiritual integration.
- Spiritual intolerance by therapists has no place in psychotherapy.
- Spiritually integrated psychotherapy requires spiritual literacy and competence on the part of the therapist, including spiritual knowledge, openness and tolerance, self-awareness, and authenticity.

Orientation of spiritually integrated psychotherapy to the process of change

- There is a spiritual dimension of psychotherapy.
- The spirituality of the client and the therapist is affected in treatment, even when the sacred is not an explicit focus of attention.
- Psychological and spiritual change go hand in hand in psychotherapy.
- Any modality of therapy can be enriched by paying more explicit attention to the spiritual dimension.
- Spiritually integrated psychotherapy can provide new perspectives on psychological problems.
- Spiritually integrated psychotherapy can offer new solutions to psychological problems.

their client's religious or spiritual functioning. Forty-eight percent also indicated that they asked about their clients' religiousness or spirituality 25% of the time or less in their assessments. Third, clients themselves, concerned about the antipathy of mental health professionals to religion and spirituality, may be reluctant to raise spiritual concerns in psychotherapy (Worthington, 1986). Finally, there is a long tradition in psychology of reducing spiritual concerns to presumably more fundamental problems. From this perspective, anger at God becomes a sign of anger at the father, spiritual emptiness is merely a symptom of depression, and so on. Thus, even when spiritual concerns are raised in therapy, they may receive little direct attention from the therapist. Treat the underlying problem, it is assumed, and the spiritual problem will be resolved as well. There is no need to assess religious or spiritual problems, for they are merely signs of the deeper distress that represents the more appropriate target for treatment.

Spiritually integrated psychotherapy makes a different assumption: that spirituality is often interwoven with the problems of clients, and that the spiritual dimension of problems calls for clinical attention. Teasing apart the interconnections between psychological and spiritual problems is not always easy. Spiritual problems can be understood as a cause of psychological problems or the end result of psychological problems. There is evidence to support each of these points of view.

Spirituality as a Cause of Psychological Problems

Unfortunately, examples of the destructive power of spirituality are not hard to find: mass suicides among members of a religious cult, murders perpetrated by individuals who believe they are responding to the commands of God, parents who refuse to provide their sick children with potentially life-saving medical assistance, and so on. Spiritually sympathetic people might dismiss these cases as aberrations. There is, however, a small but growing body of empirical evidence that shows that spiritual problems are indeed predictive of declines in psychological status over time. In earlier chapters, I reviewed several longitudinal studies that linked signs of spiritual struggle and dis-integration (e.g., feelings of abandonment and punishment by God, anger at God) to increases in depression, anxiety, paranoid ideation, and loss of independent functioning within samples of medically ill patients and young adults with serious mental illness (Fitchett, Rybarczyk, DeMarco, & Nicholas, 1999; Pargament, Koenig, Tarakeshuar, & Hahn, 2004; Phillips & Stein, in press).

Nontheistic spiritual problems can also lead to psychological problems. Several years ago, a young couple, Ron and June, came to my office following an episode of domestic violence. The violence had been precipitated by an argument about Ron's interest in soccer. For much of his life, Ron had been passionate about soccer. Born and raised in a South American family of devoted soccer fans, Ron had played soccer throughout school and continued to coach the sport in high school. June had assumed that Ron would curtail his interest in the game after they had children, but she had been disappointed. Ron spent many evenings and weekends away from home, coaching games or scouting opposing players and teams. On the evening of their fight, June lost her patience and bitterly scolded her husband. "You're 27 years old," she complained, "but you care more about children running back and forth kicking at a ball than you do your own wife and children. When will you put this childish game behind you? When will you grow up and become an adult?" Ron responded by slapping June in the face and June responded in kind, socking Ron in the jaw.

Obviously, soccer was more than a game to this couple. For June, it represented a threat to what she valued most deeply: her marriage and her family. But what did it mean to Ron? In spite of all the time he had devoted to this sport, he had never talked to June about what soccer meant to him. When he did, he spoke movingly. Soccer was a thing of beauty, not just a game but a form of poetry that touched him at his deepest level. He recalled playing the game as a child and experiencing moments of sheer joy, as if he had left his feet and been transported to heaven. He could reexperience those feelings at times when his high school team was playing well together. By teaching other children to play the game, he believed, he was passing on the timeless gift that had been given to him. It turned out that both Ron and June were speaking the language of the sacred, though they did not mention God. They were describing aspects of their lives that were transcendent, boundless, and of ultimate concern. Their marital conflict involved more than problems in communication, negotiation, and compromise. It was grounded in spiritual discord—a difference, unarticulated, in sacred strivings.

Psychological Problems as a Cause of Spiritual Problems

Just as spirituality can lead to psychological problems, psychological problems can lead to spiritual trouble. Listen, for example, to the way one woman described the spiritual impact of her eating disorder: "My eating disorder robbed me of my relationship with God. I was in a personal anguish that shred my soul and threatened my spiritual and mortal life. I felt no love and saw no mercy. Anger consumed me. I felt abandoned and worthless. My heart turned bitter and hard. I cut God out of my life. . . . It was a downward spiral that almost led to my death" (Richards et al., 2007, p. 45).

Unfortunately, psychologists have focused far more attention on the potentially problematic roles of spirituality than on the ways in which spirituality itself might be impacted by psychological problems. Greenberg and Witztum (2001) underscore the dangers of this bias in their analysis of obsessive–compulsive disorder (OCD) among ultra-Orthodox Jews in Israel. Is it true, they ask, that ritual observance within Judaism promotes the development of OCD? Drawing on a few different lines of evidence, they suggest that the answer is no. First, Greenberg and Witztum note that, although the 613 commandments of the Torah cover virtually every sphere of life, ultra-Orthodox Jews who suffer from OCD limit their religious symptoms to four areas: prayer, dietary laws, menstrual purity, and cleanliness before prayers. If the ritual obligations of Judaism were the source of OCD, a larger array of Jewish practices should be implicated in the disorder. Second, they find that the concerns of OCD among religious individuals parallel those of nonreligious OCD patients more generally. Both groups express concerns about dirt, orderliness, aggression, and sex. However, among the ultra-Orthodox, these symptoms are expressed within a religious context. Finally, even though no studies have been conducted to compare the rates of OCD among ultra-Orthodox Jews and other religious and nonreligious groups in Israel, epidemiological studies do exist that show that rates of

OCD do not appear to differ among countries that vary in their ritualistic practices. Greenberg and Witztum conclude that OCD is not the end result of ritual involvement; rather, religious practices are "the idiom of distress chosen by ultra-orthodox sufferers of OCD" (p. 130). They are "the form OCD typically takes in patients for whom religious beliefs and practices predominate" (p. 133). Religion, then, is not the source of this pathology. It is another aspect of life that is negatively affected by psychological problems.

In a similar vein, psychologist William Hathaway (2003) has described how psychological disorders can result in "clinically significant religious/ spiritual impairment (CSRI)." CSRI is defined as a "reduced ability to perform religious activities, achieve religious goals, or to experience religious states, due to a psychological disorder" (Hathaway, 2003, p. 114). To illustrate his point, Hathaway and his colleagues developed the Faith Situations Questionnaire to assess the impact of disruptive behavior disorders, such as attention-deficit/hyperactivity disorder (ADHD) and oppositional defiant disorder (ODD) on the spiritual/religious functioning of children (Hathaway, Douglas, & Grabowski, 2003). They administered their questionnaire to 98 parents of children with ADHD or ODD and found that symptoms of ADHD and ODD were associated with more indicators of religious/spiritual impairment in the child, such as problems during family devotions, difficulty preparing for religious services, difficulty attending religious services, and saying prayers. Hathaway offers a case example, a 7-year-old diagnosed with ADHD who was difficult to control in public settings. Asked by the researchers whether their son's behavior had impacted their religious lives, the parents responded emotionally: "[Our religion] is very important to us but we have not been able to go to temple for the last few years because our son is too disruptive. We can't find anyone to watch him and we want him to go. . . . But other people keep getting upset with us for his behavior and it is just too much" (Hathaway, 2006, personal communication). The researchers also asked whether the parents had ever spoken to mental health professionals about the effects of their son's disorder on their religious lives. The parents answered "No," adding, "We didn't think you were supposed to talk about these things with psychologists" (Hathaway, 2006, personal communication).

Generally speaking, psychological and spiritual distress often go hand in hand. But moving beyond this general conclusion, we may be able to make finer differentiations, for specific types of psychological problems may be linked in distinctive ways to specific types of spiritual problems. Unfortunately, there is relatively little information about the ties between particular psychological and spiritual problems (see Loewenthal, in press; Miller & Kelley, 2005, for reviews). However, clinical observations and some empirical research point to a few connections between the two domains.

1. *Depression.* Depression has been associated with perceptions of sacred loss, spiritual self-degradation, and feelings of alienation from, punishment by, and anger toward God (Elkins, 1998; Exline, Yali, & Sanderson, 2000; Fitchett et al., 2004; Pargament, Koenig, et al., 2004).

2. *Anxiety.* Anxiety has been linked to spiritual confusion and doubt, an insecure relationship with God, spiritual rigidity and narrowness, as well as to beliefs in a small god who accepts no less than perfection (Greenberg & Witztum, 2001; Kooistra & Pargament, 1999; Nielsen, Johnson, & Ellis, 2001).

3. *Addiction.* Addiction to alcohol, drugs, or sex can be understood as forms of idolatry in which false gods have rushed in to fill the vacuum left by sacred loss (Coleman et al., 1986; Yau, 2003).

4. *Eating disorders.* Eating disorders have been theoretically connected to perceptions of a punishing God, feelings of spiritual unworthiness and shame, fear of abandonment by God, difficulty with spiritual surrender, and devotion to a false god (Richards et al., 2007).

5. *Marital problems.* Marital conflict can be tied to unresolved differences in the sacred strivings of each partner (e.g., Ron and June), as well as to spiritual discord, intolerance, and inflexibility (Butler & Harper, 1994; Yanni, 2003).

6. *Violence.* Violence has been associated with perceptions of desecration, interpersonal spiritual conflicts, spiritual extremism, small gods, demonization, and narcissism (another form of idolatry) (Mahoney, Pargament, Ano, Lynn, et al., 2002; Pargament, Trevino, Mahoney, & Silberman, 2007; Peck, 1998).

7. *Serious mental illness.* Serious mental illnesses are, at times, accompanied by perceptions of sacred loss and violation, feelings of being punished by God or diabolical forces, a lack of religious support, and spiritual confusion and doubts (Lindgren & Coursey, 1995; Phillips & Stein, in press).

With further research, we should develop more insight into the relationships between distinctive types of psychological and spiritual problems. The insights gleaned from this emerging study of spirituality and psychopathology will be invaluable in our efforts to tailor spiritually integrated therapy to the needs of specific groups of people. But until additional longitudinal studies are conducted, it will be difficult to determine whether spirituality is the cause or the effect of psychological problems. Perhaps, most often, both processes are at work: spirituality is both a cause and an effect. In either case, spiritually integrated psychotherapy underscores the importance of attending to the spiritual dimension of psychological problems, a dimension that is significant in and of itself.

The Spiritual Dimension of Solutions

Though spirituality can be intertwined with psychological disorders, we have to be careful here not to fall into the stereotypical view that spirituality spawns psychopathology. Empirical evidence shows otherwise. Overall, spirituality appears to serve more as a force that prevents or mitigates psychological problems than a force that causes disorders (see Koenig et al., 2001; Pargament & Park, 1995). To put it another way, spirituality is more often involved in resolving psychological problems than in promoting them. Even people facing the most severe mental illnesses often report that spirituality was central to their recovery (Fallot, 1998).

In earlier chapters, I reviewed a wide range of spiritual resources: spiritual pathways for sustaining and enhancing a relationship with the sacred (e.g., knowing, acting, relating, and experiencing), spiritual methods of coping to conserve the sacred (e.g., spiritual support, benevolent spiritual reappraisals, spiritual purification), and spiritual methods of coping to transform the sacred (e.g., sacred transitions, revisioning the sacred, centering the sacred). I also noted that people often draw on these resources to sustain or transform themselves. For many, if not most, people in the United States, there is nothing unusual about bringing spirituality to bear on life's problems. Therapists, however, have been reluctant to access the spiritual resources of their clients in psychotherapy. In contrast, spiritually integrated psychotherapy makes the assumption that the process of change will be broadened, deepened, strengthened, and enriched by paying more explicit attention to spirituality as a source of solutions to problems.

For instance, let's return to the case of Ron and June, the couple fighting about soccer and family. The spouses had not realized that theirs was a spiritual conflict, a struggle over differences in their sacred dreams. That recognition was a turning point in therapy. Their conflict as a couple had grown out of a spiritual problem, and so it called for a spiritually sensitive solution. I spoke to Ron and June about the importance of treating sacred matters with care, respect, even reverence. The couple was responsive. Over the next few months, as each member of the couple began to acknowledge, tolerate, and ultimately affirm the spirituality of the other, they were able to arrive at a shared dream, one large enough to include a place for marriage, family, and soccer. In the chapters to follow, I examine many other ways that spiritual resources can be introduced into the therapeutic process.

The Spiritual Dimension of Resistance to Solutions

Of course, change is never easy. Resistance to change in therapy is the norm, as any therapist well knows. Although spirituality can be a resource for change, it can also be an impediment to change, even when the problem is not spiritual in nature (Eriksen, Marston, & Korte, 2002; Lovinger,

1996). One client resists any recommendation that is not explicitly linked to a sacred text; another client is uncomfortable talking about himself in therapy because it leaves him feeling self-centered and sinful. One client remains married to an adulterous husband because she believes this is what God has willed for her; another client, convinced that he is truly worthless and deserves to suffer, resists every effort to adopt a more balanced self-image. Spiritually based obstacles to change such as these may be especially difficult to deal with. As one therapist exclaimed after a session in which her client rejected an intervention because God would not approve, "It's happening again! I can't do battle with God!" (Eriksen et al., 2002, p. 48). Although battles with the client's understanding of God are not likely to be effective in therapy, it is necessary at times to address the client's spiritual resistances. In the chapters that follow, I consider ways to draw upon spiritual resources to help resolve not only problems, but also the impediments to resolving problems.

The Spiritual Dimension of the Client's Context

Clients do not enter psychotherapy as isolated beings. They are accompanied by a way of looking at the world that is, in part, the product of a larger context, made up of many ingredients: gender, ethnicity, age, family, friends, congregation, community, and culture. This point is especially important to stress in the spiritual realm. Modern-day definitions emphasize the private, interior, subjective character of spirituality. Readers are reminded repeatedly that they can be "spiritual" without being "religious." While it is true that people can reject a traditional religious identification, they cannot disconnect their spirituality from a greater context. As I noted in earlier chapters, the search for the sacred always unfolds within a field of larger forces, even if the client is unaware of these forces or reacts against them. The context that is rejected by the client continues to play as critical a role in spirituality as the context that is explicitly accepted.

For example, in Chapter 5, I introduced Rachel, the 35-year-old, single woman who had come to therapy for help with depression that, as it turned out, was connected to her traumatic experience of having been gang-raped 10 years earlier. Although Rachel had never described herself in religious or spiritual terms, she did speak of the rapes as a desecration. Prompted by her use of spiritual language, I decided to learn more about Rachel's religious background. She described a happy childhood as the youngest in a large, Italian, Roman Catholic family. She had been particularly close with her grandmother, who called Rachel "her little angel." The two would often go to mass together and then return home to bake sweets. I asked Rachel whether she continued to be active in the church and she answered no, she had lost interest in her teens and now thought of herself as nonreligious. This was puzzling. Why, I asked Rachel, had she separated herself from the church when it had been such an important part of her life as a child and such an important part of her relationship with her grandmother?

A long silence followed. Then Rachel began to cry. "I hadn't thought about this for years," she said. "I thought I had put this stuff behind me." Rachel then recounted this story: At 14 she had become pregnant. When she disclosed her pregnancy to her mother, her mother told Rachel to keep it a secret. Rachel's mother then arranged for an abortion. As the result of a complication during the procedure, Rachel was hospitalized for a few days. While she was hospitalized, her grandmother suffered a heart attack and died.

Rachel believed that, in the eyes of the Catholic Church and God, she had committed an unforgivable act. She had taken an innocent life. The death of her grandmother, she felt, was God's punishment for the life she had taken. Rachel remembered feeling horribly guilty for quite a while, though she shared her feelings with no one. And yet, as time passed, Rachel began to wonder. What kind of church, what kind of God, she asked herself, would have such little compassion for a young girl? If her religion would have nothing to do with her, she would have nothing to do with it. So Rachel walked away, believing that she had left her religion behind her. Of course, she hadn't. Over the course of therapy, Rachel began to see that the rapes and her subsequent infertility had triggered many of the same questions she had struggled with unsuccessfully as an adolescent. Had God taken her grandmother as a result of Rachel's sins? Had God allowed her to be desecrated through the rapes because she had committed violations of her own? More recently, was her infertility another case of divine retribution seemingly tailored to the crime of her abortion? Would the God that she had denied continue to punish her for the remainder of her life?

Church, Catholicism, sin, punishment, guilt, forgiveness, and grace—all concepts that Rachel felt were things of the past—had been at work in her mind all along. I will discuss more of my work with Rachel in a later chapter. Here, let me simply note that Rachel's recovery from her depression was linked with the resolution of her spiritual struggles and the integration of religion, faith, and spirituality into her life.

The client's religious identification or lack of religious identification is one critical part of the larger context he or she brings to psychotherapy. Weisbuch-Remington, Mendes, Seery, and Blascovich (2005) conducted a study relevant to this point. They presented Christian and non-Christian undergraduate students with positive religious symbols (e.g., images of Christ ascending to heaven, images of Christ's healing powers) and negative religious symbols (e.g., satanic symbols, images of demons) outside of their awareness. The students were then asked to plan and deliver a speech on one of two topics: thoughts regarding their own death or a visit to the dentist. While the students were planning and delivering their speeches, their cardiac performance was monitored. As predicted, in response to the mortality speech task, the Christian students showed fewer signs of cardiac distress when they were exposed to the positive religious symbols and more signs of cardiac distress when they were presented with the negative religious symbols. In contrast, the non-Christian students were unaffected by the positive and negative religious symbols. The authors believe that the positive and negative religious symbols increased and decreased the value of religion, respectively, as a coping resource for the Christian students faced with a spiritually threatening task. The same symbols, however, failed to affect the non-Christian students one way or another because the symbols were not meaningful to them.

Distinctions between Christians and non-Christians gloss over important denominational differences within Christianity. Robert Lovinger (1996), a clinical psychologist who has written extensively on this topic, notes that "denominations differ widely, as does their impact on the person's attitudes, values, and worldview. . . . Denominations have central qualities that they impart to their members, or that attract those who find these qualities important" (p. 328). Differences among these denominations are particularly important for therapists to understand because they shape the character of problems and solutions. For example, some research suggests that questions and doubts about basic religious tenets and doctrines may be the source of considerable anxiety and distress among conservative Protestants, while the same kinds of questions may be less problematic among Roman Catholics who are less doctrinally oriented (Kooistra & Pargament, 1999). On the other hand, three studies indicate that spiritual forms of coping that emphasize faith, religious commitment, and trust in God may be more helpful to Protestants than to Catholics, particularly in the face of uncontrollable life situations (Alferi, Culver, Carver, Arena, & Antoni, 1999; Park, Cohen, & Herb, 1990; Tix & Frazier, 1998). The Protestant emphasis on faith and acceptance, Crystal Park and her colleagues (1990) suggest, may be especially well suited to those times of life when people are pushed beyond the limits of their control.

There is a danger of stereotyping in speaking so generally of different religious groups. These stereotypes misinform and mislead. Not all fundamentalists are close-minded, not all Catholics are "recovering" from their experiences in the church, not all Jews are ridden with existential angst. Though denominations take their members down different pathways of acting, thinking, relating, and experiencing (see Richards & Bergin, 2000, for a review), within any tradition we find wide differences among members in the ways they understand and practice the teachings of their faith. Thus, important as an understanding of religious denominations is, this understanding does not replace the need for close and careful attention to the way each client lives out his or her tradition.

Spirituality is embedded in a context larger than religious denomination. Gender, age, ethnicity, family, community, and culture are also parts of the context clients carry with them to psychotherapy, and each of these factors may shape spirituality in subtle or not-so-subtle ways. For example, Annette Mahoney and I (2004) have noted how Christian men and women may experience a spiritual conversion quite differently. For men, spiritual conversion involves a fundamental shift in strivings and priorities from a life revolving around the gratification of self to a life centered on God. Pride, from this perspective, is the most basic sin that separates men from God. In contrast, Mahoney and I argue, the primary problem for many women is not self-exaltation, but self-negation: "Here excessive dependence on others for one's identity displaces God from the center of one's life. Sin, in this case, involves placing other people at the center of an individual's life, effectively allowing other people to function as God. This cuts a person off from authentic relationships with God and others" (p. 485). Spiritual conversion in this case involves "neither 'shattering' of self as by an authoritarian father-judge nor a quietistic 'acceptance' as by an understanding mother, [but rather] a profound affirmation of self as capable of living in co-union with God. . . . The 'great surrender' in this context means forsaking the depressed and empty self, and discovering self-worth in companionship with God" (p. 486). Spiritually integrated psychotherapy directs our attention to the power of gender and many other forces that define the larger context of the client, shaping the ways in which spirituality is experienced and expressed.

THE ORIENTATION OF SPIRITUALLY INTEGRATED PSYCHOTHERAPY TO THE THERAPIST

Many years ago, I attended a conference on religion and mental health. The keynote speaker was one of a handful of Jesuit priest-psychiatrists in the world. I was looking forward to hearing how he integrated religion into his approach to treatment. But, to my surprise, he didn't even mention religion. In fact, his talk could have been given by many therapists trained in psychoanalysis. After his address, I raised my hand and asked him how he dealt with his own role as a priest within psychotherapy. He responded, "Oh, before I walk into the therapy room, I always take off my collar. I keep clear boundaries between my religion and my psychotherapy." What a shame, I thought. Here was someone in a unique position to bridge the worlds of psychology and religion, yet he insisted on disconnecting the two. More than that, I wondered, how could he possibly keep "clear boundaries" between two inseparable aspects of living?

If clients do not check their spirituality at the door to psychotherapy, neither do therapists. Like the Jesuit priest-psychiatrist, many clinicians try to separate spirituality from therapy or maintain a therapeutic neutrality. But separation and neutrality are impossible, particularly in the spiritual realm, for spirituality speaks to the most fundamental assumptions of life, the deepest of beliefs, and the most sacred of matters. Attempts to cover or hide the spiritual dimension may only draw more attention to it, like an embarrassing blemish made more noticeable by too much makeup. Knowingly or unknowingly, the spirituality of the therapist permeates his or her understanding of people, problems, and change. Spiritually integrated psychotherapy makes explicit the importance of the therapist's own orientation to spirituality. Therapists, like everyone else, vary in their own degree of spiritual integration. Especially important is the therapists' level of *professional* spiritual integration, for this will affect their helpfulness most directly. The spiritually dis-integrated therapist may overlook valuable opportunities for change or unwittingly exacerbate the client's problems. In contrast, the spiritually-integrated therapist can draw on his or her understanding of and approach to spirituality as a powerful resource for change.

The Spiritually Dis-Integrated Therapist

Two types of spiritual dis-integration are particularly dangerous for therapists: spiritual intolerance and spiritual illiteracy.

Spiritual Intolerance

Spiritual intolerance can reveal itself in two therapeutic orientations to spirituality: rejectionism and exclusivism (see Pargament, 1997, for extended discussion). Rejectionism assumes that spirituality is inherently problematic, a source of pathology that must be challenged, discouraged, or replaced with a healthier perspective. There is, unfortunately, a deep tradition of spiritual rejectionism within psychotherapy. As I noted in Chapter 1, Freud (1930/1961) viewed religion as a childish response to feelings of helplessness and insecurity. It works, he said, by "distorting the picture of the real world in a delusional manner . . . by forcibly fixing [adherents] in a state of psychical infantilism and by drawing them into a mass-delusion" (p. 36). Education to reality rather than support of delusion, he argued, was the correct attitude toward religion in treatment. More recently, Albert Ellis (1986), the founder of rational-emotive therapy, expressed similar sentiments (although he has since moderated his views; see Ellis, 2000). Religion, he maintained, "is, on almost every conceivable count, directly opposed to the goals of mental health" and, as a result, "the sane effective psychotherapist should not . . . go along with the patient's religious orientation and try to help these patients live successfully with their religions, for this is equivalent to trying to help them live successfully with their emotional illness" (pp. 12, 15).

Rejectionism on the part of practitioners can assume several guises in therapy. It may take the form of blatantly antagonistic statements toward a client's religious beliefs. Nielsen et al. (2001) illustrate (and discourage) a few of these statements: "Where is the evidence that any God exists? Prove to me that any supernatural being gives a damn about you or ever will? In my view, believing your body is a 'temple' to any other being is both crazy and helping you to feel miserable" (p. 111). Less overtly hostile therapists may regard spiritual experiences as signs of immaturity that should be supplanted by more adult behavior. Consider, for example, the response of one therapist to a bereaved mother who described her experience of a visitation by her dead child: "Well, you've healed enough that you don't need that any more" (Brotherson & Soderquist, 2002, p. 77). Rejectionism may also reveal itself in clinical insensitivity. For example, Schreurs (2002) describes the case of a conservative Christian child who was offended by the continual swearing that took place on her inpatient psychiatric ward. When the child complained to her psychiatrist, he responded by treating it as her problem rather than as the hospital's problem. In addition, rejectionism can manifest itself in the refusal to take spiritual matters seriously. Assuming that spiritual issues are expressions of more fundamental problems, many therapists shift the focus of the conversation when spiritual issues arise in an effort to "reduce" the spiritual topic to what is ostensibly more basic.

Regardless of the form it takes, spiritual rejectionism promotes a number of problems. First, I have reviewed evidence throughout this book that spirituality can be a significant resource to people, one that is distinctive and not fully reducible to other seemingly more fundamental psychological or social processes. Rejectionism overlooks the distinctive value of spirituality in psychotherapy. Second, spiritual rejectionism is inconsistent with the ethical guidelines of psychologists, psychiatrists, social workers, and nurses. For example, according to the "Guidelines for Providers of Psychological Services to Ethnic, Linguistic, and Culturally Diverse Populations" (1993), published by the American Psychological Association: "Psychologists [should] respect clients' religious and/or spiritual beliefs and values, including attributions and taboos, since they affect world view, psychosocial functioning, and expressions of distress" (p. 46). Third, spiritual rejectionism is likely to create a therapeutic misalliance with the large number of clients who see the world through a spiritual lens and seek therapists who will be respectful of their most basic beliefs and values (e.g., Keating & Fretz, 1990).

Spiritual intolerance is also often associated with another therapeutic orientation to spirituality: spiritual exclusivism. This orientation rests on the assumption that there is a single absolute truth and a single best way to approach it. Spiritual exclusivism is not invariably tied to spiritual intolerance. It becomes intolerant without benefit of the balancing virtues of humility (e.g., "I believe my way is the truth, but I am only human and my understandings are imperfect") and compassion (e.g., "I believe my way is the truth, but I can value and respect you as a person of God") or an appreciation for paradox (e.g., "I believe my way is the truth, but many things can be true at the same time").

On the face of it, exclusivism on the part of the therapist would seem to be the direct opposite of rejectionism. Yet both exclusivism and rejectionism can prompt expressions of spiritual intolerance. While rejectionism reflects an intolerance toward any kind of spiritual belief or practice, unmitigated exclusivism represents an intolerance toward any spiritual expression other than that which the therapist holds to be true. Similarly, exclusivists reject solutions to problems other than those that grow out of their own particular spiritual orientation.

Exclusivism is not restricted to one particular religious tradition. It can apply to the traditionally religious therapist or to the nontraditional spiritually oriented therapist. What marks exclusivism at its most extreme is the failure to respect the diversity of pathways that may lead to the sacred. For instance, Christian writers Bobgan and Bobgan (1987) maintain that human suffering is the result of "separation from God because of the sinful condition of mankind and the presence of sin in the world after the Fall" (p. 207). "Jesus," they conclude, "is the only means to reestablish relationship between God and man and to enable people to live by faith in God" (p. 207). Other pathways to change, including secular psychological counseling, Bobgan and Bobgan insist, may only mislead the person: "Psychological systems of counseling may lead a person along the broad way which leads to destruction. . . . The entrance into new life through faith in Jesus is the small gate" (p. 225).

Like rejectionism, spiritual exclusivism has serious problems. For one, exclusivists are likely to hold a narrow spiritual perspective and, as a result, to overlook potentially valuable spiritual resources that fall outside their own particular spiritual orientation. Second, exclusivists may be able to influence only those who share their particular spiritual worldview. In this vein, Lewis and Epperson (1993) had nonevangelical and evangelical Christian college students read descriptions of a nondirective counselor and a Christian counselor. While evangelical students stated that they were equally willing to see both counselors, the nonevangelical Christian college students indicated that they would rather see the nondirective counselor than the Christian counselor. Finally, spiritual exclusivism raises ethical concerns because it fails to respect diverse spiritual perspectives and runs the risk of imposing a particular spiritual worldview on the client.

Spiritual Illiteracy

Even though we can find examples of spiritual intolerance among therapists, I believe they are fairly uncommon. Relatively few therapists are totally dismissive of spirituality, and relatively few therapists presume that they hold an exclusive claim to the truth. The bigger problem for therapists is lack of knowledge about spirituality. In the early 1990s, only 5% of clinical psychologists reported any professional training on religious or spiritual issues (Shafranske & Maloney, 1990). Though the picture has begun to improve, the problem remains. Recently, Brawer et al. (2002) surveyed directors of APA clinical psychology training programs and found that only 17% of the programs offered coursework, supervision, and research in the area of religion and spirituality. Without education, many psychotherapists are left, in essence, spiritually illiterate, unable to understand spirituality, uninformed about spiritual pathways and destinations, unappreciative of diverse religious traditions, unfamiliar with the empirical literature in the psychology of spirituality, unequipped to evaluate spirituality, and unskilled in addressing the spiritual dimension in psychotherapy. How, we might ask, can a spiritually dis-integrated therapist, a therapist whose understanding of spirituality is shallow, narrow, incoherent, and misinformed, help clients who bring spiritual matters to psychotherapy?

The Spiritually Integrated Therapist

Spiritually integrated psychotherapy is grounded in spiritual literacy and competence on the part of the therapist. By spiritual literacy and competence, I am not referring to the therapist's level of personal spiritual maturity. Recall the Jesuit priest-psychiatrist who tried to keep clear boundaries between his personal religion and his clinical practice. Just as personal mental health does not qualify an individual to be a mental health professional, personal spiritual maturity does not qualify an individual to become a spiritually integrated psychotherapist. Adept as the therapist may be within his or her own spiritual tradition, any therapist who wants to practice spiritually integrated psychotherapy must go beyond his or her own personal spirituality and develop a well-integrated professional spiritual perspective. Spiritual knowledge, openness and tolerance, self-awareness, and authenticity are four essential qualities of the spiritually integrated therapist.

Knowledge

Spiritually integrated therapy calls for knowledge about spirituality that transcends any particular set of spiritual teachings, beliefs, and practices. Spiritually integrated therapy also involves more than knowledge about spirituality and knowledge about therapy; it rests on wisdom about how to put the two together. I hope that many of the topics addressed in this book—the wide array of spiritual pathways and destinations, how spirituality works, how to evaluate when spirituality is part of the problem and part of the solution, how to assess spirituality, how to access spiritual resources, and how to deal with spiritual problems in therapy—contribute to this body of knowledge.

Openness and Tolerance

Of course, no therapist can be expert on every form of spirituality, just as no therapist could ever hope to master every area of physiology, emotions, behavior, or relationships. But with an openness to learning, the therapist can expand his or her understanding of spirituality over time. Education can come not only from readings and personal experience but from clinical work itself. Every client has the potential to teach the therapist something new and valuable about spirituality. As we will see in the next chapter, the willingness to be taught by the client is a prerequisite for the formation of a strong therapeutic relationship. An openness to learning also calls for tolerance of diverse spiritual expressions. There is no room for the intolerance that can be found in rejectionism or untempered exclusivism in spiritually integrated psychotherapy. The therapist must be able to communicate genuine respect for the many ways people understand and relate to the sacred. I am not suggesting that the therapist must affirm every spiritual pathway or destination. As we have seen, some forms of spirituality can be destructive. At times, then, the spiritually integrated therapist may need to challenge aspects of the client's spirituality. But these challenges should unfold in a milieu of sensitivity and respect for the client's deepest values and ultimate right to choose his or her own spiritual direction in life, even if the client's values run counter to the therapists' spiritual values.

Self-Awareness

There is, of course, the potential for coercion in any form of psychotherapy, including spiritually integrated psychotherapy. After all, client and therapist are not equal partners in the therapy room. By virtue of their training, education, and experience, therapists are in a position of greater power and authority than their clients and, as a result, may, knowingly or unknowingly, intrude on their client's autonomy and right to choose. Are there any antidotes to this danger? One antidote is spiritual self-awareness, insight into the therapist's own spiritual worldview and the way it may shape the therapeutic process.

In a short introspective piece, Edward Shafranske, a spiritually oriented psychoanalytic therapist, demonstrates this kind of self-awareness (in Sperry, 2001). He is able to articulate the role of religion in his own life:

> In terms of my daily life, I find that my essential religious *practice*, originating in and sustained by the beliefs and sacraments of Roman Catholicism, is *simply allowing* the door to stand ajar. I accentuate *practice* and

simply allowing to place emphasis on what I consider a particular form of spiritual discipline which involves the conscious intent to allow associations of a spiritual nature to emerge and to take root in consciousness. (p. 174)

Shafranske's personal spiritual approach is clearly reflected in his clinical practice. Here too he *simply allows* spiritual material to emerge from the narratives of the client:

Lying beneath ordinary awareness, religious narrative shapes meaning and, for many, is the predominant cognitive-affective influence that organizes experience, influences emotion, constructs meaning, and governs behavior. I do not assume that spirituality will either predominate nor be absent from a given course of psychological treatment; rather, I attempt to listen to and provide a space for the elucidation of religious sentiment. (in Sperry, 2001, p. 175)

Shafranske is well aware of the core assumptions of his personal spiritual orientation and the ways they manifest themselves in therapy:

My spiritual orientation therefore impacts my clinical practice of psychology and psychoanalysis. . . . That we are made in the image and likeness of God, that we live in a universe larger than what we can apprehend, that we are called to the courage to be, that neither suffering nor ecstasy are pointless, that the construction of meaning supercedes ordinary happiness— each of these personal beliefs orients my sitting with the person across from me. (in Sperry, 2001, p. 176)

With spiritual self-awareness of this kind, the therapist is in a better position to identify his or her own values, strengths, vulnerabilities, biases, and blind spots, and, ultimately, to reduce the likelihood of coercion in treatment. Self-awareness also sets the stage for greater authenticity on the part of the therapist.

Authenticity

A few years ago, I worked with a middle-aged women, Ruth, who had been assaulted by a coworker on the job. Although the coworker had been arrested and was awaiting trial, Ruth was petrified with fear that he might escape and attack her again. She was unable to go to work and felt virtually imprisoned in her own home. It took all her strength, she said, just to come to therapy. Prior to the assault, I learned, Ruth had enjoyed her work, close relations with family and friends, and participation in her church, but since the attack she felt she had lost herself.

One session was particularly memorable. Ruth was feeling very discouraged. "I feel as though I have descended into a pit and I've been emptied out," she said. "There is nothing left of me but fear and pain." In spite of her words, Ruth did not appear to be empty to me. She was able to smile in therapy, ask about my well-being, and talk about the people in her world with care and concern.

So I asked Ruth, "Imagine you are in the pit and you have learned that your mother has become ill and needs you. What would you do?"

"Well, I would go to her," Ruth responded immediately.

"Perhaps, then, you're not as empty as you feel," I suggested. "There does seem to be a 'you' left," I said. "You still have your spiritual core—your love and caring for people and the world—but maybe you're not able to reach it. It seems as though you've become stuck in your fears, as if they were quicksand."

Ruth paused for a while and then said, "I do feel stuck and it does feel like quicksand, but are you saying I shouldn't be afraid?"

I answered, "You have every right to feel afraid, with everything you've been through. But I think you should keep a perspective on your fear so you don't lose yourself in it, so you can still reach your spiritual core."

Again, Ruth waited and then said, "You make it sound so easy. Can you do it yourself?" This was a tougher question. I felt that Ruth was asking me whether I was sharing "book sense" or something that was more deeply and personally meaningful. I could have shifted the focus from Ruth's direct question or given an overly positive response (e.g., "Yes, I can"), but neither response would have been authentic.

This time I was the one who paused, gathered my thoughts, and finally said: "I don't mean to make it sound easy because it's not easy at all. It's something I struggle with—how to hold on to myself, my spiritual core, when I face terrible pain. I've learned that trying to make the pain go away or pretend that it's not there doesn't work. But getting lost in the pain is no answer either. Even though I know that, I still mess up sometimes. Holding on to your spiritual core when you are hurting takes lots and lots of practice, but it is something you can get better at."

This conversation was, I believe, pivotal for Ruth. She became more adept at talking about her fears without losing herself in them. And she began to take the risk of leaving her house, returning to work, and reengaging in the world. "I'm doing a better job of holding on to myself," she said later in therapy. I attribute part of the change to the authenticity she experienced in therapy. Authenticity means speaking to the truth as one comprehends it. Authenticity also entails a willingness to share one's most basic understanding of life in ways that are respectful of the client's values and autonomy. Authenticity involves self-disclosure in careful, measured ways that advance the clinical relationship, not the clinician. And authenticity creates the conditions for communication at the most profound levels. It too is an essential element of spiritually integrated psychotherapy.

Spiritual knowledge, tolerance, self-awareness, and authenticity are all critical ingredients of spiritually integrated psychotherapy. Armed with a broad, deep, flexible, and coherent perspective on spirituality; an appreciation for the richness and diversity of spirituality; an awareness of the role of spirituality in the lives of client, therapist; and process of therapy, and a willingness to share oneself authentically in treatment, the spiritually integrated therapist becomes another powerful resource for the client, a resource capable of facilitating profound change.

ORIENTATION OF SPIRITUALLY INTEGRATED PSYCHOTHERAPY TO THE PROCESS OF CHANGE

Psychotherapy involves a meeting of two worlds. As I observe my client for the first time sitting in the waiting room, I begin to enter his or her world. As I introduce myself and bring the client back to my office, he or she begins to enter mine. As we get to know each other, we begin to share our worlds and, through this process, each of our worlds begins to change. There is a spiritual dimension to this unfolding relationship, whether or not the client and therapist are aware of it. We meet, share, and change not only as psychological, social, and physical beings, but as spiritual beings as well.

Even when the sacred is not an explicit focus of therapy, the spirituality of client and therapist is affected over the course of treatment. Psychodynamic therapist James Jones (1991) provides one illustration in his work with Sylvia, a 27-year-old woman who had been raised in a family from Eastern Europe that was suspicious of anyone who fell outside of their subculture, which included membership in a Pentecostal church. Sylvia suffered sexual abuse and incest as a child, but when she spoke of it to her mother, her mother told her she was "dirty" and washed her mouth out with soap. Sylvia began to withdraw deeper into herself, which led only to further rejection and, eventually, shunning by her family and church. She came to therapy struggling with anger and guilt, feelings of isolation and alienation, and fears that she could never be understood or accepted. In the process of therapy, Jones tried to provide Sylvia with a safe haven, a place where Sylvia could be accepted and understood without conditions. This sense of acceptance was the key to Sylvia's recovery. At termination, she told Jones:

> For hours and hours you struggled with me, fighting with me, battling with my defenses against your acceptance. Finally I had to say to myself, you must care or you wouldn't fight so hard. Fighting you made me realize

how I repel others' acceptance. You kept questioning that. Finally, you got me to question why I did that. That was the biggest change in therapy, now I accept others' care and compliments. (p. 72)

Sensitive to the spiritual dimension, Jones noted how Sylvia's change in her own sense of isolation and view of herself led to changes in her image of God: "God," she said later in therapy, "is no longer a judge. I used to prefer judgmental religion; now I feel it does harm, it's not good. I see God as more forgiving. I see parts of scripture about God's love that I never saw before" (p. 72). Changes in Sylvia's relationship with the therapist were also paralleled by changes in her relationship with God. As Sylvia became more accepting of the therapist's empathy and compassion, she became more accepting of God's love: "At first when I would pray to God, I would hear God address me simply as 'my child.' Later, as 'my little child.' And now I hear God call me 'my little wounded child' " (p. 73).

Consistent with case studies such as this one, empirical studies have shown that even presumably secular psychotherapies result in changes in clients' images of God (e.g., Tisdale et al., 1997). Other studies have found that changes in spirituality and psychological symptomatology go hand in hand. For example, in a study of 251 women being treated in an inpatient program for eating disorders, improvements in spiritual well-being were significantly tied to improvements in body image, healthier attitudes toward eating, less conflict in relationships, and reductions in psychological symptoms (Smith, Hardman, Richards, & Fischer, 2003).

Spiritually integrated psychotherapy makes explicit the spiritual dimension of the encounter between therapist and client. It is, in the words of Elkins (1998), a process of "soul meeting" and "soul making." This meeting can take place within any therapeutic modality or approach to change, as long as it is respectful of clients' spirituality. In this sense, spiritually integrated psychotherapy is neither a self-contained form of therapy nor a competitor to other types of treatment. Rather, it is a therapeutic approach that extends and enriches many forms of therapy by focusing more explicit attention on the spiritual dimension of people, their problems, their resources, and the process of change. One way spiritually integrated psychotherapy can enhance other modes of treatment is by providing another perspective on psychological problems.

Adding a Spiritual Perspective on Problems to Psychotherapy

Consider a case described by psychiatrist Irvin Yalom. Thoughtful, sensitive, and articulate, Yalom has been a pioneer in the development of existential therapy (see Yalom, 1980). He is also courageous, one of the all-too-rare practitioners willing to share failures as well as successes in psychotherapy. I focus on one of his cases from his book *Love's Executioner*, not to illustrate how spiritually integrated therapy can reduce the number of therapeutic errors (I continue to make my fair share) or to demonstrate the limitations of existential therapy (an approach I admire), but to illustrate how spiritually integrated psychotherapy can offer a slant on human problems different from one of many therapeutic orientations.

Yalom (1989) tells the story of Thelma, a disheveled 70-year-old woman who announced in the first session that she was "hopelessly, tragically in love" (p. 15). Yalom admits his surprise. "How could love ever choose to ravage that frail, tottering old body, or house itself in that shapeless polyester jogging suit," he asked himself (p. 15). Perhaps sensitive to his disbelief, Thelma proceeds to show Yalom pictures of herself as a former dancer and a far more attractive woman 10 years earlier. She then goes on to describe a 27-day love affair that she had had with her therapist, Matthew, eight years earlier. Since then, she had been despondent much of the time, staring out the window of her home, unable to sleep, and devoid of any interest other than thinking about why her therapist had ended the affair and dreaming that someday he might return. In despair, she had collected her medications, overdosed, and come close to death. Suicide continued to preoccupy Thelma in her work with Yalom.

Yalom approaches the case as one of obsession, and with good reason. Thelma complains:

> "For eight years I haven't stopped thinking about him. At seven in the morning I wonder if he's awake yet, and at eight I imagine him eating his oatmeal. . . . I keep looking for him when I walk down the street. . . . I dream about him. I replay in my mind each of our meetings together. . . . In fact, most of my life goes on in these daydreams—I scarcely take note of what's happening in the present. My life is being lived eight years ago."
> (p. 21)

From Yalom's existential perspective, Thelma's obsession is a way to avoid a confrontation with the more fundamental existential concerns of aging, isolation, and death. This obsession, Yalom believes, "had to be eradicated" (p. 31) and replaced with an appreciation for the "impoverishment in her life that [had led her to] the obsession in the first place" (p. 32). Yalom tries to convince Thelma that her love for Matthew was not truly love. "His experience and your experience were very different," Yalom insists. "You cannot re-create a state of shared romantic love, of the two of you being deeply in love with one another *because it was never there in the first place*" (p. 58). But Thelma rejects Yalom's interpretation, just as she rejects his efforts to discover what he insists are the deeper roots of her problem. Ultimately, Thelma terminates therapy, reconnects with Matthew, and reports a sharp improvement in her mental health.

This brief summary does not do justice to Yalom's portrayal of this rich and complex case. Reading this story, I was struck by Yalom's honesty and courage in sharing his frustrations and critical self-analysis. Who is to say whether another therapist could have been more successful with Thelma? What I can say is, in my reading, the spiritual dimension of Thelma's problem and relationship with Yalom fairly jumped off the pages at me. In almost every account of her relationship with Matthew, Thelma is describing a relationship with what she perceives to be sacred. She speaks of him in terms of divine qualities. He touches her at her deepest levels: "He *really* cared, he *really* accepted me. No matter what I did, what horrid things I thought, I knew he'd . . . confirm me—No, *validate* me" (p. 17). She describes him as a guiding and directing force in her life: "He taught me to care for all living things. He taught me to think about the reasons I was put here on earth" (p. 17). She experiences a mystical merging with Matthew: "It was an out-of-the-body experience. I had no weight. It was as though I wasn't there. . . . I just stopped thinking and worrying about me. I became a *we*" (p. 39).

Certainly, this relationship is destructive; Thelma has elevated a very human, indeed unethical, therapist to the status of the divine. In the process, she has created an idol, a person and a relationship unable to bear the weight of the sacred. When the relationship fails, Thelma is left with a terrible sense of spiritual emptiness and loss. Unable to fully accept this loss, Thelma clings to the memory of their relationship and the hope that one day it might blossom again. Yalom, however, largely overlooks the sacred character of this relationship. Inadvertently, he commits a desecration in the eyes of Thelma when he tries to convince her that her love for Matthew is, in fact, pathological. She responds forcefully in defense of the sacred:

> When people think that we really hadn't loved one another, it belittles the love that we had. It takes away the depth—it makes it into nothing. The love was, and is, *real. Nothing has ever been more real to me.* Those twenty-seven days were the high point of my life. Those were twenty-seven days of paradise, and I'd give anything to have them back! (p. 39)

In this context, Thelma's decision to leave therapy and renew her relationship with Matthew through "monthly chats" is understandable. Through these actions, the sacred bond remains inviolable.

From a spiritual perspective, Thelma's problems take on a different appearance. I would suggest that at the root of her problems is a yearning for the sacred, a yearning that has attached itself inappropriately to a false god. While existentialists might insist that this longing serves only to protect the individual from a confrontation with the more basic conditions of life, I would argue that Thelma's yearning for the sacred is a primary irreducible human motive. True, it has expressed itself in a destructive way, but the solution is not to "cut through" the spiritual motive. Rather, Thelma could be helped to realize her motive more constructively. Therapy could have focused on articulating and affirming Thelma's sacred yearning, acknowledging what she perceived to be the divine character of her relationship with Matthew, helping her to grieve the loss of the sacred, and assisting her in the search for new and more viable ways to experience sacredness in her life.

Let me reiterate: any therapeutic approach can look good when it is applied to difficult cases retrospectively. My goal here was not to critique a powerful approach to psychotherapy and a gifted therapist, but to suggest that spiritually integrated psychotherapy can offer another valuable perspective on human problems, one that may prompt change in new and unexpected ways.

Adding Spiritual Resources to Change in Psychotherapy

Spiritually integrated psychotherapy also points to spiritual resources that could be drawn upon more fully within various models of psychotherapy. Let's take one example. Rebecca Propst (1988), one of the early leaders in the development of spiritually integrated psychotherapy, discusses a number of ways in which spiritual resources add an important and distinctive dimension to cognitive-behavioral psychotherapy. Particularly rich are her examples of the therapeutic use of spiritual imagery and visualization to foster a sense of spiritual support among her clients. One case involved a severely depressed Christian woman, Ann, who had been physically abused by her mother as a child and later sexually abused by her foster father. Although Ann had been in treatment sporadically with a number of therapists, she had never been able to overcome her shame and share her abusive history. She was certain that she was worthless, no good, and unlovable. With time, Ann was able to reveal her history in treatment. Her therapist responded by encouraging Ann to develop an "image of the healing Christ" (p. 137) and then to reexperience the pain of her abuse within the context of this larger supportive vision. Together they practiced the following visualization:

> THERAPIST: Imagine [Jesus Christ] after his crucifixion. As you see his brown eyes and hair, can you see his wounds? What do they look like?
>
> CLIENT: He has deep cuts in his hands and feet and scars on his back and legs.
>
> THERAPIST: What kind of facial expression does he have?
>
> CLIENT: He is in pain.
>
> THERAPIST: Is there any other expression?
>
> CLIENT: His eyes still look warm.
>
> THERAPIST: What lets you know he is in pain?

CLIENT: His eyes have some tears in them, and his mouth is tense.

THERAPIST: Now, Ann, I want you to switch to the image of you with your mother. Tell me what you see.

CLIENT: I see myself sitting on the floor as a young child crying.

THERAPIST: As you are crying, what else is happening?

CLIENT: My mother is angry at me, and tells me to be quiet.

THERAPIST: What happened then?

CLIENT: She turned on the kitchen stove and held me down on the stove. (*She started sobbing at this point.*)

THERAPIST: Ann, imagine now that Christ, whom you saw earlier, comes into the kitchen now. What would he do?

CLIENT: He walks over to the stove and takes me off the stove.

THERAPIST: Then what happened?

CLIENT: He is telling me that he understands what I feel, he has lots of scars too.

THERAPIST: Ann, imagine what Jesus's eyes look like as he tells you that he understands.

CLIENT: He has tears in his eyes, and they are very warm.

THERAPIST: Ann, just allow yourself to look at Jesus's eyes. (pp. 137–138)

In some ways, this form of visualization is nothing new. Changing the images and meanings of traumatic events by reexperiencing them in a more benevolent context is a central part of cognitive-behavioral therapy. But the use of spiritual resources to support and assist this process of change is new for many psychotherapists. Even though other positive images (e.g., supportive figures in Ann's life other than Jesus Christ) could have been used in this visualization, the image of the crucified Jesus had extraordinary power for a woman steeped in this narrative. Through this visualization Ann was likely able to experience a sense of reassurance that she is not truly alone, that someone else has shared her pain. She was also able to witness a model of hope and resilience in the face of suffering. And she could gain a sense of support that, in spite of her pain and guilt, she was still worthy of someone's love. In this way, Propst was bringing a distinctive resource to the process of psychotherapy.

Spiritually integrated psychotherapy is multimodal. It draws on many mechanisms of change from many traditions and can be integrated into a wide range of therapies, not only cognitive-behavioral, but psychodynamic, existential, marital/family, interpersonal, humanistic, experiential, rational-emotive, and acceptance and commitment therapies as well (see Shafranske, 1996). I will consider other examples shortly. But it is important to stress here that spiritually integrated therapy is not simply one more set of techniques that can be piggybacked onto other therapies. It grows out of a different way of thinking about problems, solutions, and human nature more generally. And the process of attending more fully to the spiritual dimension is likely to change the character of any therapy. Michael Mahoney (2000), a noted cognitive-behavioral therapist, commented that his style shifted to "deeper authenticity, compassionate witnessing, and developmental nurturance rather than clever engineering and technical solutions" (pp. 53–54) as his therapy became more spiritually oriented. Clients themselves are also likely to experience spiritually integrated psychotherapy differently, as we will see in the chapters to follow.

CONCLUSIONS

Early in my career, I was doing some work as a consultant to a police department in eastern Maryland. On my way to an appointment with a police lieutenant, I lost my way and ended up in a market. Reluctantly, I called the lieutenant, told him I was lost, and asked him for directions to the police station. Naturally enough, he asked me where I was. I had to admit that I was so lost I had no idea where I was. He paused for a moment and then said, "Well, son, I can't tell you how to get here if you don't know where you're coming from." Perhaps the lieutenant was a student of existentialism. Whether he was or not, his message was quite profound and has stayed with me over the years. It applies to many contexts including this one. Before we can help our clients get to where they want to go, we have to know where they and we are coming from. In this chapter, we have reviewed the basic assumptions of spiritually integrated psychotherapy about the client, the therapist, and the process of change. These assumptions ground and orient the therapist in treatment. With these assumptions in mind, we turn now to the first step in spiritually integrated psychotherapy: forming a relationship with the client and the process of assessment.

10

Initial and Implicit
Spiritual Assessment

Before we can address the spiritual dimension in psychotherapy, we have to understand it. Much of this book has focused on providing the reader with a way to do that. With understanding, half of the work in becoming a spiritually integrated psychotherapist is done, for a clear perspective on spirituality is the foundation for assessment and treatment. In this chapter and the next, we build on this foundation and consider how to assess the role of spirituality in the lives of specific clients: their problems, their pathways and destinations, their critical life events, their larger context, and the degree to which their lives are well integrated. Keep in mind that spiritual assessment is not an intellectual exercise, nor is it an end in itself. The goal of spiritual assessment is to develop a concrete plan of action for addressing spirituality in psychotherapy. A dry set of intake questions or a few formal tests of spirituality in the first session or two will not provide the clinician with the information that is needed to move from assessment to intervention.

In fact, a mechanical approach to spiritual assessment should be avoided for a few reasons. First, spirituality is deeply personal. Many clients are unwilling to share such an intimate part of themselves early in treatment. Years ago, I surveyed a group of church members regarding their images of God. One woman returned her survey to me unanswered, but with a note boldly written in the margins saying, "I don't know you well enough to share something so personal with you." Recall, too, the case of Alice from the first chapter, my client with bipolar illness, who had never spoken about her spiritual experiences in her decades of psychological treatment. "Why not?," I had asked. "Because they already think I'm crazy," she had answered. Only with time and trust was she able to open up to me about her spirituality. Second, spirituality is difficult to put into words. Many clients have a difficult time articulating their view of the sacred, their spiritual experiences, their spiritual struggles and dreams. Problems in the expression of spirituality should not be dismissed as signs that spirituality is unimportant, however. Clients may simply need additional help to give a voice to their spirituality. Third, the measurement of spirituality is still in early stages of development. Although there is no shortage of measures of spirituality and religiousness (see Hill & Hood, 1999), many of these measures are not clinically relevant because they are functionally disconnected from the life of the individual. Questions about how often people go to church, their religious affiliation, whether they believe in God, and the importance of spirituality in their lives say little about how these practices, identifications, beliefs, and commitments express themselves or fail to express themselves in day-to-day life. As the sole tool for spiritual assessment, structured interviews and measurement instruments run the risk of freezing spirituality into lifeless forms.

It takes a process to know a process. To capture a client's distinctive search for the sacred requires a process of assessment, one fully interwoven into the larger therapeutic task of forming a relationship with the client. Spiritual assessment is the process of getting to know the spiritual dimension of the client's life. It is part of getting to know the client more generally. The process of spiritual assessment evolves over the course of therapy as the relationship between client and therapist develops. In the remainder of this chapter and in the next, I focus on the critical elements of this process: setting the stage for spiritual dialogue, initial spiritual assessment, implicit spiritual assessment, and explicit spiritual assessment (see Figure 10.1).

SETTING THE STAGE FOR SPIRITUAL DIALOGUE

I have described psychotherapy as a meeting of two worlds. It is, however, a peculiar kind of meeting, an asymmetrical encounter in which the client shares his or her personal pain, hopes, and dreams, while the therapist shares a professional perspective. Why should any client participate in this unequal exchange? In part, because nothing else has worked. For most clients, psychotherapy is not the first helping option they choose when they face psychological problems. Quite the contrary, it is often their last resort. And yet few clients enter psychotherapy so desperate that they will immediately disclose their deepest secrets and longings to a stranger. They check their therapists out, and with good reason. Before sharing the most sensitive aspects of their lives, they want to know whether they are speaking to

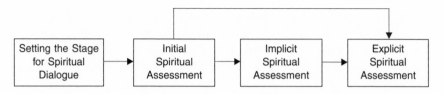

FIGURE 10.1. The process of spiritual assessment.

someone who is safe, someone who will respect their deepest confidences, someone who can be trusted to be sensitive yet honest, and someone who can help.

To enter the world of the client then, the therapist must receive an invitation. It is an invitation that often has to be earned. How? First, by communicating an openness to learning and, second, by communicating an openness to sharing.

Openness to Learning

"I know what God is like for you because I know your religious denomination. . . . I know what God is like for you because I know what your language about God means. . . . I know what God is like for you because your image of God is a reflection of your early attachment" (Griffith & Griffith, 2002, pp. 212–218). These are a few of the ways that therapists communicate their sense that they already know about their client's spirituality and, as Griffith and Griffith (2002) note, these are also a few of the ways that clinicians can shut off spiritual dialogue from the start. In contrast, the therapist earns an invitation to enter the spiritual world of the client by conveying his or her deep interest in seeing life as it looks through the client's eyes and, perhaps most importantly, a willingness to be taught by the client, especially in the spiritual realm. There is no crime to admitting a lack of knowledge—far from it. A little dose of therapeutic humility can empower clients who, by the time they come to therapy, often feel they have little to teach anyone. By conveying a willingness to be taught, the therapist sets the stage for a partnership in the process of learning.

Take, for example, the case of Karen, a single 50-year-old woman who came into therapy for long-standing depression. An MBA, she had held a series of jobs over the years, none fulfilling. She dreaded going to work and felt too exhausted in the evenings to do anything other than eat, watch television, and go to sleep. "What kept you going?," I asked. "Well," she replied, "you do what you have to do." Life, for Karen, was about fulfilling obligations: to her job, to her aging parents whom she visited regularly, to her church that she attended weekly. With her shoulders hunched, her face drawn, and her hands clenched, Karen looked as though she had been carrying the weight of the world on her shoulders for a long time. Thus I was surprised in the middle of one session to see Karen sit up, break out in a smile, and, amazingly, giggle. Following her eyes, I saw her looking intently at two squirrels playing outside my window. This led to the following exchange:

KAREN: I love watching animals.

K.I.P: Do you get a chance to do that very much?

KAREN: Oh, no. (*pause*) I used to when I was a little girl.

K.I.P: I'd like to hear more about that.

KAREN: It's silly. We lived on a farm and I used to love walking outside, looking at the flowers and trees, listening to the birds and insects. It was like a spiritual experience for me.

K.I.P: What do you mean by that?

KAREN: You know, a spiritual experience.

K.I.P: I'm not sure I understand. Could you tell me what your spiritual experience was like for you?

KAREN: Oh, I remember feeling like nature was just so amazing—none of the leaves on the same tree was exactly alike. I'd stare at the creek on our farm for hours and wonder how the water never seemed to end, how it always looked the same but always looked different. I used to lie down in the fields and listen to the insects. I thought they were talking to me.

K.I.P: (*pause*) Wow! It seems as though the farm was a magical place for you. Outdoors, you were enchanted by the wonder and beauty of it all. You felt so much a part of nature that you could hear the insects talking to you. Is that right?

KAREN: Yes. [By this point, Karen's physical demeanor had changed. She seemed less burdened and more at peace with herself.]

K.I.P: How did your parents respond when you came inside the house so excited?

KAREN: (*pause*) Well, my parents were very busy, you know. It takes a lot to run a farm. My mother would tell me to stop being so foolish and do my chores.

K.I.P: Your mother felt that your spiritual experiences were foolish?

KAREN: Well, yes. They were pretty silly. [Karen had begun to look more uncomfortable.]

K.I.P: And yet, as you describe your experience, it sounds like it was very moving for you, it touched you.

KAREN: I don't know . . . I guess so . . . I don't remember. Anyway, as my mother says, "I'm not sure what this has to do with the price of eggs." Can we move on?

K.I.P: Sure. I'm glad we had a chance to talk about your experience. Maybe it will come up again, maybe not. Anyway, let's talk about what's on your mind right now.

In my responses to Karen, I was trying to set the stage for spiritual dialogue in several ways. First, when Karen raised a spiritually relevant topic, I let her know about my desire to learn more. I shared my lack of knowledge and asked her to educate me. Second, I did not assume that I understood Karen's spiritual language. Terms such as "religious," "spiritual experience," and "born again" have very different meanings to different people. Even therapists from the same religious traditions as their clients must be careful not to assume that they share the same worldview, since there are many varieties of spiritual meaning within any denomination. Third, recognizing that I was just beginning to learn about this side of Karen, I phrased my own responses and interpretations tentatively. Fourth, I communicated my interest in and respect for spiritual matters. I did not project the notion that spirituality was silly, foolish, or irrelevant to Karen or to psychotherapy. Finally, I respected Karen's right to control the agenda. After she grew uncomfortable talking about her mother's response to her spiritual experiences (perhaps I had pushed too quickly), I let Karen know that I was willing to move on if she chose. I did, however, leave the door open to further conversation. Later, Karen would invite me into her spiritual world. This conversation was merely the first of many that focused on her spiritual longings. Over time, Karen was able to make dramatic changes in her life by drawing more fully on her spirituality. Willingness to be taught, appreciation for differences in spiritual meaning, tentativeness, interest in spiritual matters, and respect for the client's right to address spirituality as he or she chooses come together to convey an openness to learning about the client's spiritual world.

Openness to Sharing

Spiritual dialogue must be a two-way street. To encourage that dialogue, therapists must be willing not only to learn from the client, but also to share parts of themselves with the client, both personally and professionally.

Personal Sharing

The idea of *personal* sharing with clients may raise a few eyebrows among my readers. In graduate school, we are taught to deflect personal questions with a gentle question of our own ("I wonder why that is important to you?"); a reflection ("It sounds like you are having some questions about me."), or a less-than-gentle admonition ("We are here to talk about you, not me"). But our concerns about self-disclosure may be overdrawn. Few therapists would respond to a client's complaints by replying: "You think you've got problems? Let me tell you about the day I had." We are generally well aware that the personal life of the therapist is not the focus of therapy. Certainly, therapists must be careful concerning their decisions about when and how much to self-disclose. As Farber (2006) recommends, self-disclosure by the therapist should be used judiciously and infrequently, and should be focused on the needs of the client. Nevertheless, personal disclosure, including spiritual self-disclosure, by the therapist can be quite appropriate in some instances, particularly when the therapist is setting the stage for spiritual dialogue.

One of these instances involves disclosure that will facilitate the client's choice of a therapist. Clients have the right to select a therapist who comes from a similar or a different religious tradition. Their reasoning may be well conceived or not, but regardless, the choice of therapist is theirs. Just as clients have the right to find a male, female, older, younger, cognitive-behavioral, psychodynamic, or recovering alcoholic therapist, they have the right to seek out a therapist with a particular religious (or nonreligious) affiliation. So when a potential client asks me about my own religiousness, I tell him or her that I am Jewish. But I don't stop there, for the client's question opens up the possibility of a spiritual conversation. I ask the client how he or she might feel about working with a Jewish therapist. Some say that's fine, they just wanted someone who would not dismiss their beliefs in God. Others say they would prefer to work with a Christian therapist. In those cases, I do everything I can to facilitate a referral to a Christian therapist in the area. And still others ask questions: Have I worked with people from other religions? Can I be sensitive to and respectful of their tradition? Will I somehow try to convert them? In these cases, I try to respond in straightforward fashion: Yes, I have quite a bit of experience in working with people from other religions. Yes, I enjoy helping people from other religions and try to be respectful and appreciative of their faith. And no, I will not try to convert them; instead, I would hope to learn something about the role that spirituality plays in their lives. In responding to these questions, I do not try to convince the client to see me. Nor do I delve deeply into his or her underlying fears or possible misconceptions about psychotherapy or spirituality. This initial spiritual conversation will not be extensive. I simply try to give potential clients enough information to decide whether they want to work with me in counseling.

Self-disclosure by the therapist is also appropriate in order to help clients determine whether the therapist can help them realize their goals for counseling. Before proceeding with therapy, the client may want to know about the therapist's own positions on morally sensitive issues, such as abortion, divorce, extramarital affairs, or homosexuality. These kinds of questions may be motivated by several underlying concerns.[1] Perhaps, most often, the client is, in essence, asking whether the therapist will be able to help the client make his or her own decision. Once again, I believe this is a very appropriate question, one the therapist should address. There are three possible responses. In the first and easiest case, the therapist may not have strong personal views on a topic and will feel quite comfortable in helping the client move toward whatever goal he or she chooses.

In the second case, the therapist may have strong personal views, but may still feel able to help the client make an independent choice. In this case, however, there is a danger of subtle influence or coercion by the therapist, particularly when the therapist feigns moral neutrality. To protect against this danger, I believe therapists should disclose their personal positions on issues of moral and spiritual relevance to clients. As Allen Bergin (1985) puts it, "It is vital that we be more explicit about values because we use them, however unconsciously, as a means of therapeutic change . . . being explicit actually protects our clients. The more subtle our values, the more likely we are to be hidden persuaders. The more open we are about our view, the more choice clients will have in electing to be influenced or not to be influenced" (p. 107). It is important to recognize that Bergin is speaking of a particular kind of explicitness, one designed not to manipulate the client's morals, but to protect the client's right to choose, even if those choices run counter to the therapist's own values and preferences.

Finally, in the third case, as a result of the therapists' strong personal feelings, he or she may be unable or unwilling to accept the client's goals for counseling in some cases. Several years ago, following a workshop I had given to clergy, a pastor came up to me and asked if he could speak with me privately for a few minutes. A handsome man in his early 50s, he told me that he was the leader of a large successful church, married, and the father of seven children. In a low, shaky voice, he told me that he had been having an affair with a married member of his congregation for a few years. The affair was causing him tremendous anxiety and he asked whether I would be willing to see him in therapy. As he spoke to me, I tried to empathize with the pain he must be going through. The guilt and shame at what he was doing to his wife, his family, the other woman, and his church, I imagined, must be overpowering. I told him I would be glad to see him, help him deal with his pain, and resolve the affair. I was way off base, how-

---

[1]In some instances, the client may be involved in a moral conflict with family members and seeking a therapeutic ally. In other cases, the client may be hoping to avoid a difficult choice and looking for a therapist who will make the client's decision for him or her. The therapist must let these clients know that the therapist's job is not one of moral arbiter.

ever. Shaking his head, the pastor told me that he wasn't interested in resolving the affair. He was anxious because his lover wanted to end their liaison. It was she, not he, who was having difficulty reconciling the affair with her commitments to her marriage and her church. The pastor was unapologetic in his request. He wanted me to give him some "pointers" about how to persuade his lover to remain in their extramarital relationship. After the few moments it took me to get over my shock and finish kicking myself for my naïveté, I told the pastor: "I won't help you try to convince your lover to stay with you. I think what you are doing is wrong and damaging to yourself and the people in your life. If I saw you in therapy, I would help you figure out how you got into this situation and how you could extricate yourself from it, but I would not help you continue doing something wrong." Once again, he surprised me. He asked me if I could refer him to someone else who could help him convince his lover to stay. I told him I couldn't do that either. That was the last I saw of this pastor. I was sorry that he didn't pursue therapy (at times, I imagine him continuing to wreak havoc on his family, church, and himself), but I did not regret my openness; it was, I believe, the most therapeutic response I could have offered him.

Professional Sharing

There is a second kind of sharing that helps sets the stage for spiritual dialogue, assessment, and treatment. This is the sharing of the clinician's professional perspective on spirituality and its place in psychotherapy. How does this kind of sharing fit into counseling? It fits in two ways.

Many clients come to therapy without an awareness of how spirituality may be intertwined with their problems, and some may not be open to spiritual dialogue in treatment. As a prelude to any discussion about spirituality in treatment, then, the therapist should inform the client that spirituality appears to be emerging as an important topic, and solicit the client's willingness to talk about it. In essence, the therapist seeks the client's informed consent for addressing spirituality in counseling (Hawkins & Bullock, 1995). Although some therapists have recommended obtaining written, informed consent about spiritual discussions from all clients at the beginning of therapy, I prefer to seek informed consent verbally as issues arise in the course of treatment when the client is in the best position to give this consent. This approach also avoids the potential problems that arise in seeking informed consent for spiritual dialogue in cases in which spirituality is not a relevant concern. Thus, when spirituality seems to be salient in treatment, I will say to the client something like "It seems as though there may be a spiritual dimension to your problems" or "It sounds like spirituality may be a potential resource for you in dealing with your problems." Then, I would ask, "How would you feel about exploring the spiritual side of your situation?" These kinds of statements and questions are merely starting points. As we move further into spiritual conversation, and the client develops a greater awareness of the role of spirituality in psychotherapy, the issue of informed consent may be revisited.

Once they have obtained initial informed consent, therapists can then share their professional perspective on spirituality; this sharing may include remarks concerning their understanding of what spirituality is, how it may be a part of the person's problems, and how it may be a part of the person's solutions. In sharing their spiritual perspectives, therapists open the door to conversation. For example, a number of years ago, a 40-year-old conservative Protestant woman was referred to me by a colleague, herself a Christian therapist. The therapist knew that I am Jewish and felt that her client could benefit from both another clinical perspective and work with a male therapist. Mary was an attractive but intense-looking woman. She spoke in clipped no-nonsense sentences occasionally punctuated by brief, oddly out-of-place smiles. Although she was successful in her career as a lawyer, Mary felt like a failure interpersonally. Over the past 20 years, she had had a series of unsuccessful relationships with men. The pattern was consistent: she would meet someone who she was certain was the answer to her dreams, fall desperately in love, experience a few months of total bliss, develop feelings of betrayal prompted by some inconsiderate or insensitive act on the part of her lover, and end the relationship. Though many of these relationships had occurred years ago, Mary continued to harbor deep bitterness toward the men who had hurt her.

After only a few sessions of treatment, Mary came in to my office with a bright smile and told me that I was the best therapist she had ever worked with. Uh-oh, I immediately thought. I knew my time was limited; at any moment I could make a mistake, fall off my pedestal, and become the newest entry on Mary's long list of betrayers. I decided to share my assessment of the problem with Mary, from both a psychological and a spiritual perspective.

K.I.P.: Mary, it seems to me that you see two types of people in the world: saints and sinners.

MARY: No, there are two types of people in the world, but I call them angels and devils.

K.I.P.: Okay. We can go with that. But I think you're missing another group.

MARY: Who's that?

K.I.P.: Human beings. (*pause for a moment*) You see I haven't come across a lot of pure angels or pure devils. From my own point of view as a psychologist and someone who's Jewish, I think most of us fall in the category of human beings, with a bit of the saint and a bit of the sinner in them. What do you think about that?

MARY: I hadn't thought about it that way before.

For most of the remainder of the session, Mary and I had a spiritual conversation. Could people make mistakes without being devils? Isn't it hard trying to live like an angel? Mary had no problem articulating her spiritual feelings; she had thought about angels and devils for many years. Human being, though, was a new concept for her. Even so, Mary seemed to be receptive. Toward the end of the session, feeling that I had little time to waste, I decided to push things further and leave Mary with the possibility of a spiritual solution to her problem.

K.I.P: Can I ask another question?

MARY: Yes.

K.I.P: It seems to me that you have a great resource from your religious tradition that might help you see people as human beings, and I'm wondering where that fits in your life.

MARY: What's that?

K.I.P: Forgiveness.

MARY: *(another long pause)* I've never been very good at that.

K.I.P: Maybe that's something we could talk about.

MARY: Okay.

This was a key session for Mary. In sharing my own professional spiritual perspective, I encouraged a critical spiritual dialogue that led to important change. Within a short time, Mary was able to develop a more differentiated spiritual system for assessing people; where she once saw angels and devils, she now saw angels, devils, and human beings. She began to consider how she might show more compassion and forgiveness in her life to others as well as herself. And in this process she became visibly more relaxed and softer in appearance. The next time Mary met a man, she was able to remain in the relationship (even after his inevitable fall from the pedestal), work through their differences, and eventually marry.

In sum, few clients are willing to share the most intimate aspects of their lives in psychotherapy until the therapist has proven him- or herself trustworthy. This point holds true for spirituality, the most intimate dimension of life for many people. Therapists are most likely to receive an invitation into the client's world when they communicate their openness to learning and their openness to sharing. This openness sets the stage for spiritual dialogue and further spiritually integrated assessment.

INITIAL SPIRITUAL ASSESSMENT

The first session in therapy is generally the busiest. The therapist has to answer a host of questions in a short period of time. Why is the client seeking help? Why now? Are there any crises that require immediate attention? How has the client tried to deal with his or her problem in the past? What has worked before and what hasn't worked? What is the client's medical status? Does he or she use drugs or alcohol? What about family, friends, and work? Who provides the client with support and who makes matters worse? The idea of adding questions about spirituality to the already lengthy list of questions in the first session may sound anything but inviting.

From the outset, let me stress that the first session is not the time to do extensive interviewing or testing about spirituality. Think of spirituality as simply one more dimension that deserves some attention in the process of assessment. The therapist cannot afford to focus in too great detail on any single facet of the client's life in the first session, be it psychological, social, physical, or spiritual. But neither should any of these dimensions be overlooked. Every clinical intake, I believe, should include an initial spiritual assessment.

Initial spiritual assessment takes the form of a few basic questions that address four important areas: the salience of spirituality to the client, the salience of a religious affiliation or community to the client, the salience of spirituality to the problem, and the salience of spirituality to the solution (see Table 10.1). The first set of questions is: Do you see yourself as a religious or spiritual person? If so, in what way? Clients' responses will provide some inkling of whether they see their lives through a sacred lens and whether they will be comfortable addressing sacred matters in treatment. In addition, their responses may shed some light on clients' preferred spiritual pathways and spiritual destinations—that is, whether spirituality is primar-

---

TABLE 10.1. Questions in the Initial Spiritual Assessment

- The salience of spirituality to the client
  Do you see yourself as a religious or spiritual person? If so, in what way?
- The salience of a religious affiliation to the client
  Are you affiliated with a religious or spiritual denomination or community? If so, which one?
- The salience of spirituality to the problem
  Has your problem affected you religiously or spiritually? If so, in what way?
- The salience of spirituality to the solution
  Has your religion or spirituality been involved in the way you have coped with your problem? If so, in what way?

ily a way of thinking, feeling, acting, relating, or coping, and what they hold sacred in their lives.

The second pair of questions is: Are you affiliated with a religious or spiritual denomination or community? If so, which one? For most people in the United States, spirituality is nested within a particular religious context. It is important for the clinician to learn whether the client sees his or her life through the larger lens of a specific religious institution. Of course, a growing number of people do not moor themselves to a religious tradition. Nevertheless, it is equally important to learn whether the client has left a religious community. As I have stressed throughout this book, spirituality is always affected by a larger religious context, be it one that the client has accepted or one that he or she has rejected. The client's response to this pair of questions will help alert the clinician to the spiritual pathways and destinations that are a part of the client's world as well as those that are alien to it.

The third pair of questions is: Has your problem affected you religiously or spiritually? If so, in what way? These questions offer initial insight into whether the client conceptualizes the problem in spiritual terms. Perhaps the problem is perceived to be a spiritual threat or loss, or a violation of the sacred. These questions can also open the door to a discussion of the *spiritual* impact of a psychological problem. And these questions can elicit the first reports of spiritual struggle by the client. Table 10.2 presents some illustrations of spiritual struggles reported by clients. As I noted earlier, people who voice these kinds of struggles are at greater risk for psychological and physical problems, including greater risk of mortality (Fitchett et al., 1999; Pargament et al., 1998, 2000). However, spiritual struggles may also represent a step in the direction of valuable transformation. More extensive spiritual assessment is needed to determine whether these signs of struggle are leading the individual toward spiritual integration or dis-integration.

The final pair of questions is: Has your religion or spirituality been involved in the way you have dealt with your problem? If so, in what way? The answer to these questions will indicate whether spirituality may be a potential resource in the problem-solving process. It may also provide early insights into the specific pathways clients take in their search for the sacred as well as the pathways the clients have overlooked. Both types of information resources may prove to be helpful in treatment. Table 10.3 presents some of the spiritual resources clients describe in response to these questions. Once again, these responses offer only a first glimpse into the place of spirituality in the client's world.

The therapist should not separate these initial questions about spirituality from other questions in the first session. The process of assessment goes more smoothly when these spiritual questions are integrated into the flow of conversation. For instance, the first and second pairs of questions

TABLE 10.2. Signs of Spiritual Struggle

Divine struggles

- *I feel like I am being punished by God.*
- *I feel angry with God for what has happened.*
- *I feel like God has abandoned me.*
- *I wonder whether God really loves me.*
- *I wonder whether the devil has anything to do with this situation.*
- *I feel I have let God down.*

Intrapsychic struggles

- *I am having doubts about my faith.*
- *I am not sure what I really believe anymore.*
- *I know what's right but I keep doing what's wrong.*
- *I don't know why I am alive.*
- *I feel guilty about the way I think, feel, or act.*

Interpersonal struggles

- *I feel my church has abandoned me.*
- *I disagree with what my church wants me to believe.*
- *I disagree with family or friends about spiritual matters.*
- *I feel like family or friends are spiritual hypocrites.*
- *I argue with family or friends about whose side God is really on.*
- *I hope God will have his vengeance on the people who hurt me.*

on the personal salience of spirituality and religious affiliation can be broached in the context of other questions regarding the client's roles and identity, such as his or her status in the family, occupation, and dreams for the future. The third pair of questions on the salience of spirituality to the client's problems flows nicely out of the larger question about the impact of these problems on the client, psychologically, socially, and physically. The fourth pair of questions on spiritual coping follows easily from the general question of how the individual has tried to deal with his or her problems. Of course, it may become apparent early on that the client is not religiously or spiritually involved. In these cases, it is not necessary to ask all four pairs of questions.

Let me give an example from one particularly memorable first session. Tim, a 23-year-old college student, came to therapy after a horrific accident. Several months earlier, he had had too much to drink one night, fallen asleep while smoking, and set his bedroom and himself on fire. Although Tim was severely burned, his roommate was able to rush him to the hospital in time to save his life. Tim was terribly scarred and disfigured, particularly on his face; one eye had been fused shut, his nose appeared to have melted away, and he had only the smallest hole for a mouth. On top of all that, he was being fed through a tube, spoke with great difficulty, and was

TABLE 10.3. Signs of Spiritual Resources

The pathway of knowing

- *I study the Bible or other sacred texts.*
- *I try to learn more about my faith.*
- *I watch religious television.*
- *I read books to grow spiritually.*
- *I take religious or spiritual classes.*
- *I am guided by my religious beliefs.*

The pathway of acting

- *I try to live morally and ethically.*
- *I treat my life as sacred.*
- *I engage in activities that I would call spiritual (e.g., walking, knitting, cooking).*
- *I engage in regular religious rituals (e.g., prayer before meals, lighting candles on Sabbath).*
- *I try to be less sinful.*
- *I meditate regularly.*
- *I pray regularly.*

The pathway of relating

- *I am part of a spiritual community (e.g., church, synagogue, mosque, temple).*
- *I turn to my pastor for help.*
- *I participate in spiritual groups (e.g., prayer groups, meditation groups).*
- *I feel a spiritual connection with people in my life (e.g., family, friends).*
- *I treat other people as sacred.*
- *I try to make the world a better place.*
- *I feel a spiritual connection with people who have died.*

The pathway of experience

- *I feel connected to something larger than myself when I meditate.*
- *I am able to detach myself from everyday concerns when I pray or meditate.*
- *I feel close to God when I pray.*
- *I have spiritual experiences everyday.*
- *I see life as sacred.*
- *I experience the sacred in many ways (e.g., music, nature).*

The pathway of coping

- *I look to God for strength, support, and guidance.*
- *I try to find the lesson from God in the problems I experience.*
- *I do what I can and put the rest in God's hands.*
- *I work together with God as partners in problem solving.*
- *I ask for forgiveness for my sins.*
- *I try to give spiritual strength to other people.*
- *I seek a new higher purpose in life.*
- *I try to build a stronger relationship with a higher power.*

facing a series of painful surgeries over the next few years. How, I wondered, would he ever be able to recover from this trauma, not only physically but psychologically and socially? How in the world would I be able to help this man when it was difficult even to look at him?

Tim made it relatively easy for me. I asked him how he was dealing with his situation and Tim responded immediately and enthusiastically. He spoke about his "good luck" in being discovered by his roommate in time to save his life. He focused on the fact that one of his eyes was undamaged, that there were no signs of neurological impairment, that his appearance would improve with plastic surgery. In short, Tim was grateful to be alive and hopeful about his life. As best I could tell, he was not denying the problems in store for him. He was able to talk about the horrified looks he was receiving from other people, the painful surgeries that lay ahead, and his uncertainty about his future.

Raising the topic of spirituality felt neither awkward nor out of place. Rather, it seemed only appropriate to ask Tim how religion or spirituality was involved in his coping. Again, he answered without hesitation. God, he said, had given him a "new lease on life," an opportunity to replace the empty life he had been living with a life devoted to something more meaningful. With that knowledge, he felt he would be able to handle anything that came his way. We spent a few more minutes talking about the place of religion and spirituality in Tim's life, including the support he was receiving from the clergyman and members of his small Lutheran church, but this was only the first session and I was only beginning to learn about Tim, his life before the accident, and his spirituality. Nevertheless, it was clear to me that spirituality was playing a central role in the coping process, helping Tim not only to sustain himself through this tragedy, but also to transform his life in totally new directions. It was also clear to me that spirituality would likely become a vital part of the psychotherapy process.

Spiritual assessment begins with the first session, but it does not end there. Like assessment in general, spiritual assessment is an ongoing part of psychotherapy. Throughout the course of treatment, the therapist assesses, forms a plan of action, implements the plan, reassesses how well the plan has worked, forms and implements a modified plan, reassesses, and so on. Thus, spiritual assessment is not restricted to the first session. That is only a start. At times, it might be quite obvious by the end of the first session that spirituality is a significant part of the individual's life, problem, or solution to the problem (as in the case of Tim), but spiritual assessment does not stop there, for a more thorough evaluation of spirituality is still required. The focus must shift to a process of more explicit and more extensive assessment. At other times, however, the initial assessment may suggest that spirituality is not relevant to the case. Even here, though, the process of spiritual assessment does not come to a close. Recall once again the story of Alice from Chapter 1. Some clients, like Alice, are unwilling to disclose such personal information until they develop a more trusting relationship with the therapist. Other clients are simply unaware of the significance of spirituality in their lives. Not until later in treatment may spirituality emerge as a salient factor. It follows that the therapist must remain alert to the potential significance of spirituality for even the most avowedly nonspiritual client. One way to determine whether there may be underlying and undetected spiritual issues that deserve consideration in treatment is to conduct an implicit spiritual assessment.

IMPLICIT SPIRITUAL ASSESSMENT

Most clinicians have clients they dread seeing. Joe was mine. There was no good reason for my dread except that Joe was very boring. A 39-year-old accountant, Joe was of average build, average appearance, and average disposition. In fact, everything about Joe seemed to be average. He had come to therapy a few months earlier complaining about depression. Though he had a stable job and marriage, he felt as if he were just going through the motions. There were no highs or lows in Joe's life. His days were marked by a sameness and a grayness that left him feeling as if he were living in a perpetual fog. Over the past 15 years, he had tried antidepressants, different forms of therapy, meditation, reading, and exercise, but nothing had altered the dreariness of his life. I went through my own litany of therapeutic activities in an effort to help him generate a spark in his life, to no avail. The sessions were mirroring his life. "How did your week go, Joe?," I would ask, trying to inject some enthusiasm in my voice. "SOS, same old stuff," Joe would invariably reply in a monotonically average voice. Yet, in spite of our lack of progress, Joe came like clockwork to his therapy sessions. Though I tried to attend to the real meaning of SOS (the universal distress signal) to remind myself that here was a man in pain, I came to dread seeing Joe, the man I had labeled "My Boring Client."

One day, feeling sleepy, ineffective, and rather desperate, I asked Joe, "Have you ever had a time in your life when you felt deeply and fully alive?" Joe paused to consider. I awaited what I assumed would be another lifeless response. Instead, Joe answered, "Well, there was the time in college when I flew jets." I almost jumped out of my skin. "You flew jets, Joe?," I shouted. "Well, tell me about it." It seems that Joe's parents had given him flying lessons for his 21st birthday. He loved the experience and spent his free time in his college years flying and qualifying for more and more technically sophisticated planes. "Joe," I said, "I never knew you were a pilot. What was it like to fly a jet?" "It was unbelievable," he said. "That sensation of power taking off. Never knowing quite what to expect. Feeling like I was testing myself. And the experience of flying—racing through the clouds, a speck in the skies. Man, I was in Heaven, soaring with the angels. I told you I'm not a religious man, but if there's a God, well, that's the closest I've come to Him." This was not the Joe I knew. Eyes bright, voice animated, perched precariously on the edge of his seat, Joe had transformed himself from My Boring Client to an incredibly interesting guy.

"Have you ever had a time in your life when you felt deeply and fully alive?" My question had helped uncover a sacred spark in Joe that had been hidden for many years. Now the question was whether Joe could fan that spark into a flame. "Why did you stop flying?," I asked Joe. "Oh, I moved away, got a job, things came up, you know," he responded. "But, Joe," I exclaimed, "When you talked about flying just now, you came to life. You took off in here." With a very unaverage, embarrassed grin, Joe admitted, "Yeah, it did feel good." "Well," I told him, "Our time's almost up, but I want to leave you with a question I'd like you to think about. How about flying again?" For the first time, I was sorry to see a session with Joe come to a close.

Flying became the focus of our subsequent sessions, not only flying airplanes, but "flying" in other areas of his life. Using this potent metaphor, we talked about ways Joe could take the skills and qualities of a pilot—mastery, planning, self-confidence, courage, an adventurous spirit—and apply them to his job, his relationships, and his life more generally. And Joe did "take off." He began to fly airplanes once again and he began to approach his life with a new enthusiasm.

Nothing in my initial assessment of Joe had suggested that spirituality would be a relevant part of his case. While other clients wait to disclose spiritual material until they have established a trusting relationship with their therapists, Joe was not holding back. Like many others, he had never made the connection between his situation in life and his spirituality. Spirituality emerged as an important concern not by hitting Joe over the head with questions about God, the church, or prayer, but by a more implicit, indirect effort to reveal a deeper, spiritual dimension to his life.

An implicit spiritual assessment is made up of two vital ingredients. First, the clinician raises questions that hint at the possibility of a deeper dimension for the client. Table 10.4 contains several illustrations of implicit spiritual questions that I have found useful over the years to assess the client's resources, destinations, and struggles and transformation. A number of these questions have been drawn or adapted from the excellent book by James Griffith and Melissa Griffith (2002) entitled *Encountering the Sacred in Psychotherapy: How to Talk with People about Their Spiritual Lives.* As you can see, the questions do not refer directly to higher powers, religious institutions, or religious practices. Instead, they make use of "psychospiritual language," psychologically meaningful concepts carrying rich, emotionally powerful connotations that invite spiritual exploration. Em-

TABLE 10.4. Questions for the Implicit Spiritual Assessment

Resources and pathways

- *From what sources do you draw the strength and courage to go on?*[a]
- *Where do you find peace?*[a]
- *Who truly understands your situation?*[a]
- *When you are afraid or in pain, how do you find comfort and solace?*[a]
- *For what are you deeply grateful?*[a]
- *What sustains you in the midst of your troubles?*

Destinations

- *What are you striving for in your life?*
- *Why is it important that you are here in this world?*[a]
- *What legacy would you like to leave behind in your life?*
- *How would you like people to remember you when you are gone?*
- *To what or whom are you most devoted?*[a]
- *Who is your true self?*
- *Who or what do you put your faith and hope in?*
- *To whom, or what, do you most freely express love?*[a]
- *When have you felt most deeply and fully alive?*

Struggles and transformation

- *What are the deepest questions your situation has raised for you?*
- *What causes you the greatest despair and suffering?*
- *How has this experience changed you at your deepest levels?*
- *What have you discovered about yourself that you find most disturbing?*
- *How has this situation shaken your faith?*
- *What has this experience taught you that you wish you had never known?*
- *What are your deepest regrets?*
- *What would you like to be able to let go of in your life?*
- *When in your life have you experienced forgiveness?*

[a]Drawn or adapted from Griffith and Griffith (2002).

bedded in the psychospiritual questions are words that contain sacred qualities, such as "peace," "courage," "solace," "sustenance," "devotion," "faith," "hope," "love," "letting go," "forgiveness," "regrets," "despair," and "suffering." Even though none of these terms is explicitly religious, some clinicians may find these kinds of inquiries unscientific and merely sentimental. It is true that the questions depart from the traditional, clinical, linear, no-nonsense language of practitioners. It is also true that some clients will not respond to these questions. But the language does resonate for other clients, like Joe, whose search for the sacred may be taking place beneath the surface of their own awareness. And they may respond to these psychospiritual questions with spiritual language of their own.

Clinicians should be sensitive to spiritual responses from their clients. In essence, practitioners must turn on their "spiritual radars." This is the second vital ingredient of an implicit spiritual assessment. With their spiritual radars on, clinicians are attuned to several signs of spirituality. First, they listen for their client's spiritual or psychospiritual language. For instance, for Joe, flying was a spiritual experience: he was a speck in vast skies, soaring with the angels, and as close to God as he would ever be on earth. Other clients will speak in psychospiritual terms of their own that open the door to further spiritual exploration. Along these lines, Nash (1990) encourages clinicians to listen for psychospiritual language, "major polarities," that point to deeper spiritual struggles. These include the contrasts between brokenness and wholeness, curse and blessing, foolishness and wisdom, bondage and freedom, revenge and mercy, arrogance and humility, and faithlessness and faithfulness. Second, therapists attend to changes in the atmosphere of the room. My first hint of something spiritual in my work with Karen, the depressed woman described earlier in this chapter, came when she looked out the window and, for the first time, smiled and giggled as she watched some squirrels at play. As it rises to the surface, spiritual material can elicit a variety of emotions: pleasure, solemnity, awe, profound sorrow, terrible fear, gripping excitement. It does not, however, elicit boredom. Third, with their spiritual radars on, clinicians are alert to "spiritual-like" processes, processes that parallel spiritual practices, relations, beliefs, or experiences. For instance, in the last chapter, I noted how Yalom's client, Thelma, was treating her former therapist and lover as if he was a god. Similarly, Schreurs (2002) notes that "one may hear in other people's anger their disappointment about the general injustice of life, indicating that even though they do not believe in God, they deep down still relate to life itself as if it were a supreme judge who should administer justice but neglects to do so" (p. 121). Finally, therapists are sensitive to the sacred qualities their clients may project onto them (Pattison, 1982). Earlier I noted that when my client Mary told me that I was the best therapist she had ever worked with, I knew my time with her was limited. I was becoming one more "angel" in her life. Unless I was able to help her develop a more differentiated spiritual view, I would shortly become one more "devil" to be rejected in the search for a true and perfect God.

Through the process of implicit spiritual assessment, the therapist offers the client an opportunity to explore the spiritual domain. To the client who may have been reluctant to broach the topic of spirituality, the implicit spiritual assessment may represent a welcome invitation to enter into a spiritual conversation. To the client whose life has been shaped by the spiritual dimension in unrecognized ways, the implicit spiritual assessment may be the first step in revealing the character of this domain. Of course, implicit spiritual assessments do not inevitably point to the salience of spirituality for psychotherapy. Oftentimes, they do, however. And in some instances, as was the case with Joe, they are critical to therapeutic change.

CONCLUSIONS

Setting the stage for spiritual dialogue and conducting an initial and implicit spiritual assessment are critical steps in the process of getting to know the client spiritually. Important as they are, however, they cannot yield rich, detailed information about spirituality and the degree to which it is well integrated or poorly integrated in the client's life. For that, a more explicit and extensive spiritual assessment is required. In the following chapter, we turn our attention to the process of explicit spiritual assessment.

11

Explicit Spiritual Assessment

When conducting an explicit spiritual assessment, the clinician focuses directly and extensively on the place of spirituality in the client's life. In what ways does spirituality contribute to the client's problems? In what ways could spirituality be a part of the solution? These are the most critical questions for the clinician. At first glance, they might appear to be relatively easy to answer. A survey or a few simple questions would seem to be all that are needed. But, as I have noted, spirituality is a rich, multidimensional process. No single spiritual belief, practice, or experience can hold the key to the search for the sacred. Whether spirituality is a part of the client's problem or part of the solution will depend instead on the degree to which the individual has integrated the varied elements of spirituality into a coherent whole.

Like spirituality itself, then, the process of explicit spiritual assessment is multifaceted. It rests on a clear, evaluative framework for the clinician, multiple assessment methods, and sound clinical judgment.

THE EVALUATIVE FRAMEWORK FOR THE CLINICIAN

Without a framework for understanding and evaluating spirituality, the practitioner is likely to find him- or herself lost when working with spiritual issues in therapy. For the clinician with a perspective in mind, though, spiritual assessment becomes manageable. Drawing on the understanding of spirituality that was presented in the first half of this book, I have summarized several important sets of evaluative questions (see Table 11.1) the clinician should ask him- or herself as he or she tries to place the client's

TABLE 11.1. Evaluative Framework for the Clinician to Guide the Spiritual Assessment

1. Locating the client in the search for the sacred
   a. Is the client in a conservational mode?
   b. Is the client going through a spiritual struggle?
   c. Is the client experiencing a spiritual transformation?
   d. Is the client spiritually disengaged?
   e. Is the client rediscovering the sacred?

2. Spiritual integration in the destinations
   a. How does the client envision the sacred?
      i. Is the client's representation of the sacred large enough to encompass the full range of life experiences, or is it constricted?
      ii. Is the client's representation of the sacred benevolent or malevolent?
      iii. Does the client recognize the limits in his or her understanding of the divine, or does the client confuse representations of the divine with the divine itself (i.e., idolatry)?
      iv. Does the client accept his or her darker side or project these qualities onto demonic forces in others?
      v. Do the client's various understandings of the sacred blend together or do they clash with each other?
      vi. Is the client aware or unaware of the place of the sacred in his or her life?
   b. Where does the sacred fit into the client's strivings?
      i. Is the client engaged or disengaged in the search for the sacred?
      ii. Is the sacred central or peripheral to the client's strivings?
      iii. Is the client's spiritual motivation internally based or externally based (e.g., guilt, social pressure)?

3. Spiritual integration in the pathways
   a. How broad and deep are the client's spiritual pathways?
      i. Does the client integrate the spiritual pathways into his or her life or does he or she compartmentalize them?
      ii. Does the client take a number of spiritual paths or follow one spiritual pathway to the exclusion of others?
      iii. Does the client have a long or a short history of spiritual involvement?
      iv. Is the client disciplined or undisciplined in following the spiritual pathways?
      v. Is the client's relationship with the sacred secure or insecure (e.g., anxious, hostile, self-degrading)?
      vi. Is the client aware or unaware of the spiritual pathways he or she is taking?
      vii. Is the client familiar or unfamiliar with the variety of spiritual pathways that are available to him or her?
   b. How flexible are the client's spiritual pathways?
      i. Is the client flexible or inflexible in selecting and following the spiritual pathways?
      ii. Is the client working through or stuck in his or her spiritual struggles?
   c. How well do the client's spiritual pathways fit with the problem, destination, and social context?
      i. Are the client's spiritual pathways appropriate to the destination or too extreme?
      ii. Is the client spiritually authentic or hypocritical?

TABLE 11.1. (*continued*)

    iii. Are the client's spiritual pathways appropriate or inappropriate to the problem?
    iv. Is the client embedded in a spiritually benevolent or malevolent context?
    v. Does the client experience spiritual support or spiritual conflict with others?

4. Spiritual efficacy
  a. How comfortable is the client with his or her spirituality?
    i. Does the client experience spiritual comfort or spiritual distress?
    ii. Does the client feel he or she is growing or declining spiritually?
    iii. Does the client feel that spirituality is a part of the solution to his or her problems or a part of the problem?
  b. How does the client's spirituality affect his or her life?
    i. Does the client's spirituality lead to connection with or disconnection from the sacred?
    ii. Does the client's spirituality increase or decrease his or her health and well-being?
    iii. Does the client's spirituality enhance or detract from the well-being of others?
    iv. Does the client's spirituality lead to benefits in many areas of life or are some of the benefits accompanied by costs for the client or those in his or her life?

5. The place of spirituality in treatment
  a. Is spirituality a part of the solution or a part of the problem?
  b. What spiritual resources can the client draw on in therapy?
  c. What spiritual problems should the client address in therapy?
  d. What spiritual obstacles are likely to arise in treatment?

---

particular spiritual story into the larger spiritual framework. Admittedly, these evaluative questions are complex, but it is important to stress that they are not questions to be asked directly of the client. Rather, they are designed to orient and guide the clinician's own thinking through the process of explicit spiritual assessment.

Let me briefly review these guiding sets of questions. First, the clinician should locate where the client is in the search for the sacred. For example, some clients come to therapy in the midst of a spiritual struggle and potential transformation. Others enter therapy with a spirituality that has been stable and sustaining to them for much of their lives. Still others come to therapy spiritually disengaged, but in the process of rediscovery. Second, the clinician assesses the degree to which the client's spirituality is well integrated. To that end, it is important to consider several aspects of the client's spiritual destination and pathways: the client's vision of the sacred; the place of the sacred in the client's strivings; the breadth, depth, and flexibility of the client's pathways; and the fit between the client's pathways with his or her destinations, problem, and social context. Third, the clinician should be able to evaluate the efficacy of the client's spirituality, including his or her level of spiritual comfort and the degree to which spirituality leads to valuable outcomes. Finally, the clinician should come away from the assessment process with a sense of the role spirituality can play in therapy, how it might be a part of the problem, how it might be part of the solution, and how it should be addressed in treatment.

GATHERING INFORMATION ABOUT SPIRITUALITY

How does the therapist gather the information that he or she needs to answer these questions about spirituality? The clinician gathers information in several ways: by eliciting the client's spiritual story, by attending to the client's nonverbal behavior, by collecting information from the client through the use of quantitative measures, and by placing the client in context.

Eliciting the Client's Spiritual Story

Many people find it hard to talk about spirituality. Thoughts, feelings, and actions in this realm of life seem elusive, and everyday language seems inadequate to the task of communication. Spirituality is, instead, best conveyed through narratives. For thousands of years, the world's greatest religious figures and their teachings have been passed down from generation to generation through epic accounts of people striving toward sacred ends. These stories, filled as they are with images, symbols, and metaphors, point beyond themselves to deeper meanings and larger forces at play in the universe. Stories are also uniquely able to capture the drama that is played out in the search for the sacred. We hear of people trying to discover the sacred, attempting to hold on to the sacred in the face of threats and challenges, and struggling with their faith in ways that may lead either to powerful transformation or disengagement from the quest. Past, present, and future are all embedded in the client's spiritual narrative because it speaks to where the client has been, currently is, and plans to go. By eliciting the client's spiritual story, the clinician can also assess the degree to which spirituality is well integrated and efficacious, for stories vary both in their coherence and in their outcomes. In short, the best way to gather information for an explicit spiritual assessment is by eliciting the client's spiritual story.

Unfortunately, there is no simple way to elicit a spiritual story. The clinician who relies on a structured, invariant set of questions is more likely to interfere with the unfolding of the client's tale than to promote it. The story must grow out of the conversation of therapy. This is not to say that the therapist cannot encourage clients to share their accounts. Over the years, I have found a number of open-ended questions to be valuable in this regard (see Table 11.2). These questions prompt clients to tell their stories, but, more than that, they are designed to assess spirituality in its richness and

TABLE 11.2. Open-Ended Questions to Elicit the Client's Spiritual Story

Taking a history, taking a future

- *Describe the spiritual/religious tradition you grew up in. How did your family express its spirituality?[a]*
- *When did you first discover or learn about the sacred?*
- *How did you envision the sacred?*
- *What sort of spiritual experiences stood out for you when you were growing up?[a]*
- *How did you try to foster your relationship with the sacred when you were younger?*
- *Have you had periods in your life when you feel like you've lost the sacred?*
- *How has your understanding or experience of the sacred changed since you were a child?*
- *How have your spiritual practices and beliefs changed since you were a child?*
- *How would you describe your current spiritual orientation?[a]*
- *What do you see yourself striving for now and where does the sacred fit in?*
- *How do you see yourself changing spiritually in the future?*

Sacred destinations

- *Why do you think you're involved in spirituality?*
- *What do you hold sacred in your life?*
- *What do you feel God wants from you?*
- *When do you feel the presence of the sacred in your life most strongly?*
- *When do you feel the sacred is not there?*
- *What do you imagine that God feels when he sees you going through this difficult time?[b]*
- *How do you feel your problems have affected what God wants from you?*
- *Do you ever experience a different side of the sacred than what you are experiencing now? What is that like?[b]*
- *Do you ever have mixed thoughts and feelings about the sacred? What are they like?*

Sacred pathways

- *What has helped nurture your spirituality?*
- *What has been damaging to your spirituality?*
- *Who supports you spiritually? How so?*
- *Who does not support you spiritually? How so?*
- *What spiritual rituals or practices are especially important to you?*
- *What aspects of your spirituality are particularly uplifting?*
- *What spiritual beliefs do you find especially meaningful?[a]*
- *Where do you go to practice your spirituality or feel the presence of the sacred?[b]*
- *In what ways has your spirituality helped you understand or deal with your problems?*
- *In what ways has your spirituality been less helpful or even harmful in the ways you have tried to understand or deal with your problems?*
- *What gets in the way of your spirituality?*

(continued)

TABLE 11.2. (*continued*)

Spiritual efficacy

- *How has your spirituality changed your life for the better?*
- *How has your spirituality changed your life for the worse?*
- *In what ways do you feel you may have grown or failed to grow spiritually?*
- *To what degree has your spirituality given you pleasure? Meaning? A sense of connectedness to others? A sense of closeness with the divine? Hope for the future? Confidence in yourself? A feeling of being loved? Compassion for others?*
- *To what degree has your spirituality been a source of pain? Guilt? Anger? Confusion and doubt? Anxiety? Fear? Feelings of personal insignificance? Feelings of alienation from others?*

[a]Drawn or adapted from Hodge (2001).
[b]Drawn or adapted from Griffith and Griffith (2002).

depth. The questions go beyond a focus on the "what's" of spirituality (e.g., Do you believe in God, Do you pray, Do you meditate, Do you attend church) to the "why's," "where's," "when's," and "how's" of spirituality. These questions rest on some assumptions: that people may have mixed and conflicting experiences of the sacred; that people experience periods when the sacred is absent from their lives as well as periods when it is present; that spirituality can change a life for the better or for the worse; that it is as important to take a "spiritual future" as it is to take a spiritual history. Again, it is important to stress that the open-ended questions and probes in Table 11.2 should not be used as a structured interview. Instead, they should be freely adapted to each client and interwoven into the clinical conversation and larger life story of the client. Consider the following example.

Eliciting the Spiritual Story of Agnes

"So, tell me," I asked Agnes, "how did you lose your soul?" This is not the first question that usually comes to mind when I am conducting a spiritual assessment, but it seemed fitting for this client. Agnes had come to my office a few months earlier. A tall, thin, 50-year-old woman, dressed in a severe black skirt and grey blouse, she reminded me of a schoolmarm or a former nun perhaps, sitting so perfectly erect that her back never touched the chair, enunciating each carefully chosen word with precision. With her hair pulled back tightly off of her face, there was a tautness and brittleness about her. Agnes was seeing me after a stay in an inpatient psychiatric unit. She had voluntarily committed herself to the hospital one evening after she and her husband, Peter, had finished doing the dishes. Walking behind him with a kitchen knife in hand, she told him matter-of-factly that she thought it would be best if he took her to the hospital. She was thinking of killing him or herself.

Over the next few weeks, I learned that Agnes had spent much of her adult life living in the shadow of her husband. A charismatic figure, active in charity work, and by all appearances a successful businessman, Peter was well known and respected in the community. Repeatedly, Agnes was reminded by family and friends how fortunate she was to be married to her spouse. Yet she herself seemed invisible, a person that others saw through as if she were made of cellophane. Once, she and her husband had accompanied another couple to a restaurant only to learn that the couple had made the reservation for three people, forgetting to include Agnes in the tally.

Only Agnes knew, though, that her husband was a terribly ineffectual businessman. Over the years, Peter had failed to generate new accounts, spent more time socializing than working, and made a number of poor decisions that had brought them to the brink of bankruptcy. Agnes was, in fact, keeping the business afloat, bringing in the lion's share of the business and attending to its day-to-day operation. Even so, her accomplishments were hidden from others, and she herself took little pleasure from them for she had little interest in the business. As she put it, "It's not what I want to be doing in life." Her remark led to an exchange in which I began to elicit Agnes's spiritual story:

K.I.P.: What is it you that you *would* like to do?

AGNES: I just don't know. I can't get any traction. There's nothing to grab hold of inside of me. I feel such an emptiness in my core. I feel soulless.

K.I.P.: So tell me, how did you lose your soul?

AGNES: I've often thought about that. I met Peter before I left for Europe to study the cello. Going to Europe was probably the most radical thing I had ever done. My parents discouraged me from going, telling me I could never support myself with music, and I had never been off on my own. But I won a scholarship to study music in Paris and I had a wonderful time. I was going to stay another year, but over the summer Peter proposed to me and said he wanted me to come home to be with him. I hesitated. My parents wanted me to return too. On top of that, they were charmed by Peter and reminded me that I wasn't much in the looks department. Oh, and of course I wasn't getting any younger. I left my music and came home to Peter.

K.I.P.: You stopped playing the cello?

AGNES: Yes. (*long pause and deep sigh*) It's funny. Even though music was the heart and soul of my life, I didn't miss it at first. You have to understand that I adored Peter. He was utterly beguiling and I was incredulous that this fascinating man would have any interest in me. I worshipped him.

K.I.P.: How did you worship him?

AGNES: I just put everything else aside. My art, my music and I devoted myself to him. Whatever Peter wanted, I supported. Wherever he went, I followed. I made allowances for him. I covered for him. I allowed him to live the life he wanted to live.

K.I.P.: And what about you? Did you have other objects of devotion in your life?

AGNES: No, I gave everything to him . . . (*pause*). And he took it all, without even a thank-you.

K.I.P.: You feel like he took your soul?

AGNES: (*pause*) Maybe, but I was complicit in it. I was willing to give it up, to sacrifice even my soul for him.

K.I.P.: We're talking about sacred matters here and I hate to stop, but we're coming to the end of our time today. I'd like to leave you with a question to consider for our next session. You said that you feel soulless. Here's the question. Have you lost your soul or have you lost touch with your soul?

[Next session.]

AGNES: Well, I thought about your question. Actually, I thought about it quite a bit. My first reaction was that I've lost my soul completely, but I am wondering now whether there might be a little of me left inside. I used to think of my soul as a lantern, lighting my way in life, but for a long time I felt that the light had died out. Now I wonder whether there might be a little flicker of light left.

K.I.P.: Are there times when you feel a bit of warmth from the light?

AGNES: Yes, I notice that there are times when I feel something stir inside of me.

K.I.P.: When does that happen?

AGNES: Oh, when I listen to a piece of music, go to an art museum, or lose myself in poetry. I've never been beautiful on the outside, but something inside of me has always been receptive to beauty.

K.I.P.: And that part of you is your soul?

AGNES: I think so. You see, God to me is all about creation and beauty. Those are the things that are truly immortal. I used to be able to create beautiful things. I don't do that anymore, but I can still appreciate beautiful things and that's the closest I can come to God.

Eliciting Agnes's spiritual story was not difficult. It flowed directly out of her larger life story. My questions were designed not to bracket spiritual matters from the dialogue of therapy, but rather to encourage spiritual conversation in the context of her problems, life history, social relationships, and vision of herself. Thus, my queries and comments were tailored to Agnes; it is doubtful that I would ever pose precisely these same questions to another client. But the questions served their purpose. They helped draw out Agnes's spiritual narrative, yielding important information for an explicit spiritual assessment.

What was I beginning to learn? Agnes was suffering not only emotionally, in the form of a major depressive disorder, but spiritually as well. In terms of the major categories of guiding questions in Table 11.1, I was struck first by the signs of spiritual dis-integration in destinations and pathways of Agnes's life. She had given up a spiritual pursuit, her love for the cello, to devote her life to the worship of her husband. As charming as he was, Peter could not bear the weight of the sacred. He was painfully human, unable to care for Agnes financially, emotionally, or spiritually. Family members were equally unsupportive in her spiritual journey. Agnes's spiritual pathways were narrow and constricted. For years, she had sacrificed her own dreams to advance those of her husband. In the process, she had become a gaunt shadow figure, unknown to others, unknown to herself, unable to nourish herself spiritually. With respect to the guiding question of spiritual efficacy in Table 11.1, it was clear that spirituality for Agnes had become increasingly destructive. As she grew more aware of her poor choice in gods and the high price she had paid in her own life, she began to teeter on the edge of spiritual extremism. She came close to killing Peter, the idol who had accepted her sacrifices and failed to care for her in return. And she came uncomfortably close to killing herself, in part for her foolishness and in part to put an end to the emptiness she felt inside.

Clearly, spirituality was an important part of Agnes's problem, but there were signs that it might be part of the solution too. Agnes was spiritually flexible, open to exploring other sources of sacredness in her life. Perhaps she hadn't lost her soul, but had simply lost touch with it. She was able to identify a source of light and warmth within herself, her lantern. And she was beginning to broaden and deepen her approach to the sacred. Through her appreciation of creativity and beauty, she might turn up the light in the lantern from a flicker to a flame. Through my explicit spiritual assessment, I was able to locate where Agnes was in her search for the sacred and consider the role spirituality might play in treatment. I concluded that Agnes was emerging from a long period of deep spiritual struggle and entering a period of spiritual transformation. I saw her moving from a false god to a more authentic sense of her own spirituality and from self-derogation to more fulfilling ways to nurture her soul. She had little external support for the spiritual steps she was beginning to take, but I could offer her some of that in therapy. Facilitating Agnes's transformation toward a more fully integrated and effective spirituality would become a central part of our work together in therapy.

Attending to the Nonverbal

There is more to explicit spiritual assessment than asking questions and listening for answers. Because spirituality is difficult to put into words and because people may be unaware of the part spirituality is playing in their lives, the clinician must look beyond what is said to what is not said, the feelings that are conveyed, and the congruence between words, feelings, and actions.

Attending to What Is Not Being Said

In Chapter 10, I talked about a woman, Mary, who placed her romantic partners on a pedestal, only to see them fall and shatter her dreams. God, as she understood him, expected people to make the most of their gifts and emulate the life of Jesus. Mary expected no less of the men in her life. As I noted earlier, Mary suffered from an undifferentiated spiritual perspective. She could see only two types of men: angels and devils. But my assessment of Mary's problem came less from what she was saying (she expected people to live up to high spiritual standards), and more from what she was not saying. Although Mary could talk about angels and devils, she did not have a way to talk about humanness, a way of coming to terms with human frailty that could lend some balance and compassion to her high standards. Mary could also admit that she was unfamiliar with the language of forgiveness. "I've never been very good at that," she said when I broached the topic with her. It turned out that the key to Mary's clinical progress lay in what was not being talked about. The same point often applies to other cases. Thus, it is important for the clinician to "listen" to what is not being said in the explicit clinical assessment: the kind of God who is not there for the person, the spiritual pathways the individual is not taking, the ways in which the sacred is not integrated into the individual's life, and the satisfactions the individual is missing from his or her spirituality.

Attending to Emotions

Spirituality is as much felt and experienced as it is understood and practiced. In the search for the sacred, people encounter the full range of emotions, positive and negative: peacefulness, gratitude, excitement, joy, awe, anger, sadness, fear, jealousy, and shame. These emotions often contain important clues about the client's spiritual status. For example, sadness or anger can hint at sacred loss or violation; excitement and joy can point to sources of sacredness; peacefulness and calm can suggest powerful spiritual resources. Conversely, the absence of emotion often suggests spiritual disengagement. To repeat a point I made earlier, spirituality can be many things, but it is never boring.

Negative experiences and emotions are especially important to consider. They have tremendous potency in people's lives, even greater potency, some have argued, than positive experiences. Paul Rozin and Edward Royzman (2001) offer this graphic illustration: "Brief contact with a cockroach will usually render a delicious meal inedible. The inverse phenomenon— rendering a pile of cockroaches on a platter edible by contact with one's favorite food—is unheard of" (p. 296). Negative experiences and emotion are no less powerful in the spiritual domain. A single negative encounter in a church can undo years of supportive and sustaining interactions with fellow church members and clergy. One moral infraction, such as an extramarital affair, can topple what had once been a strong and stable marriage. Though it takes years to become "holy" or "saintly," according to most religious traditions, it takes only a few sins to compromise this status. It is far easier to pollute oneself than to purify oneself, Rozin and Royzman note.

Consistent with these assertions, our research studies have shown that positive spiritual experiences and emotions far outnumber negative ones. Nonetheless, infrequent as they are, negative experiences are often the more powerful predictor of physical and mental health. For instance, in our study of medically ill elderly patients, we found that the patients were far more likely to draw on positive forms of spiritual coping with their illnesses than voice any spiritual struggles (Pargament et al., 2001). Yet reports of spiritual struggle were tied to significantly greater risk of dying over the next two years and these effects were not offset by positive religious coping.

There is an important practical message in these findings. Clinicians must pay close attention to signs of spiritual struggle and emotional distress in the spiritual arena. The signs may be subtle, for many people feel shame and guilt about their spiritual conflicts or fear that their conflicts would meet with disapproval from others (Exline & Martin, 2005). Nevertheless, signs of struggle may hold a great deal of significance for the client's health and well-being. This is not to say that spiritual struggles are necessarily problematic. As I have stressed in this book, spiritual struggles can also be a prelude to spiritual growth and development. During the process of explicit spiritual assessment, the clinician should delve more deeply into signs of spiritual distress to determine whether the client is stuck in these struggles or working through them.

Attending to the Incongruous

A few years ago, I saw a man in therapy who was quite upset that his wife was planning to leave him after 35 years of marriage. He admitted that he had been emotionally abusive to her for much of their marriage, but he wanted me to help talk her into staying. I told him I couldn't do that, but that I would be willing to help him share his feelings with his wife if she were willing to come in for a session. The wife agreed. My client took full advantage of the session by trotting out a list of reasons why she should stay with him: he still loved her and would change his ways, the divorce would hurt their children and grandchildren, the divorce would be costly, and they would lose many of their lifelong friends. But none of these arguments was convincing to his wife, who sat unmoved through his entreaties. Finally, he told his wife, a long-time churchgoer, that he was most worried about her spirituality. "We pledged our eternal love to each other before God," he said, "and now you are breaking that vow. That vow means something to me even if it means so little to you." He then added, "I'm just concerned about your soul."

The words and the feeling behind the words didn't add up to me. My client seemed to be speaking more out of anger and desperation than husbandly concern. Lurking beneath the surface appeared to be a final and perhaps ultimate threat that to leave him would endanger his wife's soul. So I asked his wife whether she could feel her husband's concern for her spiritual well-being. She was blunt in her response to her husband's insincerity. "No," she answered, "he's just pulling out all the plugs now. He's still trying to control me. He never had much interest in religion before now. I could never get him to go to church. And now he's telling me he's worried about my soul? I don't think so." At that point, there was a quiet in the room and my client visibly sagged in the chair. With a defeated look, he spoke more honestly: "I'm sorry. I don't know what I'm doing. I just get so frightened about you leaving that I'll do anything to get you back." Painful as it was, this session helped my client face the reality that his marriage was indeed over.

As important as words are, they do not always tell the full story. There are instances in which people purposely use their spirituality to achieve destructive ends, such as the pedophile who enters the ministry to gain easier access to potential victims or the televangelist who schemes to bilk people of their savings. More often than not, though, people are simply unaware of the part that spirituality is playing in their lives. In this case, for instance, I don't believe the husband was conscious of how he was using the language of spirituality to coerce his wife back into the marriage. But the inconsistency between his words and feelings made clear to me and, more importantly, made clear to his wife that his spiritual concerns were less than genuine. In the process of explicit spiritual assessment, the clinician must not only attend to what is said and what is felt, but also to the congruity between words, actions, and feelings.

Gathering Spiritual Information Quantitatively

Whether eliciting spiritual stories, attending to nonverbal behavior, or evaluating the degree to which spirituality is well integrated and efficacious, the process of explicit spiritual assessment is not a totally objective business. As a result, there is a danger of bias and loss of perspective on the part of the therapist. What is to prevent the clinician from seeing only that which aligns with or fails to align with his or her own spiritual mind-set? More generally, what is to prevent the clinician from reaching faulty conclusions? One potential check on the clinician's own biases and preconceptions could come from quantitative information about the client's spiritual life. In the best of all worlds, the practitioner would be able to draw on well-established measures of spiritual integration and well-being and compare the client's level of spiritual functioning to that of an appropriate normative sample. Instruments such as these could also provide another valuable perspective on the client's spiritual progress over the course of treatment. Not that these measures would replace other ways to gather spiritual information, but quantitative information could supplement what the clinician has learned through conversations with the client.

It is unfortunate that, until recently, most measures of spirituality have been quite limited in their clinical applicability (see Hill & Pargament, 2003). One problem comes from the fact that most of these measures have been developed and normed with theists, most specifically, Christians, in mind. Though most people in the United States are theists and Christian, many are not. Measures that use traditional theistic language (e.g., God, Supreme Being) are, at best, irrelevant and, at worst, offensive to those who see the sacred in less personal terms. The same point holds true when measures grounded in Christian language (e.g., "church," "born again," "Jesus Christ") and concepts (e.g., grace, sin) are applied to non-Christians. A second and perhaps even more important problem that limits the applicability of spiritual measures grows out of the simplicity of the scales themselves. Most measures of spirituality are descriptive in nature, addressing which denomination people belong to, whether they believe in God, how often they pray or attend church, or the degree to which they see themselves as religious or spiritual. Items such as these provide very little in the way of useful information to the clinician who is more interested in assessing spiritual integration, spiritual efficacy, and the ways in which spirituality may be a part of the client's problem or a part of the client's solution. For these reasons, quantitative measurement has not generally been integrated into spiritual assessment by most clinicians, myself included.

Recently, however, this picture has begun to change. Researchers and practitioners have developed a number of measures that have clinical promise. Some of these measures are illustrated in Table 11.3.[1] In contrast to global spiritual measures, these scales are designed to assess spirituality in

---

[1]This table includes only measures that are explicitly linked to the sacred. Thus, although researchers and practitioners have developed a number of measures of spiritually related psychological constructs, such as facets of mindfulness (Baer, Smith, Hopkins, Krietemeyer, & Toney, 2006) and various virtues, such as forgiveness (R. P. Brown, 2003) and gratitude (Emmons & McCullough, 2003), these measures are not included in Table 11.3 because they are not directly tied to the sacred.

TABLE 11.3. Promising Instruments for Assessing Spirituality in Psychotherapy

Dimension	Scale (author)	Scale description	Sample item
Spiritual pathways	NIA/Fetzer Short Form for the Measurement of Religiousness and Spirituality (Idler et al., 2003)	33 items that assess 10 spiritual pathways: public and private activity, congregation support, coping, intensity, forgiveness, daily spiritual experience, spiritual beliefs and values, commitment, and religious history	"Because of my religious or spiritual beliefs, I have forgiven those who hurt me." (Forgiveness)
Spiritual pathways (breadth and depth)	Spiritual History Scale (Hays, Meador, Branch, & George, 2001)	23-item scale assessing degree to which religion has been source of support and conflict over the lifespan	"For most of my life, my social life has revolved around the church (synagogue)."
Spiritual pathways (breadth and depth)	Spiritual Assessment Inventory (Hall & Edwards, 1996)	36 items that measure four dimensions of individuals' quality of relationship with God: instability, grandiosity, defensiveness/ disappointment, realistic acceptance	"God recognizes that I am more spiritual than most people." (Grandiosity)
Spiritual pathways (flexibility)	Quest Scale (Batson & Schoenrade, 1991)	12-item scale of open, changeable approach to religion	"As I grow and change, I expect my religion to grow and change."
Spiritual pathways	Hindu Spiritual Pathways Scale (Tarakeshwar et al., 2003b)	27-item scale assessing degree of involvement in four Hindu pathways: devotion, ethical action, knowledge, and restraint	"How often do you perform *puja* in honor of your deity?" (Path of Devotion)
Spiritual destinations	Christian Religious Internalization Scale (Ryan et al., 1993)	12-item measure of internalized religiousness vs. religiousness based on guilt or social approval	"When I turn to God, I most often do it because I enjoy spending time with Him." (Internalized)
Spiritual destinations	Age Universal I-E Scale (Gorsuch & Venable, 1983)	20-item scale that assess intrinsic and extrinsic religious orientations	"My whole life is based on my religion." (Intrinsic)
Spiritual destinations	Spiritual Strivings (Emmons et al., 1998)	Coded spiritual responses to list of 15 personal strivings ("an objective you are typically . . . trying to obtain")	Sample spiritual strivings: "To approach life with mystery and awe," "To deepen my relation with God," "To achieve union with the totality of existence."

TABLE 11.3. (*continued*)

Dimension	Scale (author)	Scale description	Sample item
Spiritual destinations	Spiritual Strivings (Mahoney et al., 2005)	Ratings of degree to which each of 10 personal strivings is perceived as a manifestation of God or holding sacred qualities	"This striving reflects what I think God wants for me." (Manifestation of God)
Spiritual destinations	Adjective Ratings of God Scale (Gorsuch, 1968)	Scale consisting of 91 adjectives that are rated for the degree to which they describe God	Sample adjectives: "comforting," "distant," "mythical," "infinite," "weak."
Sacred loss and desecration	Sacred Loss and Desecration Scale (Pargament, Magyar, Benore, & Mahoney, 2005)	23-item scale that assess appraisals of negative events as sacred losses and desecrations	"A sacred part of my life was violated." (Desecration)
Spiritual coping (conservational)	Positive RCOPE (Pargament et al., 2000)	40 items assessing positive methods of spiritual coping (e.g., spiritual support, benevolent spiritual reappraisals, collaborative spiritual coping)	In coping with my negative event, I: "Looked to God for strength, support, and guidance."
Spiritual coping (conservational)	Religious Problem-Solving Scale (Pargament et al., 1988)	36-item scale assessing degree to which individual collaborates with God, defers to God, or solves problems independently	"In carrying out the solution to my problem, I wait for God to take control and know that somehow He'll work it out." (Deferring)
Spiritual coping (conservational)	Positive Religious Detriangulation Scale (Yanni, 2003)	Seven-item scale assessing degree to which individual views God as "on the side" of the relationship	When I differ with my mother/father/child: "I ask us to pray together to God to understand one another."
Spiritual struggles	Negative RCOPE (Pargament et al., 2000)	35 items assessing divine, interpersonal, and intrapsychic spiritual struggles	In coping with my negative event, I: "Wondered whether God had abandoned me."
Spiritual struggles	Religious Strain Scale (Exline et al., 2000)	13-item scale assessing alienation from God, religious fear and guilt, and religious rifts with others	To what extent are you currently experiencing: "Bad memories of past experiences with religion or religious people."

(*continued*)

TABLE 11.3. (*continued*)

Dimension	Scale (author)	Scale description	Sample item
Intrapsychic spiritual struggles	Religious Doubts Scale (Altemeyer, 1988)	10-item scale measuring doubts about traditional religious teachings	"A feeling that the overall religious teachings are contradictory or that they don't make much sense."
Interpersonal spiritual struggles	Negative Religious Triangulation Scale (Yanni, 2003)	Seven-item scale measuring efforts to triangulate spirituality into familial conflicts	When I differ with my mother/father/child: "I suggest that my mother/father/child is rejecting God's will."
Spiritual transformation and disengagement	Spiritual Transformation Scale (Cole et al., in press)	50 items that assess spiritual changes and disengagement following a major trauma	Since your trauma: "I more often see my own life as sacred."
Spiritual efficacy	Religious Comfort Scale (Exline et al., 2000)	13-item scale assessing experience of comfort through religion	To what extent are you currently experiencing: "Feeling comforted by your faith."
Spiritual efficacy	Penn Inventory of Scrupolosity (Abramowitz et al., 2002)	19-item scale measuring religious obsessive–compulsive symptoms	"I worry I must act morally at all times or I will be punished."
Spiritual efficacy	Spiritual Experience Index (Genia, 1991)	38-item scale assessing spiritual maturity	"My faith gives my life meaning and purpose."
Spiritual efficacy	Spiritual Support Scale (Maton, 1989)	Three-item scale assessing experience of support from God	"I experience God's love and caring on a regular basis."
Spiritual efficacy	Hindu Religious Outcome Scale (Tarakeshwar et al., 2003b)	20-item scale assessing degree to which involvement in Hindu pathways leads to valued outcomes	"Practicing yoga/ meditation brings me mental peace and stability."
Spiritual efficacy	Religious Well-Being Scale (Paloutzian & Ellison, 1982)	10-item global measure of perceptions of religious well-being	"My relationship with God helps me not to feel lonely."
Spiritual efficacy	FACIT-Spiritual Well-Being Scale (Peterman, Fitchett, Brady, Hernandez, & Cella, 2002)	12-item scale assessing spiritual well-being following illness	"I find strength in my faith or spiritual beliefs."

greater depth. They attempt to tap into elusive aspects of spirituality, such as an individual's deepest strivings, the motivations underlying the spiritual search, spiritual flexibility, and the quality of an individual's relationship with God. Measures are also beginning to appear that have utility for non-Christians, such as Tarakeshwar's scales to assess the spiritual pathways and outcomes of Hindus (Tarakeshwar, Pargament, & Mahoney, 2003b). In addition, scales have been constructed to assess the role of spirituality in appraising and coping with serious problems in living.

Once again, quantitative instruments are no substitute for the other methods of spiritual assessment, for there are limits to how well people will be able to report on their own spirituality. Furthermore, some problematic forms of spirituality, such as spiritual hypocrisy and extremism, will likely remain difficult, if not impossible, to measure directly. Nevertheless, quantitative measures can provide another significant source of information in the explicit spiritual assessment. In addition, they can be used to evaluate the efficacy of treatment as well as the client's progress in therapy. As a case in point, Nichole Murray-Swank (2003) developed a psychospiritual intervention for women who had been sexually abused as children. To help Murray-Swank to assess their progress in individual therapy, the clients completed a set of spiritual measures at several intervals. Figure 11.1 presents the scores of five of her cases on a measure of positive religious coping. As can be seen, most of the women made more use of positive religious coping methods over the course of treatment. Interestingly, several experienced a dip in positive religious coping early in their therapy as they were struggling with difficult spiritual issues. Data such as these converged with other sources of evaluative information to yield a clearer picture of the role

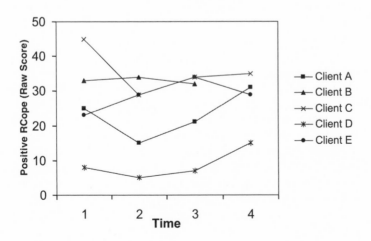

FIGURE 11.1. Changes in positive religious coping across clients.

of spirituality in the lives of these women and the impact of this new mode of treatment.

In sum, promising strides have been made toward the development of more sophisticated and clinically useful quantitative measures of spirituality. This work is still in its early stages, but with further development instruments such as these may become invaluable tools to the clinician seeking answers to critical questions about spiritual integration and efficacy.

Placing the Client in Context

I have stressed the idea that spirituality grows out of a larger field of social forces made up of family, friends, congregations, communities, and culture. These contexts are as diverse as the people who inhabit them. Like individuals, social contexts can be adaptive or destructive. On the one hand, the social milieu can support and encourage the individual's spirituality and general well-being. On the other hand, this environment can contribute to the individual's spiritual discord and dis-integration. Furthermore, the client's social milieu plays a crucial role in defining "normal" and "abnormal" spiritual expressions. For example, though they are not characteristic of mainstream religion in the United States, feelings of being possessed by the devil and participation in methods of deliverance from evil spirits are commonplace among some religious subcultures (Csordas, 1994). Similarly, Miller and Kelley (2005) have pointed out that "in some African communities, a person would be considered insane *not* to believe that the spirits of the dead actively influence an individual's life" (p. 471). Thus no assessment of spirituality would be complete without attending to the client's larger spiritual context.

To place clients in a spiritual context, the therapist can gather information about this larger milieu from clients themselves as well as from external sources. Clients can be asked about the forces that shaped their spiritual development, for better or worse. Clients can also be encouraged to represent their own spiritual journey in visual form. They could construct a spiritual genogram that elaborates on elements of a family genogram by depicting the religious structure of the family (e.g., religious affiliations, interfaith marriages), spiritual emotional dynamics in the family (e.g., spiritual rifts and conflicts), inspirational models and antispiritual models, and critical spiritual events, both positive and negative (Sperry, 2001). In addition, clients could create a spiritual lifemap which makes use of a timeline to describe how spiritual events, experiences, relationships, practices, and ideas have evolved over the course of a client's life. Clients who enjoy writing could also be encouraged to author their own spiritual autobiographies.

Because the client can offer only one (admittedly important) perspective on his or her spiritual context, it is important to supplement the client's point of view with information gathered from other sources. By visiting other congregations and reading about other religious traditions, therapists may learn that their clients have neglected important resources within their tradition or distorted some of its teachings. A number of texts are currently available that offer cogent summaries of diverse religious traditions as well as commentaries about the particular challenges that often arise in working with diverse clients (e.g., Lovinger, 1984; Richards & Bergin, 2000). Sensitivity on the part of the therapist to larger cultural shifts in religiousness and spirituality can also help place a client's behavior in context. For example, in a 22-year retrospective study of medical records, Atallah, El-Dosoky, Coker, Nabil, and El-Islam (2001) found that the religious content of symptoms among Egyptians diagnosed with schizophrenia waxed and waned with increases and decreases in religious fundamentalism in Egypt. Finally, therapists can develop a more fully dimensional picture of the place of spirituality in the life of the client by gathering information from members of the client's family or spiritual community, if the client is willing to provide the appropriate release of information. In some cases, the therapist may then decide to work directly with a married couple or the family as a whole to encourage spiritual support or to reduce spiritual conflicts. In other cases, the therapist may look to the clergy or members of the client's religious community for help in assessment and treatment.

Littlewood and Lipsedge (1989) present a striking illustration in their clinical work with Evadne Williams, a 45-year-old woman who had come to Great Britain from Jamaica when she was 30. In London, Williams became involved in her local Pentecostal church. Several years later, she was hospitalized "in a state of ecstasy," sobbing, rolling on the floor, singing gospel hymns, speaking incoherently, and complaining that she was being treated poorly because she had been trying to spread the word of God. In an effort to make sense of this behavior, Williams's psychiatrist wondered whether Evadne was simply "speaking in tongues" and, more generally, acting in ways consistent with her tradition. To test out this possibility, the psychiatrist met with several of Evadne's friends from her church who, to the surprise of the psychiatrist, agreed that William's behavior was "nothing like speaking in tongues" and that she was "sick in the head" (p. 173). Williams was treated with medications, responded positively, and later agreed that she had had a "breakdown." It would have been impossible to assess Williams outside of her social context, the psychiatrist concluded.

THE IMPORTANCE OF CLINICAL JUDGMENT

There is no simple method of assessment. This is probably one of the chief reasons why it takes so many years of clinical education and experience to become a competent practitioner. If assessment merely required gathering information about a few important variables and the application of a few standard treatments based on the results, then psychotherapy would be a matter of simple technology rather than a complex approach to change. But people and problems come in too many shapes and sizes to be summarized so neatly. In reality, clinicians must gather information on a host of variables from a variety of sources and then weigh these variables not singly but in interaction with each other, for every individual presents distinctive configurations of strengths and weaknesses. No formula can fully capture the uniqueness of an individual. Neither can formulas replace the need for clinical judgment, in spite of its limitations, in the process of assessment and psychotherapy. This point holds particularly true for new approaches to treatment, such as spiritually integrated psychotherapy. Consider, for instance, these questions: At what point do spiritual openness, flexibility, and questioning become confusion, aimlessness, and a lack of resolve? At what point do commitment, faith, and tenacity constitute an arrogant conviction of the truth? At what point does love for a partner become idolatrous? At what point does regular spiritual practice become compulsive? At what point does spiritual commitment to growth become an oppressive and hopeless pursuit of perfection? In the process of spiritual assessment, clinicians will often find themselves wrestling with thorny evaluative questions such as these. Answers to some of these questions may come from further research in the psychology of spirituality. But, important as such studies are, I doubt that research findings will ever be able to eliminate the need for sound clinical judgment in treatment.

CONCLUSIONS

In the last two chapters I have described spiritual assessment as a process that grows out of the relationship between client and therapist. Direct questions about spirituality before a relationship has been established may yield little or misleading information. Instead, spiritual dialogue flourishes in an atmosphere of trust, respect, and openness to listening and sharing. Though it is important to ask some initial questions about spirituality, keep in mind that spirituality may emerge as a critical issue in treatment for even the ostensibly nonspiritual client or nonspiritual problem. Thus, the clinician must remain alert to signs of spirituality that lie beneath the client's own awareness. In the process of implicit spiritual assessment, the practitioner probes for underlying and undetected spiritual issues, and provides the client with an invitation to enter into a spiritual conversation, one that may lead to more extensive discussion of spiritual matters. In the process of explicit spiritual assessment, the therapist elicits the client's spiritual story, attends to nonverbal behavior, draws on quantitative instruments, places the client in context, and relies on his or her clinical judgment—all in an effort to evaluate the degree to which the client's spirituality is well integrated and efficacious.

Spiritual assessment is not a distinct and separate stage of psychotherapy; rather, it is an ongoing part of treatment—assessment leads to intervention, which leads to reevaluation and further assessment, which leads to intervention once again, and so on. In this sense, spirituality is not an end in itself. It is a vital part of therapy, a process that should lead the clinician to a sense of where the client is in the search for the sacred, how spirituality might be a part of the solution to the client's problem, and how spirituality might be a problem in and of itself. The answers to these questions will guide the way in which spirituality is best addressed in treatment. Thus, as we turn our attention now to spiritually integrated interventions, we will not be leaving spiritual assessment behind.

12

Drawing on Spiritual Strivings, Knowledge, and Experience

Ron, a 45-year-old pastor of a Methodist church, came to my office because he was having difficulty coping with a separation from his wife of 15 years. A few weeks earlier, she had moved out of their home, after telling her husband that she needed some time apart to decide whether she wanted to stay married. Her decision came as a surprise and, in spite of his repeated efforts to learn what his wife was unhappy about, Ron hadn't a clue. How had he hurt her? Was she having an affair? Was she clinically depressed? In response to his questions, his wife simply said, "I just need time to think." Now Ron was having trouble concentrating at work, eating, and sleeping. "I feel as though I'm on a train that's racing down the tracks," he said, "and no one's at the controls." Over the course of the next few weeks of uncertainty, I helped Ron keep himself together. We talked about people who could be supportive, ways he could fill his time with meaningful activities, and how he could hold on to the rhythm of his daily life. What we didn't talk about, though, was spirituality. When I broached this topic as another potentially valuable resource, he stopped for a moment and then said, "I hadn't thought about that."

The notion of a minister who overlooks his spiritual resources while in the midst of an intensely painful crisis may sound far-fetched. We might wonder whether this was a sign of a deeper spiritual ambivalence or spiritual dis-integration on the part of the minister. In Ron's case, however, the problem was not spiritual. I was to learn that he had a reasonably well-integrated faith that had helped guide and direct him in the past. The shock of the separation, however, seemed to result in a type of spiritual amnesia. Ron simply forgot about the spiritual methods of coping that had proven valuable to him in other difficult situations. A few reminders were enough to help Ron recall and reconnect to his spiritual resources to help him deal with the stress of marital separation.

This is not a singular case. In times of emotional distress, it is not uncommon for people to lose touch with the resources that normally sustain them in their lives. On a personal note, many years ago, I recall racing to the hospital with my wife, who was about to deliver our second child. As she was whisked away to the delivery room, I was left behind at the front desk, fretting and frazzled, as I faced the questions of the intake receptionist. Though I was able to give her our names, I had trouble when the questions got tougher. My memory finally gave out when the receptionist asked me for our home phone number and address. This was not my finest moment.

Helping clients identify and draw on their own resources is one of the most important services therapists can offer. In most cases, there is no need to start from scratch. Clients generally come to therapy with psychological, social, financial, and medical resources that have proven invaluable to them in the past. Therapists regularly help their clients tap into these assets as a basic part of treatment. Spirituality is another critical resource that can be accessed in psychotherapy. This chapter and the one to follow focus on the ways in which therapists can help clients draw on their spiritual resources in therapy. Because spiritual resources come in so many shapes and sizes, this review is intended to be illustrative rather than comprehensive. Let's begin by considering a few basic rules of thumb (see Table 12.1).

BASIC RULES OF THUMB FOR HELPING CLIENTS DRAW ON THEIR SPIRITUAL RESOURCES

First, it is important to tailor spiritual resources to both the particular case and the particular problem. For instance, many clients may gain strength and support from religiously based rituals. Not all will do so, however. Survivors of clergy sexual abuse, for example, are often unable to disentangle religious rituals from the abusive clerics who enacted them. For these survivors, religious rituals are likely to reawaken memories of trauma rather than to offer solace. Similarly, though meditation may help allay anxiety for many clients, other clients rooted in conservative religious traditions will find some forms of meditation, such as transcendental meditation (TM), quite alien. Thus, when it comes to spiritual resources, one size does not fit all. Part of the challenge for clinicians is to help clients identify and draw on those resources that are best suited to their distinctive needs and preferences.

TABLE 12.1. Rules of Thumb to Help Clients Draw on Their Spiritual Resources

1. Tailor spiritual resources to the specific client and problem.
2. Remind the client that it takes time and practice to benefit from spiritual resources.
3. Recognize and respect the sacred character of spiritual resources.
4. Work with spiritual resources from within one's own professional and personal boundaries.
5. Help clients identify and overcome barriers to using their spiritual resources.

Second, remember that it takes time and practice to reap the benefits of spiritual resources. The client must be ready to tap into a spiritual resource. According to Hasidic thought, "It is not within the power of human beings to place the divine teaching directly in their hearts. All we can do is place them on the surface of the heart so that when the heart breaks they drop in" (Domback & Karl, 1987, p. 192). Practice is important too. Proficient figures from diverse religious traditions agree that spiritual mastery does not happen overnight. Repetition, hard work, and discipline, they maintain, are essential to the development of spiritual practices and virtues, from prayer and meditation to forgiveness and compassion. Yet many clients, including some who follow disciplined regimes in diet, exercise, and work, expect immediate, even miraculous, results when it comes to spirituality. Clinicians therefore need to remind their clients that practice is as important to progress in spirituality as it is to progress in other spheres of life.

Third, handle with care. Spiritual resources should not be treated as just more techniques for treatment. Remember that spiritual resources are designed with a spiritual purpose in mind: to facilitate the individual's relationship with the sacred. To the spiritually-minded, spiritual resources are trivialized when they are removed from their sacred context and treated merely as psychological tools. Therapists must demonstrate respect, sensitivity, and care in their work with spiritual resources. These are, after all, sacred matters. Although some might argue that the use of spiritual resources in psychotherapy necessarily reduces spirituality to a technique in the service of psychological rather than spiritual ends, I believe that there is no sharp dividing line between psychological and spiritual goals. As I noted earlier, people often sanctify seemingly psychological goals, from becoming a better parent to searching for peace of mind to seeking meaning and purpose in life. Thus, it is important not to think about spirituality narrowly as if it were distinct from or opposed to other aspects of life. Working with spirituality in psychotherapy provides the therapist with an opportunity to help people spiritually, psychologically, socially, and physically.

Fourth, clinicians must work within their own professional and personal boundaries. While therapists can help their clients reach out to their formal religious resources, they must not confuse their roles with those of clerical figures. Most therapists are not ministers. They are not legitimated by religious traditions to offer sacraments, give blessings, or speak with the authority of a particular denomination. Just as clinicians can talk about the physical health of their clients, but not as if they were physicians, clinicians can and should talk about spiritual issues in therapy, but only from their position as mental health professionals.

Clinicians should also work within their own personal boundaries as they help clients draw on their spiritual resources. For example, though I encourage many of my clients to pray, I do not pray together with my clients in therapy—not because I believe prayer has no place in counseling, but because one-to-one prayer is not a part of my own religious tradition and background. To pray together with a client would be inauthentic for me. Though therapists can find ways to expand their own spiritual comfort zones, they should not try to help their clients in ways that feel "spiritually dystonic."

Finally, therapists should be alert to spiritual problems that pose a barrier to spiritual resources. Among the most common of these barriers is mild, stress-induced spiritual compartmentalization of the kind experienced by Ron. A lack of spiritual breadth and depth is another common barrier. Often people are unaware of the spiritual resources that are potentially available to them. For example, a rabbi told a joke about a Jewish woman who had been deeply moved by the Twenty-third Psalm of the Hebrew Bible, and then told him, "I wish we had something like that in our tradition." In some cases, it can be relatively easy to help some people overcome their spiritual barriers, reconnect with old spiritual resources, or identify new ones. In other cases, however, the barriers reflect more fundamental spiritual problems that must be dealt with more directly in treatment as significant issues in and of themselves. I examine how clinicians can address these spiritual problems in the next chapter.

With these rules of thumb in mind, I now review some of the ways in which clinicians can help their clients gain access to different kinds of spiritual resources in psychotherapy. This chapter examines spiritual strivings, spiritual knowledge, and spiritual experience. Chapter 13 focuses on spiritual practices, spiritual relationships, and spiritual coping methods.

HELPING CLIENTS DRAW ON SPIRITUAL STRIVINGS

Many people find it increasingly difficult to locate the sacred in their lives today. As Thomas Moore (1992) wrote, "The great malady of the twentieth century . . . is 'loss of soul' " (p. xi). Social scientists have offered a variety of explanations for this "malady": the loss of compelling religiously based explanations for the cosmos, the increasingly private nature of religious life, the rise of scientific frameworks that view the world in materialistic terms, the disconnection of people from family and community, and the frenetic pace of daily life that distracts people from the sacred. But whatever the reasons, many people are left with the feeling that they are missing something, a spiritual center that could lend direction and vitality to their lives. Some of these people find their way into psychotherapy, presenting problems attributable in one way or another to that lost sense of the sacred, such as the depression that grows out of spiritual emptiness, the anxiety that accompanies the feeling of life being lived inauthentically, and the pursuit of false gods such as consumerism, workaholism, narcissism, nihilism, hedonism, and alcoholism—those destructive "isms" of our times.

In helping clients recognize and pursue their spiritual strivings, we need to maintain the important distinction between losing one's soul and losing touch with one's soul. Since we have no instruments that detect the presence or absence of soul, the question of whether people can, in fact, lose their souls must be left to theologians. Conceptually, it is difficult to understand how people could lose their souls if the term is understood to encompass a sacred quality of ourselves, one marked by transcendence, boundlessness, and ultimacy (Hillman, 1975; Moore, 1992). Certainly, on clinical grounds, it seems more useful to think of people losing touch with their souls than of losing their souls entirely. Framed in this fashion, therapists have a hopeful message they can offer their clients who feel "soulless." What seems lost *can* be found. Clients do have spiritual resources within themselves. With help, they can reconnect to their sacred core, identify the hopes and dreams that lie in this spiritual center, and call upon these spiritual strivings in ways that provide them with direction and coherence in life (Miller, 2005).

Helping clients identify their spiritual strivings is the biggest challenge in working with people who appear to be spiritually lost. Toward achieving this end, clinicians should keep three points in mind. First, it is hard for people to think spiritually when they are caught up in the distractions and demands of their everyday lives. To identify their own deepest strivings, clients must take a step back from the everyday and examine their lives from a broader perspective. The therapist can facilitate this process by assigning the client several types of tasks. For example, the therapist can ask clients to write two obituaries: one as it would be written if they continue in the current way in which they are living, and another as it would be written if they were to change course and pursue the way in which they would ideally like to live (Yalom, 1980). Not only does this task encourage people to step back from day-to-day experience and specify what is truly most important to them, it also confronts people with their own finitude and the urgency of living fully and authentically.

Another task that serves the same purpose is to have clients imagine meeting their future, fully mature selves at the age of 120, the biblical age of wisdom and accomplishment. Schachter-Shalomi and Miller (1995) describe this meditative exercise:

> To visit your future self, sit quietly, take a few deep, calming breaths, and then count slowly from your actual physiological age to 120. . . . At the same time, visualize walking up a path that leads to the door of your realized self. At the end of your ascent, when you reach 120, enter his or her abode and look into your Inner Elder's compassionate eyes, feeling reassured about your progress so far. As a pilgrim confronting your highest potential for growth, ask for a word of guidance or a blessing for proceeding on your path. Then after resting in silence for a while, take leave of your future self and return to normal consciousness, knowing that you can return again for continued guidance. (p. 129)

Yet another task involves homework for the client. Ask the client to set aside a quiet time during the week to think deeply and carefully about 10–15 of his or her most important personal strivings, those goals that direct and determine what he or she does everyday (Emmons, 1999). The client's list of strivings can raise important questions for therapy, such as: Which, if any, strivings does the client hold sacred? How much time and energy is the client putting into his or her most important strivings? To what extent are the client's strivings self-determined or externally imposed? Are there sacred dreams and strivings that the client has avoided or been unable to pursue?

This last question leads to a second key point. Clients often need help distinguishing "true" from "false" strivings. Separating what others want for the client from what clients want for themselves is part of our job. Discerning the underlying motivations for various choices in life is another. In the following hypothetical case, one client, a scientist and mother who recently gave birth to a baby who is mentally retarded and physically handicapped, struggles with these issues:

> The pediatrician, my family doctor and my husband all insist on having me put the child into an institution. They reason that it will be cared for in a professional way I cannot compete with if I were to care for the child personally. They also point out that I would jeopardize my marriage and my development as a person and as a scientist if I undertake the all-consuming task of taking care of my child. . . .
>
> Nevertheless, I have a strong feeling that I have to look after my child personally. The pediatrician attributes this to false and unnecessary guilt feelings for having "failed" to produce a healthy child. . . . I have considered this advice seriously but I still feel a strong inner conviction that my life lies with this child even though this means giving up my career and putting my marriage at risk. (Schreuers, 2002, p. 139)

In cases such as this one, therapists can raise critical questions to help their clients tap into their spiritual core when they are facing difficult life decisions. With respect to the mother above, Schreurs (2002) poses a number of central questions: "Should she decide for common sense and competent advice, or should she acknowledge her 'strong feelings' as sufficient reason for sacrificing her career and family life? What is the nature of this strong feeling? Is it indeed the false guilt mothers so easily become prey to, or could it be something else?" (p. 140). That "something else," Schreurs suggests, could be the "deep and persistent longing" for a "spiritual True self," but she goes on to note that it takes "critical self-examination to sift out the authentic from the inauthentic" (p. 159).

The final point to remember in helping clients identify spiritual strivings is that this process is more than intellectual; perceptions of the sacred often elicit powerful spiritual emotions. Attending to where clients put their energy and passion may hold the key to discerning their spiritual strivings. For example, Bill O'Hanlon (1994) recounts a story told by Milton Erickson about his work with a severely depressed woman who was, confined to a wheelchair. Entering her home, Erickson noticed that darkness and gloom pervaded the whole house. But there was one exception: attached to the house was a light-filled greenhouse, this woman's "pride and joy." There she showed off her African violets to Erickson. At that point, he told her that she had a "God-given gift" that was going to waste. Erickson went on to recommend that she give gifts of her African violets to all the members of her church who were experiencing either a sad or a happy event. When later asked about his work with this woman, Erickson replied, "I looked around her house and the only sign of life I saw were those African violets. I thought it would be easier to grow the African violet part of her life than to weed out the depression" (p. 23). Erikson was quite directive in determining this client's "God-given gift." I would prefer to help clients discover their gifts for themselves. Nevertheless, this case illustrates how spiritual strivings can be hidden in nonverbal expressions, the "signs of life" noted by Erickson. Other cases from this book reinforce the same point: the depressed woman (Karen) who laughs for the first time when she sees two squirrels playing outside, the boring man (Joe) who comes to life when he describes the experience of flying a jet, the woman (Agnes) close to suicide or homicide who feels most fully alive when she listens to music or goes to an art museum. Powerful emotions of one kind or another often provide important clues about the deepest hopes and dreams of the client.

Once their spiritual strivings have been identified, clients are often more than happy to pursue these sacred ends. Just as it took only a little bit of encouragement from Erikson for his client to share her African violets with the members of her church, it only took a little clinical nudge from me to encourage Karen to cultivate her spiritual interest (outdoor photogra-

phy), Joe to begin flying once again, and Agnes to reinvolve herself in poetry and music. In each of these cases, the results were striking. By accessing their spiritual strivings more fully, these clients added color and passion
into their lives. They experienced a lightening of their gray moods as well
as a greater sense of meaning and satisfaction in life. Of course, helping clients identify and access their spiritual dreams does not guarantee that they
will be successful in realizing them. Many obstacles can get in the way.
Nevertheless, some empirical studies suggest that these cases are not unusual. In a study of spiritual strivings among community members, Mahoney
et al. (2005) found that people reported greater satisfaction with the time
and energy they invested in their sanctified strivings than in other non-
sanctified strivings. Emmons, Cheung, and Tehrani (1998) found that people who had a higher proportion of spiritual strivings experienced higher
levels of marital satisfaction, life satisfaction, and purpose and meaning in
life.

HELPING CLIENTS DRAW
ON SPIRITUAL KNOWLEDGE

Several years ago, I worked with a woman, Denise, who came to my office
distraught after discovering that her husband of 30 years had been having a
series of affairs over the course of their marriage. What had been the center
of her life, her marriage, was shattered, as were the friendships, family relationships, and financial security that had been built around her marriage.
Denise was deeply depressed. A thin woman to begin with, she lost 30
pounds within 2 months of her discovery. She cut herself off from the people
and activities that had given meaning to her life because they only reminded
her of what she had shared with her husband and now had lost. Unable to
concentrate at work or to stop herself from breaking into tears in public,
she preferred to remain in bed. Worst of all, Denise said, was what she felt
as the loss of her spirituality. Denise had been raised in the United Church
of Christ, but did not identify with a particular denomination. Instead, she
saw herself as a spiritual sojourner, open to a variety of experiences that
put her in contact with something beyond herself. Spirituality, for Denise,
had to do with the strong connection she felt with the transcendent—a
force she experienced most powerfully outdoors or in her quiet moments of
contemplation. Denise could never remember a time when she didn't have
this sense of the sacred, until the loss of her marriage. Sadly, the opposite
seemed true now; she could not imagine ever emerging from the dark, dank
pit of isolation in which she found herself. She had even begun to contemplate suicide.

   Addressing the hopelessness that accompanied Denise's trauma and
depression was one of the central priorities of therapy. Toward this end, I

talked with Denise about how her feelings were understandable in light of the loss of what had been the centerpiece of her life. However, rather than leaving her stuck in her dark, dank pit, I offered her a different image to think about, one consistent with her view of herself as a spiritual sojourner. Perhaps, I suggested, she was going through her own wilderness period, a time in which she felt as if she were wandering aimlessly through a desert, but one in which she was actually being steeled and strengthened. We talked about other people Denise knew who had come through their own periods of struggle and had emerged stronger for the experience. Though Denise was familiar with the image of a wilderness period from her religious upbringing, she found it a powerful new image to apply to herself. The possibility that her own spiritual journey might be accompanied by periods of darkness and loss had not occurred to Denise until our conversation. She began to feel a new sense of hope in the knowledge that her current wilderness period signaled an opportunity for spiritual growth rather than the end to her spiritual quest.

Sharing knowledge is one critical ingredient of psychotherapy. Therapists share information with their clients about the varied dimensions of human behavior: emotions, relationships, development, communication, stress, and so on. Knowledge about spirituality can be shared in similar fashion. For example, the knowledge that spirituality is a search for the sacred, an evolving process rather than a static set of beliefs and practices, can be helpful to people who feel stuck in their faith. Similarly, the knowledge that spirituality encompasses the full range of human experience, from times of greatest awe and inspiration to times of struggle, desolation, and loss, can be of tremendous value to people, like Denise, who come to therapy feeling spiritually bereft.

Therapists can also help their clients call on more specific forms of spiritual knowledge that are embedded in their particular religious or spiritual tradition. Drawing on the spiritual wisdom found in religious texts can be beneficial to clients who place great store in religious writings as sources of authority. For example, Prest and Keller (1993) describe their work with the Christian parents of a 17-year-old daughter who had lost interest in school and was dating a man whom they disliked. The parents were furious with their daughter, so angry that they were contemplating making a complete emotional and financial break with her. The therapists gave the parents a homework task. Every night they were to read the following New Testament passage: "While we were yet *sinners* [italics added], Christ died for us." They returned the next week to discuss the meanings they found in this verse. Prest and Keller (1993) note that "it was this scriptural representation of God's love for humans, while they were in their most unattractive state that, according to the parents, helped them to continue to love and accept their daughter through her difficult adolescence" (p. 144).

Griffith and Griffith (2002) illustrate how to draw on religious texts to encourage clients to think about themselves and their problems in a different way. They present the case of Jack, a Southern Baptist who had repeatedly tried to stop using drugs and alcohol, but had repeatedly failed. Jack had been successful in many areas of his life: he had graduated from college, he had been more attentive to his widowed mother than his siblings, and he had been a loyal friend and a conscientious worker. But Jack dwelled more on his failures than his successes: his broken promises to God, the money he had lost to alcohol and cocaine, his string of relapses. Convinced that Jack's problems grew out of the stories of self-hatred and despair that he continually told himself, the therapist presented Jack with a biblical verse that he was likely to be familiar with: "Finally, brethren, whatsoever things are true, whatsoever things are honest, whatsoever things are just, whatsoever things are pure, whatsoever things are lovely, whatsoever things are of good report, if there be any virtue, and if there be any praise, think on these things" (Philippians 4:8, King James Version). After discussing the wisdom of this passage, the therapist encouraged Jack to "[dwell] mindfully upon stories that facilitated his recovery, not on ones that undermined it" (p. 97). Jack was receptive to this message. He began to attend more to his history of positive accomplishments than to his history of failures, and in the process he became more successful in adhering to his program of recovery.

Empirical studies have provided some initial support for the value of integrating religious texts into psychotherapy. For example, Wahass and Kent (1997) worked with three Muslim patients with schizophrenia who were experiencing auditory hallucinations, some of which were threatening (e.g., warnings of torture in the hereafter). They asked their patients to read the Koran when they were hallucinating. The therapists then drew on Islamic doctrine to counter the threatening content of their patients' hallucinations, pointing out that, according to traditional Islamic beliefs, "a person who performs good actions under what God and the Prophet ordered will be saved in paradise" (p. 356). Two of the three patients showed a sharp reduction in the number of their hallucinations over the 9 weeks of treatment. In the third case, the authors report, the therapists were unable to establish a cooperative working relationship. Larger scale studies of interventions with Muslim clients who were bereaved (Azhar, Varma, & Dharap, 1994) and diagnosed with anxiety disorders (Azhar & Varma, 1995a) yielded similar results. Psychotherapy that integrated religious texts into treatment led to more rapid improvement than drug treatment or supportive therapy alone.

Religious texts can also provide clients with valuable models of strength, compassion, hope, and resilience in the face of suffering. Sperry (2001) presents one illustration in his work with a 47-year-old Christian woman whose adult son had died of cancer 2 years after she had sought a separation from her husband. Both her ex-husband and her own parents blamed her for her son's death. She came to therapy struggling with grief, rage, and self-doubt. Recognizing that this woman had few positive female role models, Sperry encouraged her to look to Mary, the mother of Jesus, as a source of support and direction. The client was able to resonate with Mary, "a strong competent woman who, like [the client], also let go of her son at a very young age" (p. 141). This positive identification, Sperry reported, was instrumental in helping his client work through her grief.

Similarly, religious texts offer stories that serve as models for how people should treat themselves. For example, Nielsen et al. (2001) present the case of Andrew, an 18-year-old Mormon college student, who was depressed to the point of considering suicide following the breakup of his relationship with his high school sweetheart. In the following dialogue, working from a rational-emotive behavioral orientation, the therapist takes on a Socratic style and draws on the model of the biblical Job to dispute the student's belief that he cannot withstand the pain of the breakup:

> THERAPIST: Well now, Andrew, I understand your girlfriend decided not to date you anymore . . . and that you've become very depressed about that, but I'm not understanding how you got yourself from just depressed to deciding you must die rather than feel depressed.
>
> ANDREW: I don't know . . . I just can't take feeling this way. Everything sucks . . .
>
> THERAPIST: Losing the relationship is very difficult and you've gotten quite depressed about it, but do you think you could survive even with feeling depressed?
>
> ANDREW: Yeah. I don't know how long, though.
>
> THERAPIST: Can you think of anyone in the Bible who really suffered?
>
> ANDREW: You mean like Job?
>
> THERAPIST: Exactly. Job is a great example. . . . What happened to him?
>
> ANDREW: He lost everything. All his riches were gone and he threw himself down on the ground.
>
> THERAPIST: That's right. He was a prosperous man who lost everything. . . . The Bible says he was covered from head to toe with painful sores. He then sat down in a heap of ashes. He loses everything including all of his children in one day and then gets hit with painful sores. . . . Would it be safe to say Job's day sucked?
>
> ANDREW: [laughs slightly for the first time] Yeah, that would suck.
>
> THERAPIST: Okay, so Job's day really sucked, and he certainly got very depressed and could have killed himself, but didn't. Job was depressed enough to curse the day he was born, yet he didn't take his life. Instead, what did he do?
>
> ANDREW: He sat there and put up with his obnoxious friends.

THERAPIST: Yes, he sat there in intense pain, listening to his "friends" ridicule him day after day. Now if really, really intense suffering means one has to commit suicide, wouldn't Job have done it? Killed himself?

ANDREW: Probably . . . yeah, I'd say that would do it.

THERAPIST: So, does it follow that you probably can stand working through this break-up with Sarah, even if it sucks and you feel quite down for a while?

ANDREW: Yeah, I hear what you mean. I know I can survive . . . I'm not going to kill myself.

THERAPIST: Even if you feel very unhappy and even feel miserable sometimes?

ANDREW: Yes. (pp. 136–138)

Before concluding this section, I think it is important to add that spiritual knowledge and wisdom can be gleaned from modern as well as more traditional sources. For example, a number of my clients have found the recent book *The Purpose Driven Life* a valuable source of motivation and direction (Warren, 2002). Responding to a challenge in the book, one of my clients asked himself, "Since I'm not made to last forever, what should I stop doing and what should I start?" Along similar lines, clients can be encouraged to find modern-day spiritual models for themselves, not only among the famous (e.g., Mother Teresa, Nelson Mandela, the Dali Lama), but also among inspirational members of their own family and their circle of friends.

HELPING CLIENTS DRAW ON SPIRITUAL EXPERIENCE

Spiritual experience represents another potentially powerful resource that can be accessed in psychotherapy. Prayer and meditation have begun to receive particular attention as resources that facilitate spiritual experience in psychotherapy.

Prayer

Prayers are designed to sustain and strengthen the individual's connection with God. At the same time, however, prayers offer a response to very human needs and aspirations. In fact, often it is difficult to disentangle the sacred from the secular in an individual's communication with God. The critical point I wish to make is that prayer can facilitate both the spiritual and the psychological well-being of the client in therapy.

How can prayer be integrated into psychotherapy? Clients who are comfortable with prayer might benefit from the encouragement to pray in whatever way is most meaningful to them. But clinicians should always keep in mind that prayers take many different forms. Think of prayer as a channel on the television or radio. The value of the channel depends on the quality of the program that is being offered and its appeal to the audience. Similarly, clinicians should attend to the specific kind and quality of their client's prayers. Specific prayers will speak in very different ways to different clients depending on their particular problems. Rather than simply encouraging their clients to pray, clinicians can help their clients locate those prayers that are best suited to their needs. Clients who enjoy writing can be encouraged to write their own prayers that address their deepest concerns and yearnings. Clients uncomfortable with writing can be advised to seek out prayers from their religious leaders, congregations, religious bookstores, or libraries. There are numerous popular books that offer prayers tailored to the needs of people facing a variety of challenges. Some of the books are written for members of specific religious traditions (e.g., Brown, 2003), while others offer prayers that are religiously diverse (e.g., Kirvan, 1999). Still other books illustrate how well-known religious leaders bring prayer into their own lives (e.g., Castelli, 1994).

Consider a few examples of the ways prayer has been integrated into psychotherapy. A few years ago, I worked with Christina, a 60-year-old Roman Catholic Hispanic woman who suffered from bipolar illness. At her best, she was actively involved in church life and successful in her work as an accountant. Her depressed periods, though, were marked by lethargy, social isolation, and disinterest in work and church. Having witnessed several cycles of her changing moods, I learned that Christina retained little memory of the resources that helped her when she was in her depressed periods. She seemed to be continually reinventing the wheel. I encouraged Christina to create a book of resources that she could access easily to speed her recovery from her periods of depression. One important resource for Christina was prayer. Two types of prayer were especially significant for her: prayers that energized and mobilized her, and prayers that addressed her feelings of isolation and loneliness. Christina looked for these kinds of prayer in her parish newsletter and then copied them into her book. One prayer from the book was a kind of "spiritual wake-up call" with God that she recited every night before she went to bed: "Lord, I want to meet with You first thing in the morning for at least 5 minutes. Tomorrow when the alarm clock rings, I have an appointment with You." Other prayers helped address her loneliness:

> I live alone, dear Lord,
> But I am sure
> Your gaze is ever on me
> As on an only child.
> Abide in me, dear Lord,
> That I may live in you. Amen!
> (Hite, 2005, p. 1)

Along with the other resources in her book, Christina's prayers proved to be quite helpful in shortening her periods of depression.

Abramowitz (1993) describes another therapeutic use of prayer in a program for mentally impaired, elderly, Jewish men and women attending elder centers in Jerusalem. At the end of a daily program that included art, music, dance, and physiotherapy, the elders sat around a table and were led in 10–15 minutes of prayers that were long familiar to the participants. Family members were surprised by the ability of their loved ones suffering from dementia to participate in the prayer activities. Elders who had seemed unable to read or appeared unresponsive to other activities were able to follow along and join in the singing and ritualized movements that were part of the prayers. At the end of a dance session, one participant said, "Come on, let's cut the nonsense and get down to prayers" (p. 72). Like this participant, many of the elders, including those who were less religious, looked forward to the prayers as a regular activity lending some structure and orientation to their daily lives. The prayers served other functions as well. Those who were more docile were comforted by the prayers. The more agitated participants found the prayers soothing. And even though the participants were limited in their ability to make intellectual sense of the prayers, they retained a deep emotional connection to the prayers, approaching them with a sense of reverence. Thus, the prayers were well suited to the particular needs of these elderly individuals.

Prayer can be a valuable adjunct in couple therapy. Butler, Gardner, and Bird (1998) conducted a qualitative analysis of the use of prayer in times of conflict among 26 Christian spouses, and found that prayer served a number of important purposes. Prayer helped some of the couples move beyond their own point of view and see their problems from a larger, more empathic metaperspective. In the words of one wife, prayer "sometimes helps me realize that there are other ways of thinking, that my way isn't always right, and my feelings aren't the [only] ones getting hurt. And so it makes me realize that I need to be more sensitive to his [her husband's] thoughts and opinions . . . to put myself in the other person's shoes" (p. 464). Prayer also appeared to "soften" spouses' feelings of hostility, contempt, and negativity toward each other. As a wife said, "You can't hold your anger and say a heartfelt prayer . . . you gotta get rid of one to make the other work" (p. 461). In addition, prayer helped the couples place their conflicts in the context of their spiritual commitments and accountability to something larger than themselves. One husband remarked that "when you start having bad feelings in conflict the Spirit helps you remember the commitment you have made . . . through prayer . . . so [when in conflict] immediately I think that I have committed not to do these things. You know it kind of tempers your spirit" (p. 461). Other couples stressed the more concrete role of prayer in "step-by-step coaching" of what to say and what to do to improve their relation. According to one wife, through prayer "the

Spirit prompts us. Thoughts will come to your mind that help you in particular situations. Maybe to tell you, 'Now, you've said enough' or 'This is something that you may need to do' " (p. 464). Butler and his colleagues (1998) concluded with the recommendation that clinicians integrate prayer into their work with religious couples who are experiencing serious conflict.

These are just a few examples of the ways prayer can be called on as a resource in therapy. Because prayer takes so many forms and serves so many spiritually related functions—comfort, gratitude, forgiveness, protection, guidance, compassion, connection, meaning, support, pain tolerance, empowerment, transformation—it can be applied to a wide variety of people and problems. Unfortunately, researchers have yet to evaluate the efficacy of prayer as a resource in psychotherapy (see McCullough, 1995), with a few exceptions (e.g., Rajagopal, Mackenzie, Bailey, & Lavizzo-Mourey, 2002). I hope that this picture will change in the next few years.

Meditation

When we turn our attention to meditation, we find a very different situation. In contrast to prayer, meditation has received a great deal of attention from both practitioners and researchers. As I noted earlier, there are many types of meditation. Regardless of their differences, however, all forms of meditation are designed to help people experience a different kind of consciousness. Although this often involves a shift away from the stresses and strains of everyday experience, meditation should not be understood as nothing more than a way of coping. To most of its practitioners, meditation represents the path to a different way of being, one that can be applied continuously to all aspects of experience. In this vein, Jon Kabat-Zinn (2003), a leading proponent of meditation, describes mindfulness meditation (MM) as "akin to an art form that one develops over time. . . . It is not about getting anywhere else or fixing anything. Rather, it is an invitation to allow oneself to be where one already is and to know the inner and outer landscape of the direct experience in each moment" (p. 148).

The shift to a different kind of consciousness promoted by meditation may be especially valuable to people suffering from two classes of psychological problems: difficulty separating from cravings (e.g., for alcohol, for drugs, for food, for sex), and difficulty coming to terms with painful emotions and experiences (e.g., anxiety, anger, depression, physical pain, difficult life histories). In their efforts to deal with these problems, many people find themselves caught in a terrible cycle: their desperate attempts to avoid cravings or painful thoughts and feelings are followed by a loss of control and periods of immersion in the cravings or pain, which lead once again to efforts to eliminate the cravings or painful thoughts and feelings, and so on. Meditation offers an alternative. Instead of avoiding the craving or painful experience, the individual is asked to observe it. But rather than lose him- or herself in the experience, the individual is asked to attend to the experience from a more distant, detached vantage point. In my own work, I have found it helpful to ask clients to imagine themselves on a raft in the ocean. The waves that pass beneath them represent their cravings or painful thoughts and emotions. Their task is to notice the ebb and flow of the waves without flailing against them or falling off the raft into the ocean. By mastering the art of floating, people can weather virtually any storm. Therapists have suggested other helpful metaphors to capture this meditative type of consciousness, including the image of the mind as the sky that witnesses the clouds of thoughts and feelings that continuously pass by, and the image of the mind as a conveyor belt that observes the progression of thoughts and feelings coming down the line (Baer, 2003).

Meditation has been applied to a variety of psychological problems by practitioners from diverse therapeutic orientations (see Germer, Siegel, & Fulton, 2005; Hayes, Follette, & Linehan, 2005). For example, Siegel (2005) recounts his work with Beth, a woman who had been experiencing severe sciatic pain. Though she had hoped to attend her brother's wedding, her pain was so excruciating that Beth felt she would be unable to tolerate the plane flight in a cramped airline seat. Using a combination of concentration and mindfulness techniques, Siegel taught Beth to attend to the sensations in her leg: "She was asked to observe the sensations as precisely as she could, to notice whether she felt burning, aching, throbbing, or stabbing. Whenever she had a fearful or distracting thought, she was asked to return her attention to the actual sensations in her leg at the present moment" (p. 183). Initially, Beth's pain increased in intensity, but as the session progressed Beth began to notice that the pain was not, in fact, continuous; it seemed to ebb and flow. Siegel encouraged Beth to continue to attend to the details of her sensations and noted that by the end of the session she was "surprised to find that she could stay with the experience" (p. 183).

Consistent with clinical reports such as this one, a growing body of empirical research has shown that various forms of meditation, such as TM and MM, can stimulate positive physical, psychological, and behavioral changes (e.g., Alexander, Rainforth, & Gelderloos, 1991; Baer, 2003; Lazar, 2005). The efficacy of meditation has been attributed to several psychological mechanisms (Baer, 2003). Distraction is one possible mechanism. Concentration on breathing, a phrase, or an emotion can distract the individual from painful and pointless rumination. Similarly, mindfulness shifts the individual's attention from past losses and future worries to being in the present moment. Exposure is another potential mechanism. Rather than trying to avoid the pain, the individual is encouraged to reexperience the pain until it loses its capacity to elicit other negative emotions and responses. The effects of meditation have also been attributed to cognitive changes. Miller, Fletcher, and Kabat-Zinn (1995) note that "by adopting a more dispassionate, witness-like observing and self-reporting of the moment-to-moment unfolding of one's experience," the meditator develops greater cognitive mastery and an alternative to the fight-or-flight response to stress (p. 197).

Interestingly, when trying to explain the effectiveness of meditation, many researchers and practitioners have overlooked the spiritual nature of this technique or have attempted to separate the method from its connections to the sacred. For example, commenting on the therapeutic value of techniques that are rooted in spiritual traditions, Hayes (2002) goes on to add that "we must fit them into our field theoretically, without any sectarian or supernatural connotations. It may appear slightly sacrilegious to say so, but if religious and spiritual traditions are to enter empirical clinical psychology, they must be ours" (p. 105). Yet, in attempting to peel the sacred "connotations" away from meditation, clinicians may be removing one of its vital ingredients. For example, meditators often report powerful experiences and emotions filled with sacred meaning, such as deep gratitude, feelings of love and compassion, a sense of awe and uplift, and a feeling of connection to their very ground of being or a transcendent force outside of themselves (e.g., Astin, 1997; Shapiro, Schwartz, & Bonner, 1998). These sacred emotions may account for some of the beneficial effects of meditation. In this vein, Alexander et al. (1991) conducted a meta-analysis of 42 studies on the effects of TM. The practice of TM was tied to a greater number of transcendental experiences and these experiences, in turn, were associated with significant psychological and physical change. Similarly, acceptance—a critical element of meditation—may be closely connected to a spiritual dimension, for the ability to accept painful thoughts, feelings, and cravings is interwoven with the ability to accept human limitations and finitude, and the ability to let go of fruitless efforts to eliminate pain is linked to the ability to surrender control to a larger field of forces when control is no longer possible. Finally, part of the power of meditation may lie in the underlying worldview it presents to practitioners. From the perspective of Western religious traditions, meditation represents a pathway to the experience of God. Of course, it could be argued that popular forms of meditation today come from nontheistic Eastern traditions. However, these traditions also rest on ultimate and untestable assumptions about the character of existence, such as the belief that suffering is caused by false attachments to illusion and the belief that meditation helps people awaken and see the true nature of reality. Even though these ontological assumptions are not often explicitly articulated, they are embedded in meditative practices and may account, at least in part, for their helpful effects.

Some research evidence suggests that spirituality adds an important dimension to at least certain forms of meditation. For example, Amy Wachholtz has conducted studies that suggest that the spiritual content of the object of concentration in meditation can magnify the power of this practice (Wachholtz & Pargament, 2005; Wachholtz, 2005). Her findings challenge the view that "thinking about the meaning of your word during the meditative practice constitutes distraction from the exercise of the meditation, so the meaning of the word should not matter and should not come into play during meditation" (Helminiak, 2005, p. 39). In her most recent study, Wachholtz (2005) worked with 80 college students who were suffering from migraines. Students were taught one of three concentration types of meditation: meditation to a spiritual phrase (e.g., "God is peace," "God is love"), meditation to an internal secular phrase (e.g., "I am happy," "I am good"), and meditation to an external secular phrase (e.g., "Grass is green," "Sunshine is warm"). A fourth group of students was taught a progressive relaxation technique. The students practiced their meditation/relaxation method for a month. Measures of psychological, physical, and spiritual functioning were collected at three time points: before they began to meditate/relax, after 1 month of practice, and 1 month later. The results were striking. In comparison to the other three groups, the spiritual meditators reported significantly fewer headaches, less migraine headache pain, reductions in negative mood and trait anxiety, greater existential well-being, more mystical experiences, and greater pain tolerance (as demonstrated by their ability to keep their hands in ice water for significantly longer periods of time). Wachholtz's findings are intriguing and need to be extended to other clinical populations. But they hold potentially important implications for practitioners because they suggest that the effects of at least some types of meditation can be enhanced when the spiritual dimension is made more explicit.

CONCLUSIONS

Embedded within spirituality is a rich and diverse set of resources that can be applied to the variety of problems people bring to psychotherapy. In this chapter, we illustrated some of the ways clinicians can help clients draw on three of these resources: spiritual strivings, spiritual knowledge, and spiritual experience. There are others, however—too many to review in a single chapter. In the next chapter, I consider another potent set of spiritual resources for psychotherapy.

13

Drawing on Spiritual Practices, Relationships, and Coping Methods

Clients' spiritual resources can take many forms. In Chapter 12, we explored how therapists can help their clients draw on their spiritual strivings, knowledge, and experiences. Now we consider some of the ways therapists can help their clients access another set of resources: spiritual practices, relationships, and coping methods.

HELPING CLIENTS DRAW ON SPIRITUAL PRACTICES

Of all the spiritual practices, rituals have received the greatest amount of attention in psychotherapy. Why might that be? Perhaps because there is a shortage of rituals designed to mark and facilitate critical transitions in living. Underritualization is a problem in our culture today. More and more people are encountering profound shifts in their lives as a result of social and technological change. Unfortunately, religious traditions, by and large, have not kept up with these changes by offering new rituals for emerging transitions, such as divorce, unemployment, blended families, in vitro fertilization, adoption, an elder child returning home to live, menopause, retirement, entry into a nursing home, and removal from life support equipment. The frantic pace of life today has also contributed to underritualization. Caught up in the rush of day-to-day demands, we find it increasingly difficult to take a step back from it all and mark truly momentous periods of life. Who can afford the time off from work to welcome a new baby into the world or to grieve a death? Other people shy away from rituals because they arouse painful memories of conflict and loss. There is a cost, however, to underritualization.

Without the ability to make "some days and some hours special," Kushner (1989) writes, we would live in a "flat, monochromatic world, a world without color or texture, a world in which all days would be the same" (p. 206). Stripped of ritual, even the most powerful negative events go relatively unrecognized, and people are left with unresolved grief. Disconnected from rituals, people cannot participate in purposeful acts of transformation that propel them over sacred thresholds from one place in life to another. Instead, they become stuck in particular emotions (e.g., anger, shame, sadness), particular ways of life (e.g., constant work, social isolation), or particular life conditions (e.g., widowhood, unemployment). And lacking the power of ritual, people are less able to signify the sacred moments in life. Clinically, this loss of spiritual meaning may express itself through a variety of psychological problems, including depression, adjustment disorders, anxiety, and PTSD.

Drawing on rituals in therapy is one way to address this loss of significance. Rituals serve many purposes. They encourage emotional catharsis, define identity, build community, and help people make meaning of change and transition. Most importantly, however, rituals reinstill a sense of sacredness in people by placing the conditions of their lives within the context of a grand drama that expresses deeper and greater truths about existence. Rituals have a dual nature: they promote both continuity and change (Pargament, 1997). At one level, they are transformational, pushing people through sacred "hinges of time" (Friedman, 1985, p. 164) from one phase of life to another, one emotion to another, and one level of experience to another. On another level, they provide a secure grounding, reminding participants that in spite of the changes they are undergoing, some things remain constant. Because of their dual nature, rituals often have a melancholy quality about them, for they confront people with the realities of change and loss while celebrating the preservation of sacred memories, relationships, communities, identities, hopes, and dreams.

Rituals are particularly important in psychotherapy when words are simply not enough. Though words are necessary to make meaning of ritual, actions are the critical vehicle for the experience of the sacred in the ritual drama. Let's return to the case of Rachel, the 35-year-old Roman Catholic client who felt that she had committed an unforgivable sin by having an abortion at age 14. Recall that Rachel believed that the death of her beloved grandmother and the rapes and infertility she experienced later in her life were punishments from God for her transgression. Over the course of therapy, Rachel and I explored her understanding of God and the Catholic Church. Yet, in spite of our conversations, she could not rid herself of the lingering feeling that she was being punished for the unforgivable sin she had committed as an adolescent. I questioned Rachel on her belief that the sin she had committed was unforgivable in the eyes of the Church and asked her for permission to raise the issue with a Roman Catholic priest. She agreed. I called a priest who was a colleague of mine and a respected theologian, shared elements of Rachel's story with him, and asked him whether she had committed an unforgivable sin in the eyes of the Catholic Church. He responded, "Absolutely not." In fact, he said, he would be more than happy to work with Rachel so that she could receive the Sacrament of Reconciliation (also known as Penance). After some initial reluctance, Rachel agreed to meet with the priest, and over the next 6 months she moved toward participation in this sacrament. The results were noticeable. It seemed as though a burden had been lifted off of her shoulders. Rachel began to speak of God less as a punishing figure and more as a sympathetic figure who suffered alongside her. And, for the first time, Rachel could direct her anger outward at the rapists in her life rather than inward at herself. The ritual act of purification within her church had helped Rachel in a way that the conversation of psychotherapy could not.

In many cases such as this one, therapists can call upon well-established rituals from the client's religious tradition to facilitate change. Take another example. Pamela was a 50-year-old client who usually came to therapy out of breath. The reasons would vary: she had been racing from one appointment to another, she had been trying to solve the problems of friends or family, or she had been responding to one of the crises in her life that seemed to arise with regularity. Pamela was very successful as a businesswoman, wife, and mother, but she was also constantly on edge. In therapy, she was often close to tears as she voiced her feeling that she was about to fall apart. When I talked to her about the possibility of slowing down and giving herself a chance to catch her breath, literally and figuratively, she responded by saying that she was a Christian woman and knew God had blessed her with many gifts in her life. It was up to her to use all of her gifts as fully as she could. I paused for a moment and then said, "Even God rested on the seventh day. What about you?" Pamela also paused for a moment and then answered, "I hadn't thought about it that way." She came to the next session noticeably calmer, with her breath under control, and announced that she had decided to celebrate the Sabbath. Sunday, she had told her family, was now her day of rest and she was going to take resting very seriously.

At times, established rituals may need to be modified to fit changing needs and contexts. This is not as difficult as it may seem. As Herbert Anderson and Edward Foley (1998) write in their book *Mighty Stories, Dangerous Rituals*, "The standardized liturgies of our various traditions are not ceremonial cookie cutters that need to force every human situation into their mold. Rather they are resources and models of ritual wisdom that should inspire rather than constrain those who employ them" (p. 133). We can find a number of strikingly powerful examples of the creative use of rituals that can be accessed in counseling. Anderson and Foley (1998) present the case of Jack, a man dying of AIDS who was concerned about the impact of his death on his family. He wanted to leave his family with a reminder of his feelings for them, a permanent legacy that they could hold onto and use to ease their grief. With the help of his pastor, he wrote letters to each family member. On the day he died, he read the letters to the family members who were standing vigil by his bedside. "Each reading took a while, as they were frequently interrupted by tears. But the readings were not difficult for Jack, and they actually seemed to calm him. He died quietly, forty-five minutes after the last of his letters was read to his kid brother" (p. 51). At the funeral, Jack had a final letter read to his loved ones. In the closing lines, he wrote:

> I am especially grateful that you helped me die well; that in the final days and weeks together you didn't try to hold on to me, or ever make me feel guilty for having AIDS. You loved me enough to let me go when God called. Know that in my gratitude I'll be waiting for you on the other side, so that when it is your time, you too will not die alone—Love Jack. (p. 50)

Mark Molldrem, a Lutheran pastor, developed a ritual for newly divorced couples that includes their children in the process (Paquette, 2005). He notes that ritual is ideally suited for children because it relies not only on words, which may be difficult for children to understand, but also on images, symbols, and drama that children can intuitively grasp. Molldrem's divorce ritual expresses truths, hope, and affirmation of the bonds between parent and child. The ritual is conducted before the altar of a sanctuary to remind the newly divorced participants that, even though they are divorced, they continue to stand before God in a holy space. A central "marriage candle" is lit and "those assembled acknowledge the sanctity and pure intentions of the marriage, and also that those intentions have met with failure, bitterness, and despair" (p. 2). The pastor then offers forgiveness to the couple in words that parallel the marital vows: "What God has forgiven, let no one doubt; what God has set aside, let no one bring up again" (p. 2). The couple extends a hand of friendship to each other and agree to treat each other kindly. Their children are then called forward and invited to acknowledge their own pain in this transition and express their hope for happiness after divorce. A final blessing is offered: "Parenthood remains a link between husband and wife, even though they separate. Guide them . . . that in the love of each parent the children may know the joy of family" (p. 2). The ritual concludes with the divorced pair lighting two individual candles from the flame of the central marital candle, which is then extinguished.

There are many other examples. Tisdale (2003) describes how she encouraged a couple to renew their wedding vows in a ceremony designed to celebrate their success in coming to terms with the trauma of an extramarital affair. Imber-Black and Roberts (1992) describe how they helped a boy fully grieve the death of his father. He had been discouraged from attending his father's funeral at the age of 11. Imber-Black and Roberts helped him create a special individualized memorial service for his father several years later so that he could finally obtain closure. Schachter-Shalomi and Miller (1995) present a ritual to facilitate the transition of elders into the role of sacred sages by celebrating their status as patriarchs and matriarchs who have stocks of wisdom to pass on to successive generations. My colleagues and I have found this ritual particularly helpful in clinical work with depressed elders. Johnson, Feldman, Lubin, and Southwick (1995) create moving rituals for soldiers suffering from PTSD to facilitate their departure, return home, and mourning for friends who were killed in combat.

In spite of their diversity, effective rituals have several points in common. First, they are simple. They do not overexplain, they are not overly complicated, and they do not lose the interest of the participant (Anderson & Foley, 1998). Instead, they capture and express basic truths of life simply through image and symbol, action and word. Second, they are honest. They encourage people to face both the realities of pain and loss and the hopes and dreams they continue to hold for their futures. Third, rituals are public. They are enacted in relationship to other people who witness the drama, cushioning the individual through the process with their support and affirmation. And finally, they are sacred. They speak to a timeless, ultimate dimension of existence and touch people at their deepest levels of emotion and meaning. Unfortunately, researchers have not systematically examined the effects of incorporating rituals in psychotherapy. Yet clinical accounts suggest that rituals have the capacity to prompt significant transformations in psychotherapy, even when other modes of treatment have proven to be ineffective.

HELPING CLIENTS DRAW
ON SPIRITUAL RELATIONSHIPS

There is a sacred dimension to relationships that can also be integrated into psychotherapy. As I noted earlier, many people experience the divine through their encounters with others. Even nontheists may describe relationships in terms of sacred qualities. However, clients suffering from loneliness, alienation, and depression often find themselves cut off from this deeper level of connection. Therapists can help clients draw on spiritual relationships in a number of contexts.

Religious Congregations

At their best, religious congregations represent "convoys" (see Kahn & Antonucci, 1980) of support to people over the course of their lifespan. Other social resources may come and go, but churches, synagogues, mosques, and temples remain available to many people, including those whose social networks have been shaken or shattered. By cultivating ties with diverse religious communities, therapists can help these clients reconnect to a supportive group. For example, Hathaway (2004) describes his work with a 27-year-old African American woman in the U.S. Air Force who was having difficulty adjusting to her move from an urban, northern setting to a rural, southern community. The loss of her close-knit religious community was particularly hard for her. A Wiccan, the client had encountered negative reactions to the altar she had erected in her quarters. She was unaware of other Wiccan worshippers on her base. Hathaway helped this client locate a similar, supportive community through a meeting of the Society of Creative Anachronism.

Religious communities can be especially valuable resources for socially marginal clients who find themselves alienated from other networks of support. Some congregations, for instance, have developed programs to reach out and welcome people with serious mental illness. Walters and Neugeboren (1995) write that "church-based programs can become a means [for individuals with mental illness] to re-enter the normal community, remove the stigma and burdens of being a 'mental patient,' and find socialization and networking opportunities leading to client empowerment and normalization" (p. 52).

Religious Leaders

Though clinicians have often sought out referrals from the leaders of religious communities, they have traditionally overlooked clergy as potential resources in and of themselves. Yet religious leaders have their own distinctive skills and resources. In contrast to health professionals, clergy have greater access to people in difficult times, the legitimacy to reach out proactively to people who may be reluctant to seek help, the sanction of a tradition to impart its religious wisdom, and the authority to perform rituals within the tradition of a faith. In short, clergy can do some things that therapists cannot. Therapists who are able to appreciate the unique resources of religious leaders could forge invaluable collaborative ties with this group that would enrich their clinical work (Tyler, Pargament, & Gatz, 1983).

For example, Suess and Halpern (1989) describe the case of Daniel, a 19-year-old Jewish college student diagnosed with obsessive–compulsive disorder. Fearful of punishment from God, Daniel dealt with his transgressions by making promises to God that he would abstain from a pleasurable act. With time, however, he would forget the vow and then make new, negative promises to maintain his feelings of remorse and prove himself to God. Gradually, he became trapped in a series of punitive oaths that made it impossible for him to experience any pleasure or productivity in his life. Daniel's therapist thought a religious ritual might be helpful to allay Daniel's unrelenting guilt and remorse, so he sought out help from a rabbi, who suggested adapting a purification ritual used during the Jewish High Holy Days, the Annulment of Vows ("Hatarat Nedarim"). The therapist met with the rabbi to plan the ritual in a synagogue. There, standing in front of two rabbinical judges, Daniel formally petitioned for the annulment of his vows. Daniel's vows were annulled, and he was also presented with scriptural citations to remind him that Judaism emphasizes the importance of appreciating the pleasures of life (e.g., "Do not miss a day's enjoyment or forego your share of innocent pleasure" [New English Bible, cited in Suess & Halpern, 1989, p. 322]. Several months later, both rabbi and therapist reported significant improvements in Daniel's mood and behavior.

Spouses and Family

Don and Julie had been married for 10 years and had been in conflict for about eight of them. Each had accumulated a litany of grievances over the years, and each expected the other to change his or her ways. In the initial sessions, I tried to get Don and Julie to calm down, slow down, and listen to their partner's feelings and wishes. I was remarkably unsuccessful. Neither was willing to shift the focus from his or her own needs to those of the other. Like a tape stuck in replay mode, the couple kept repeating the same discordant tune:

DON: You don't give me what I want.

JULIE: Well, you don't give me what I want either.

DON: What I want is really important.

JULIE: I've given a lot to you over the years and now what I want is more important.

In the midst of another unproductive session, I asked the couple what seemed to me a perfectly reasonable question: "Why are you two still married?" Both partners seemed taken aback, and then they answered simultaneously, "We love each other!" I responded, "I have to tell you that, at least from an outside perspective, you don't seem to be showing much love to each other. Could you tell me what you mean when you say you love each other?" Again, Don and Julie appeared to be surprised by the question. In a faltering way, Don said, "You know, love, it's a feeling deep down, an intense kind of thing." Julie nodded her head in one of the first signs of agreement I had seen between the couple. I decided then to see if I could help the couple access whatever love they might hold for each other through a "love intervention," a method I have used over the years to help many couples tap into the sacred core of their marriage.

There are several steps to this intervention. I begin with an explanation to the couple. Love is defined not as an emotion, but as a behavior. Feelings of passion are not hard to come by in relationships. Love, however, is more difficult. It is defined by a partner's willingness to give what the other person wants, even if it is not what the partner wants to give. Love requires a shift from a focus on oneself to a focus on the other person, and a readiness to make this shift without resentment. Viewed in this way, love is a gift. If forced, coerced, or offered grudgingly, it is no longer love. Only when it is given freely does love have the capacity to deepen and enrich a relationship. Given freely, however, love is the heart and soul of marriage.

I then ask the partners to go home and make a list of what they want from each other. They can list as many things as they want. However, they are encouraged to phrase their needs positively and concretely (e.g., "I would like you to say 'Hello' to me when you come home from work") rather than in negative, vague ways (e.g., "I wish you would grow up"). I also ask the partners to construct their lists privately to prevent the intervention from becoming another battleground before they return to therapy.

I begin the next session by asking one partner to take the role of "speaker" and express one need from his or her list to the "listener." (It is best to avoid starting with "hot-button needs.") If the wife is the speaker, her job is to state her need as clearly as possible. The husband-listener's role is to make sure he understands what is being requested. Once the listener feels that he understands the speaker, and once the speaker feels that she has been understood, the focus shifts to the listener. I then ask the listener to consider to what extent he can respond to the request of his partner, not because he feels forced or coerced, but because he loves the other person. In the same session, I ask the couple to switch positions, and the new speaker (husband) is asked to present one need from his list to the new listener (wife).

Over the next few sessions, the partners repeat this process, moving through several items on their respective lists. One hopes that, outside of therapy, each has also begun to respond more lovingly to the needs of the other. With practice, they can begin to share their needs with each other at home too. Throughout this intervention, the therapist must work hard to break the cycle of self-preoccupation and external blame that has led to ongoing and unresolved conflict. The speaker is discouraged from slipping into a long litany of accusations, and the listener is discouraged from engaging in self-defense or changing the subject to his or her own needs. By keeping the focus on one need at a time, lowering the emotional temperature in the room, and clearly defining the roles of speaker and listener, the love intervention directs the attention of each partner to one critical question: How much do we love each other?

The love intervention proved to be quite effective with Don and Julie. It was not a panacea; it did not resolve their long lists of mutual grievances, but it did create a new cycle of giving to each other in ways that communicated sensitivity and caring. As the couple began to show more love to each other, their lists of complaints seemed to fade into the background. Even though it has not been formally evaluated, I have found this intervention to be helpful to many couples with long histories of conflict and resentment, provided that a spark of love and caring remains in the relationship.

I realize that talk of love in the context of psychotherapy may sound mawkish or corny to scientifically minded clinicians. However, it is a vital, even essential, part of a thriving marriage and, as a result, deserves greater attention. The love intervention is one way to address this aspect of marital life. It is effective, I believe, because it helps couples access the sacred dimension of their relationship. As I stressed earlier, love embodies qualities of the sacred. Love is the heart and soul of a marriage, the secure foundation on which marriages flourish or the shaky foundation on which marriages flounder. Love is the vehicle through which partners touch each other at their deepest level and elevate themselves to bring out the best in each other. And love is perceived by many as transcendent and timeless, the extraordinary quality of marriage that rises above all others and endures through eternity.

Therapeutic Relationship

The client's relationship with the therapist can also be understood as a sacred resource. Theistically oriented therapists have described themselves as conduits of divine love and care. Wayne Aoki, for example, talks about his sense that he is not working alone when he is doing couple therapy: "I am working in community with the very Creator of fidelity, of commitment, and faithfulness" (Aoki, Barsness, & Leong, 2001, p. 81). Similarly, Aoki cites another Christian therapist who writes that "If we believe that God took human form in Christ Jesus, and that through the incarnation we are Christ to one another, then God's own love comes concretely into our midst through our own interpersonal interactions" (Aoki et al., 2001, p. 82).

Other therapists have spoken in less theistic terms about therapy as a form of spiritual care (Swinton, 2001). In a clinical case study, Tricia Hughes (2001) captures the spiritual character of her relationship with Heidi, a bright young woman plagued by feelings of unworthiness and moods that vacillated from expansiveness to despair. Growing up with an intensely judgmental, highly accomplished father, Heidi worried constantly about making mistakes, rejection, and disapproval. Hughes notes that "Heidi seemed uneasy in her own skin and would often pull her limbs in close to her onto the chair" (p. 4) and later "she seemed to have no refuge, no place of rest" (p. 8). Hughes decided that she wanted to offer Heidi an experience of deep and unconditional acceptance—an experience of grace. Hughes writes: "In the midst of Heidi's own struggles to be better, to become more, to try and 'get it right' this time, I wanted to give her the experience of saying right here you are enough. There is nothing more you need to do or be or become" (p. 9). In response to Heidi's sense of fundamental isolation in her life journey, Hughes offered her a different image, the image of a "faithful companion" (see Schlauch, 1995). Hughes asks Heidi, "What would it be like to have someone with you in the midst of the struggle, along through the twists and turns of your journey?" (p. 11). These are some of the ways Hughes consciously draws on the sacred qualities of the therapeutic relationship—grace, deep acceptance, reassuring presence—to repair Heidi's sense of brokenness and instill feelings of hope and wholeness.

Thinking about the therapeutic relationship as a spiritual resource may seem strange. After all, therapists have generally avoided the spiritual life of the client entirely, not to mention the spiritual characteristics of the therapeutic relationship. Yet the sacred qualities of the connection between clients and therapists may be among the most critical of therapeutic ingredients.

HELPING CLIENTS DRAW
ON SPIRITUAL COPING METHODS

My review of the ways in which therapists can help clients reach out to their spiritual resources has already touched on several largely conservational types of spiritual coping, such as support from clergy, spiritual connection, and purification rituals. Two additional conservational forms of spiritual coping, spiritual support and spiritual meaning making, deserve clinical attention. Both of these coping resources can help many kinds of clients sustain themselves psychologically, socially, and spiritually.

Spiritual Support

Like support from congregation and clergy, support from the sacred is available when other resources are lacking. For even the most isolated and depleted clients, spiritual support can be a significant source of comfort, strength, and encouragement. A number of therapists have begun to help people seek out spiritual support in psychotherapy. Toward this end, most therapists follow three basic steps: (1) they create a relaxing context for the client; (2) they encourage their clients to identify the problem, memory, or experience that is causing them distress; and (3) they help their clients recall or imagine a spiritually supportive image or experience (Tan, 1996).

Consider, for example, the "Breath of God" visualization exercise developed by Brenda Cole (1999) as part of a group intervention for women with cancer. Designed to help these women come to terms with the uncontrollable in their lives, this exercise combines elements of spiritual support and spiritual surrender:

> Close your eyes and begin to focus your attention on your breathing. Let your body become more and more relaxed as I count to five—1 . . . 2 . . . 3 . . . 4 . . . 5. As you continue breathing deeply, and slowly, visualize God as a beautiful light surrounding you. With each breath that you take notice that you are breathing in this beautiful Holy light. This light fills your lungs and as you exhale you feel the light of God permeating your entire body, and flowing out your fingers and toes. . . . Now that you are completely relaxed continue to visualize God's presence in whatever way you prefer. And when you are ready, ask God "What do I most need to surrender to you?" [pause] What response do you hear? [pause] When you are ready to surrender what God asks, visualize placing this in God's hands. As you let go, feel yourself bathed in a circle of light, feeling acceptance, peace, and protection. Remember that the circle symbolizes wholeness, completion, harmony, and oneness with God. Allow yourself to feel the healing power of this light as you breathe it in with each breath. You may experience this deep feeling of surrender whenever you wish, by closing your eyes and visualizing the "Breath of God" entering your body. . . . (pp. 267–268).

This exercise has been applied successfully to women from a variety of religious backgrounds. However, in a sense, it imposes a particular supportive image and experience of God on the participants.

Spiritual support can be found in ways that are more closely tailored to the client's own understanding and experience of the sacred. Griffith and Griffith (2002) illustrate how to help a client identify and draw on her own spiritually supportive metaphor. The client, Mary, came to therapy struggling with the discovery that her husband of 30 years had been involved in a long-term affair. Though she felt emotionally overwhelmed, Mary noted that she had been through other hard times in her life, including a deadly tornado. This led to the following exchange:

> MARY: I will never forget what I saw. The devastation. There were bodies, dead and wounded out in the open, homes demolished. We worked for days afterward, cleaning up the debris. . . . In fact, that's more like where I feel I am now, rather than in the middle of the storm. I'm cleaning up the debris.

THERAPIST: As you are cleaning up debris, where is God?

MARY: Just beside me. Right next to me. As I pick up a board, he's picking up the heavy end, making the board somehow supernaturally lighter. (p. 54)

Mary's greatest fear was that, by remaining in her marriage with her husband, she risked another betrayal. To help her cope with the uncertainty in rebuilding her marriage, the therapist returned to Mary's metaphor and encouraged her to call upon it once again:

THERAPIST: If you were out there steadily cleaning up the debris, with God alongside you, lifting heavy ends of the boards, and, suddenly, another storm hit, then where would God be?

MARY: Where would he be? I'm not sure. But I do know that he would know what to do. If there were a ditch, he would grab me and run there. He would put me down in the ditch and lay on top of me. . . . I guess I don't really know exactly what he would do. Maybe I don't have to know, but I do know that he would know what to do. (p. 55)

Although spiritual support is most often sought from God in our culture, therapists can also gain support from other forms of the sacred. For example, recently I worked with a single, middle-aged woman, Ruth, who had come to my office suffering from depression following the death of her mother. For much of her life, Ruth had devoted herself to her mother's care. She was, Ruth said, her closest friend. When her mother died, Ruth felt as if a huge part of herself had been torn away. Most distressing of all, she could not stop thinking about her mother lying in her grave, all alone, missing her daughter. Ruth spent much of her time contemplating suicide. That way, she felt, she could join her mother and ensure that she would never be alone again.

My efforts to encourage Ruth to reengage herself in life were not successful. Finally, I asked Ruth to bring in pictures of her mother and herself. The pictures revealed her mother to be a stout, cheerful woman who seemed to radiate warmth, strength, and good humor, even though she was restricted to a wheelchair. Ruth, in contrast, appeared to be dark and somber, even as a young child. In commenting on the pictures, I asked Ruth to consider who seemed lonelier, her or her mother. Ruth admitted that she had always been the lonely one. In fact, her mother had continually encouraged her to make friends, spend more time away from home, and create a life for herself. "And if the spirit of your mother could speak now," I asked, "what would she say?" "Oh, she'd probably say the same thing," Ruth answered. "Get out of bed, get dressed, get to work, get some friends, and get started with the rest of your life." Over the next few sessions, I continued to have Ruth voice the spirit of her mother. In the process, it became clearer to Ruth that her mother was not lonely. Most of all, the mother who spoke to her wanted Ruth to take some pleasure from life. Ruth's thoughts of suicide came to an end and her depression lifted. Punctuating these changes, Ruth had a dream before the last session of therapy in which her mother came to her and said, "You've been given a new chance at life, grab it."

Spiritual Meaning Making

In the effort to make sense out of difficult life experiences, many clients find themselves confronting a crisis of meaning. Unable to assimilate painful events into their worldviews, they may repeatedly struggle with the question, Why? Or they may get stuck in explanations that leave them disheartened, confused, or unable to achieve closure. Spiritual reframing can help clients place negative life events into a larger, more meaningful, often more hopeful and benevolent context.

For example, James Magee (1994) describes the case of a widower who was part of a life review group made up of other elderly participants. The widower was grieving about a succession of losses and failures that had occurred over a period of decades. His grief was intensified by the desolate framing of his life, a desolation he captured by quoting from William Butler Yeats's The Second Coming (1920):

> Turning and turning in the widening gyre
> The falcon cannot hear the falconer;
> Things fall apart; the center cannot hold;

Other participants in the group challenged the widower to find a more compelling way to make meaning of himself and his life, and he responded to the challenge. At the next meeting of the group, the widower offered a profoundly spiritual reframing:

> I am a living tree. Together we form a forest, all rooted in a common Ground. Though we are not the Ground, we cannot live apart from the Ground. Uprooted, I am lumber, fuel, or furniture, but not a tree. I have lived so concerned about my fruits. I mean to focus now upon my roots! (p. 67)

Not all clients are capable of making spiritual meaning so quickly or so creatively. In some cases, the therapist may need to take a more active role in helping the client view his or her life from a larger spiritual perspective. For instance, I worked with a 60-year-old man, Doug, who, 3 years earlier, had divorced his wife after 35 years of marriage. She had been emotionally abusive to him for much of that time, but he had remained in this joyless relationship for two reasons: he was frightened about the prospect of living alone, and he felt divorce was wrong in the eyes of God. Only when the abuse became physical did he end the marriage. Following the divorce, Doug developed tremendous anxiety whenever he found himself alone. To deal with his anxiety, he threw himself into a frenzy of activity: boating, hunting, hiking, basketball, painting, remodeling, music, and church attendance. But the anxiety only intensified. Over the next few years, he dated a number of women. A handsome man with a comfortable retirement income, Doug had no problem attracting eligible partners. However, when these relationships became more intimate, he experienced powerful fears that he would once again find himself trapped in a loveless marriage. Much to the surprise of his partners, he would call a sudden end to these promising relationships, only to experience the anxiety of being alone once again.

The sessions of therapy reflected the cycle of anxiety in his life. When he was between relationships, Doug spoke of his fears of isolation and never "finding that right someone." When he was in the midst of a relationship, he described his fears of intimacy and what he believed to be the inevitable result: rejection. Fear, be it the fear of isolation or the fear of intimacy, was the way Doug framed his problem. But this form of meaning making didn't lend itself to a solution. In his efforts to avoid fear of one kind, he introduced fear of another kind.

Relaxation training, exposure to his fears, exploration of the childhood roots of his anxiety—none of these approaches was especially helpful to Doug. He remained locked in his fruitless attempts to avoid his fears. So I decided to try to reframe Doug's situation into a larger spiritual context. Knowing that Doug had been a lifelong Christian and deeply involved in his nondenominational fellowship, I shifted the focus of the conversation from fear to faith in the following exchange:

K.I.P.: Doug, we've talked a lot about some of the things you're afraid of. But I've been struck by some of the things that don't seem to frighten you. You haven't talked about any fears of dying. Why is that?

DOUG: I'm not really afraid of dying. That's something that's never bothered me. I know that when I die I will join my Lord and all of my loved ones who have gone before me.

K.I.P.: I wonder how you know that, Doug?

DOUG: Well, the Bible says that it's true.

K.I.P.: I respect your beliefs, Doug, but I'd like to learn a little more about them. Tell me, how do you know that what's written in the Bible is true?

DOUG: Well, I can't prove it to you, if that's what you mean. I just feel in my heart that it's true.

K.I.P.: It sounds like it's a matter of faith for you.

DOUG: Exactly.

K.I.P.: Your faith seems to have helped you push beyond any fears you might have of dying. I wonder whether you might draw on that same faith to help you break through to the other side of your fears about being alone and being in relationships.

DOUG: I don't know. I hadn't thought about it like that before.

K.I.P.: Let me leave you with this question today. What do you want to have the last word on your life, your fears or your faith?

Reframing his problem from fear to a matter of faith proved to be very helpful to Doug for a few reasons. Like other forms of successful spiritual meaning making, this one grew out of Doug's own spiritual framework. Thus, it was difficult to refute and easier for him to apply. The reframing was also freeing; by shifting the focus from fear to faith, it created new options and possibilities. Doug was able to step back from failed attempts to avoid isolation and intimacy, and to consider instead how he might live a life more fully based on his faith.

This process did not occur overnight. Initially, Doug tried to use his faith as one more method to make his fears disappear. For example, he would ask God to take his fears away. But we continued to work with this metaphor, and talked about how he might draw on his faith to help him accept anxiety in his life. Some anxiety was appropriate, for there were no guarantees that Doug would not end up alone or find himself trapped in another destructive relationship. But what was the guarantee of heavenly rewards?, I asked Doug. And if rewards in heaven and earth were absolutely certain, what need would there be for faith? By understanding his problem as a matter of faith, Doug developed greater confidence that anxiety did not have to have the last word on his life, that he could experience anxiety and transcend it at the same time.

Initial empirical studies underscore the potential value of spiritual meaning making to clients. For example, Julie Exline and her colleagues studied 15 male and female adults who had been diagnosed with PTSD following war experiences or sexual assault (Exline, Smyth, Gregory, Hockemeyer, & Tulloch, 2005). They asked their participants to write about their traumatic experiences for three 20-minute sessions. In the first session, they were asked to describe their traumatic experience in detail, including their deepest emotional reactions. In the second session, participants were encouraged to write about their experience in the form of a story with a beginning, a middle, and an end. In the third session, the participants were asked to reflect on their thoughts and feelings in writing the first two essays and retell the story of their experience while integrating their new insights. Participants were not instructed to write about religion or spirituality in any of these sessions. Exline and her colleagues coded each of the essays for religious references, and found that 80% of the participants framed their experiences in religious terms in at least one of their essays. Furthermore, those who framed their experiences through positive religious references experienced significantly greater positive mood changes over the three writing sessions. Exline et al. (2005) concluded that "to the extent that religious views help people to make sense of negative events, religious framing may have helped people to gain useful insights and to gain a sense of meaning or closure about the traumatic situation" (p. 28).

CONCLUSIONS

In this chapter and the previous one, I reviewed several ways clinicians can help their clients to make use of their spiritual resources in psychotherapy. But this review has only been illustrative. There are many spiritual resources that can be applied to clients dealing with a variety of problems. Clinical accounts suggest that these resources represent a potentially valuable adjunct to treatment. Although empirical studies have shown these resources to be helpful to people in the general population, as yet there is relatively little research evidence for the efficacy of specific spiritual resources in therapy, with the exception of meditation research and individual studies such as those by Exline et al. (2005). Practitioners, however, have started to design and test spiritually integrated therapies that draw on several different spiritual resources, and, as we will see later in the book, these initial efforts have begun to yield promising results.

In sum, spirituality is an overlooked yet potent resource in therapy. Nevertheless, there are times when spirituality cannot be accessed. Why? Because, on occasion, spirituality is more a part of the problem than it is a part of the solution. In these instances, the task for the clinician shifts to helping clients address their spiritual problems and move toward greater spiritual integration. I consider this task in the next two chapters.

14

Addressing Problems
of Spiritual Destinations

Spirituality has been described as a double-edged sword throughout this book, a part of the solution to problems on one edge of the sword, and a problem in and of itself on the other. We have considered a number of cases in which clients' spiritual problems contribute directly to the concerns they bring into therapy: the woman who continues to visit her abusive parents because she believes she must honor her father and mother as the Bible commands; the man who turns to alcohol to fill a spiritual vacuum in his life; the young bereaved mother who comes to therapy at the request of her parents, who are convinced that she is crazy because she continues to talk to her daughter in heaven; the minister who keeps his diagnosis of cancer a secret because he believes it is a sign that he has fallen out of favor with the Lord; and the woman whose compulsive attention to ritual purity prevents her from having intimate relations with her husband. It is hard to imagine how a practitioner could make much progress in cases such as these without attending to the client's spiritual problems.

In this chapter and the next, I focus on a variety of ways in which clinicians can address spiritual problems in psychotherapy and help their clients move toward greater spiritual integration. Once again, this review is illustrative rather than comprehensive. I consider how spiritual resources can be brought to bear on problems of spiritual destinations in this chapter, and how they can be applied to problems of spiritual pathways in the next.

ADDRESSING SMALL GODS

As I noted earlier, small gods create significant problems for people—be they the harsh god incapable of offering mercy or compassion, the loving god that cannot be reconciled with pain and suffering, the distant god that leaves the individual adrift in times of greatest need, or the fortress god whose support and protection encompass only those who live within the boundaries of particular religious walls. Whichever form small gods take, they are problematic because they cannot respond to the full range of human potential and life experiences. Small gods exacerbate feelings of confusion, guilt, alienation, anger, and antagonism and, as a result, often need to be addressed in psychotherapy as a significant problem in their own right.

Simply pointing out an individual's small god may be sufficient in some cases to prompt a shift to broader representations of the divine. Prest and Keller (1993) describe the case of a widower who came to therapy depressed because a new woman in his life refused to marry him. In his efforts to explain his misfortune, he raised questions about the divine: "Why has God done this to me? I thought God never brought anything on us that we were not capable of bearing" (p. 146). God, he believed, had left him to face the darkness alone. The therapist responded by suggesting that this client believed in a " 'wimpy' God, one who was only in charge of life filled with light" (p. 146). This interpretation led the client to an alternate possibility: a God who could be in charge in times of darkness as well as in times of light.

In many cases, however, addressing small gods may require more active clinical efforts by therapists. In this vein, Exline and Rose (2005) suggest a variety of methods to enlarge the individual's understanding of and relationship with a God who may be perceived as distant or hidden, including a two-way conversation with the divine in which people speak to God and imagine God's response to them through reading holy texts, imagery, or journaling. Therapists can also provide their clients with spiritual metaphors and spiritual frames that encourage them to conceive of the sacred more broadly.

For example, in a moving spiritual autobiography, Tony Hendra (2004) describes the anguish of a night when he, as an 8-year-old boy, had a vision that he had lost his God:

> I was falling, in an elevator with its cables severed, accelerating down into the blackness of the shaft . . . and I knew even as I fell that my faith was being torn from me by the slipstream of my descent. . . . I was utterly alone . . . so nightmarish was the feeling that I wasn't even sure I did exist. Which threw me into an even greater panic. (pp. 88–89)

Feeling desperate and desolate, Tony seeks out Father Joe, a kindly monk who had served as confidant, priest, and counselor to Tony. Father Joe does not discount Tony's experience, but counsels him not to confuse his feelings with a larger reality. "You may not feel your love, but God is still your loved one, your other," Father Joe says (p. 99). He then offers a powerful reframing of Tony's night of anguish:

> God gave you a great gift that terrible night, Tony dear. He gave you a vision of Hell. Not that silly fire-and-brimstone stuff. True Hell. Being alone with your self for all eternity. Only your own self to hope in, only your own self to love. . . . As you said a p-p-prison with no door. I don't think that vision will ever come to you again. You must never forget it. (p. 100)

Father Joe's reframing helps Tony extend and deepen his understanding of God, faith, and the purpose of his life. Tony leaves Father Joe with these thoughts:

> My descent into Hell had forced me to consider the deeper nature of what I professed to believe, the life I wished to choose. For a year I'd basked in my faith as if it were no more my responsibility than a fine spell of weather. Now I had to fight for it, dig deeper foundations, prove how much it meant to me. Thinking I'd been engulfed by darkness, I'd instead found enlightenment and strength of purpose. (pp. 100–101)

This example may leave the impression that people move from small gods to larger gods quickly and easily. This is usually not the case. Helping clients enlarge their understanding of God can take as much time as it takes to enlarge their understanding of their mothers, their fathers, or themselves. In most cases, therapists will need to address the topic more than once, approaching it from different angles at different times. Nichole Murray-Swank (2003) illustrates this point in her work with women who have been sexually abused as children. Based on her recognition that sexual abuse impacts people spiritually as well as psychologically, socially, and physically, Murray-Swank developed a manualized therapeutic program entitled "Solace for the Soul." One of the goals of the program is to help women move from narrow, harsh, often male-dominated images of God to larger, more empowering, more compassionate images of the divine.

Toward this end, Murray-Swank involves her clients in a variety of activities. She asks her clients to spend time writing in their journals about how they view God. She then encourages them to generate other less masculine, more comforting images of God. Murray-Swank also provides her clients with prayers that speak of God and spirituality in ways that are freeing rather than restricting, and hopeful rather than dark. In another exercise, Murray-Swank asks her clients to circle items from a list of more loving and compassionate adjectives that describe who God is to each of them: "giver of life," "friend," "holy spirit," "mother," "peace," "wind," "sister," "light," "nature," "beauty," "warmth," "love," "mystery," "wisdom." She goes on to present her clients with a visualization exercise in which they imagine God's love as a waterfall within each person:

> Picture God as a waterfall within you . . . pouring down cool, refreshing water . . . the waters of love, healing, restoration throughout your body . . . a cool, refreshing waterfall washing down over your head, your face, your shoulders, your neck, out through your arms, down your legs, out through your toes, refreshing, bringing life, quenching thirst . . . renewing, refreshing, restoring. (p. 232)

Although the program is new, initial findings suggest that Solace for the Soul facilitates a sense of connectedness with a God, who is seen as less punitive and more benevolent and empowering (Murray-Swank & Pargament, 2005).

ADDRESSING FALSE GODS

Earlier, I noted that addictions and compulsions can be understood, at least in part, as one type of spiritual problem, the problem of false gods. The list of potential false gods seems endless: drugs, alcohol, sex, anger, anxiety, physical objects, money, people, fame, power, relationships, and so on. Almost anything can become an object of worship. False gods are problematic not because they are false in the ontological sense (a judgment that goes beyond the capability of the practitioner), but because they are incapable of holding the sacred. They also become problematic when people approach them as idols, confusing symbols of the divine with the divine itself. The end result is a life dedicated to gods that diminish rather than enrich human experience.

Addressing false gods in therapy can be a difficult business. True or false, gods are objects of devotion, and people do not generally change allegiances to their gods very easily. To give up the pursuit of bogus gods and center life on more viable forms of the sacred calls for transformational coping. Practitioners have, in fact, developed several spiritually based methods over the years to facilitate this process of fundamental change, though these programs are not typically described as efforts to address false gods or spiritual interventions more generally. Twelve-step programs, for instance, promote shifts from the devotion to an addictive object to a life centered on a higher power. Similarly, forgiveness interventions encourage people to replace long-standing anger and resentment with more spiritual values, such as compassion and peace of mind (see Worthington, 2005). From programs such as these, we can glean four basic clinical steps to help clients address their false gods: naming false gods, identifying the spiritual yearning, letting go of false gods, and practicing the perception of the sacred.

Naming False Gods

In many instances, people are unaware of the forces that are, in fact, guiding their lives. By giving them a name, therapists bring these inadequate substitutes for God to their clients' awareness. Naming the false god can come as a shock, especially to clients who see themselves as religious or spiritual people, because it points to the contradictions between the faith they espouse and the faith they live by. Naming the false god also requires a strong therapeutic alliance because this kind of intervention can lead to feelings of hurt and anger directed at the therapist. Under the right conditions, however, therapists can motivate clients to change by highlighting the nature of the gods they appear to be worshipping.

James Griffith (1986) illustrates this point in his description of his work with Byron, a 20-year-old evangelical Christian, son of a physician, who was often absent from home, and a mother who was isolated and lonely. Byron was preoccupied with concerns about his mother's safety, and he often intruded in her life. Byron's enmeshment was interfering with his own functioning; he was having difficulty concentrating and performing well at school. When other efforts to create more distance between Byron and his mother failed, Griffith decided to reframe the problem in spiritual terms:

> THERAPIST: For many years, Byron, you have stepped into your father's shoes; now, you are trying to step into God's shoes.
>
> BYRON: What do you mean?
>
> THERAPIST: For many years you have been more a husband to your mother than her own husband; now, by acting as her protector against every natural disaster, you are trying to be her God.
>
> BYRON: I never thought about it that way. (p. 610)

This intervention proved to be effective. Over the next few months, Byron and his mother were able to achieve greater separation. Naming Byron's false god (in this case, himself) confronted Byron with the inconsistency between his religious commitments and his actions. In essence, he had to choose between taking on the role of a god and worshipping the authentic God. Byron chose the latter.

Naming the false god can extend beyond the god itself to the teachings sanctified by that god. Merle Jordan (1986) describes the case of one woman who identified her secular "Decalogue" in counseling, including commandments such as "Thou shalt not upset other people and hurt their feelings," "Thou shalt judge thyself harshly," and "Thou shalt not succeed for that would be sinful" (p. 36). Over the course of counseling, she created a "Revised Decalogue" consisting of a very different set of commandments to live by: "I am a spark of God which grows brighter and clearer every day," "I am a vital and integrally important part of the flow of life," and "I am honest, I am kind, I am patient" (p. 36).

Identifying the Spiritual Yearning

Naming the false god is likely to leave clients with an uneasy feeling, but uneasiness is insufficient in most cases to prompt a change. To give up a god, clients need an alternative. Unfortunately, in the pursuit of false gods, many people lose touch with their more basic spiritual yearning. They may feel as if they have abandoned or been abandoned by anything sacred in their lives. Yet beneath the surface of these feelings often lies a deeper yearning for a more profound object of devotion. Recall, for instance, Yalom's (1980) portrayal of Thelma, the client with an obsessive focus on her former therapist, an obsession which, I suggested, grew out of a more basic longing for a relationship with the sacred. Therapists can help their clients identify their spiritual yearnings.

For example, recently I worked with Mark, a 35-year-old pastor who seemed frozen into seriousness, with an expression that rarely departed from somber, a voice that sounded almost robotic, and a demeanor so stiff and tight that I often found myself stretching my own muscles in therapy. Mark had come to therapy because he had been engaging in a series of sexual relationships with other pastors. Though he felt guilty about his relationships, he was less disturbed by the guilt than by the emptiness he felt while carrying on these affairs. Mark described these liaisons as his "secondary vocation." He would spend much of his time during the day fantasizing about potential sexual partners, the art of seduction, and the possibilities of sexual pleasure. In spite of his terrible seriousness, Mark was able to form sexual connections with a number of partners. Yet these relationships left him unfulfilled and were invariably short-lived.

Exploring Mark's past, I learned that he had grown up as an only child in a home with a single mother. His father had left the family soon after Mark's birth. Mark described his mother as depressed and emotionally unavailable. Church became Mark's home away from home. There, he felt some sense of connection with other people and some relief from those feelings of emptiness that had plagued him throughout his life. I asked Mark whether he had ever experienced feelings that went beyond relief. Had he, for instance, ever experienced joy? Mark hesitated and then spoke movingly about a 2-year period in Africa when he had served as a minister in a small village. During those 2 years, he shared the joys and tragedies of the villagers' everyday lives and, in the process, felt a closeness to others he had

never experienced before. This was a different Mark. The mask of seriousness was temporarily gone, replaced by a montage of emotions: happiness,
sadness, longing, hurt, and frustration.

This discussion led to the following exchange:

K.I.P.: Have you ever had a similar experience in your sexual relationships?

MARK: No. I wish!

K.I.P.: Did you mean that? Is that what you are wishing for?

MARK: Maybe so.

K.I.P.: I'm wondering, then, whether you're looking for sexual pleasure or
something else.

MARK: What do you mean?

K.I.P.: Could it be that you're looking for something that goes a little
deeper than that . . . something you experienced in Africa—an emotional connection, a spiritual connection with other people.

MARK: (crying softly) It's what I've wanted my whole life.

K.I.P.: But maybe in pursuing these sexual relationships, you're just settling
for the foreplay. Maybe spiritual connection is what you're really looking for. The real climax.

This was a crucial point in therapy. The focus of our conversation shifted
from his devotion to the false god of sexual pleasure to the pursuit of his
deeper and more authentic spiritual yearning: greater intimacy with others.

Letting Go of False Gods

False gods pale in comparison to more genuine spiritual longings. Even so,
the process of letting go of these inadequate substitutes can be quite challenging. Old habits are hard to break. There is familiarity and pleasure to
be found in the pursuit of established goals, even those that are destructive.
Thus, the client has to be ready to shift from old gods to new ones. The
choice to change is ultimately the client's, but the therapist can encourage
and support constructive decisions by drawing on a variety of spiritual resources.

Avants, Beitel, and Margolin (2005) developed a spiritually integrated
therapy designed to help drug-dependent and HIV-at-risk clients make just
this kind of a shift. Spiritual Self-Schema (3-S) Therapy is an 8-week
manualized treatment that draws on Buddhist teachings to help clients
replace "unwholesome habit patterns of the mind (i.e., the addict self-
schema) with wholesome habit patterns that lead to 'liberation from suffering' (i.e., the spiritual self-schema)" (p. 169). Clients are taught that the

addict self, that part of the person driven by cravings and avoidance, does not reflect the individual's true nature. It is, instead, an illusion, one that prevents the person from recognizing his or her true spiritual self. Much of 3-S therapy consists of encouraging spiritual qualities and spiritually based techniques to facilitate the shift from addict self to true self. These include (1) spiritual self-affirmations and prayer; (2) mindfulness meditation to help the individual identify the activation of the addict self and the spiritual self; (3) increased awareness of the thoughts that sabotage spiritual progress; (4) transforming cravings by observing their impermanence; (5) introduction of the client to the spiritual self's five "friends" (faith, energy, awareness, concentration, wisdom) and five "enemies" (addict thoughts, addict speech, addict emotions, addict behaviors, addict self-identity); and (6) seeking out community resources that can support the client's spiritual journey.

Preliminary evaluations of 3-S therapy have yielded promising results (Avants et al., 2005). In a study of 29 cocaine- and opiate-dependent clients who had been defined earlier as "treatment failures," participants in 3-S made a number of positive changes. They demonstrated a significant shift in their schemas from the addict self to the spiritual self, as shown by a computerized reaction time task. They significantly decreased their use of illicit drugs according to self-reports and increased the percentage of their heroin- and cocaine-free urines. And they reported significant increases in their daily spiritual experiences, spiritual coping, church attendance, and private religious practices. Asked what he found most helpful about 3-S, one client answered, "The freedom. The freedom of knowing that my true self is my spiritual [self] not the addict [self]. That's a freedom itself" (p. 176). These were impressive findings for a program that was aimed at "treatment-resistant" clients. More generally, the results illustrate how spiritual resources can be used to facilitate powerful transformations in the spiritual strivings of clients, transformations from the pursuit of false gods to lives directed to more authentic forms of the sacred. Finally, it is important to note that even though 3-S is based on Buddhist philosophy, its underlying values (e.g., wisdom, compassion, morality) are consistent with those of other religious traditions. In fact, participants in 3-S are encouraged to draw on the resources of their own particular religious groups to enact these values in their lives.

Practicing the Perception of the Sacred

Clients often require additional help to solidify, broaden, and deepen the changes they have made in their lives. This rule certainly applies to changes from one form of the sacred to another. Perseverance, rehearsal, and "working the program" are hallmarks of 12-step programs, forgiveness interventions, and other spiritually oriented change initiatives.

Recently, my colleagues developed a spiritually integrated intervention specifically designed to help embed the sacred more fully in the lives of people who suffer from social anxiety (McCorkle, Bohn, Hughes, & Kim, 2005). Social anxiety, they note, is often characterized by a narrowing of the individual's attentional focus. The lives of people with social anxiety are marked by single-minded efforts to avoid threatening social situations. In this sense, the avoidance of pain becomes their object of devotion.

McCorkle and his colleagues theorized that this clinical group would be helped if they were able to place social anxiety within a larger spiritual context. The goal was not to eliminate clients' social anxiety but rather to help them to see social anxiety through the lens of the sacred. Drawing upon Rubin's figure-ground illusion from gestalt psychology (which can be viewed either as a vase in the middle of the picture from one perspective or the silhouettes of two people facing each other from the two sides of the picture from another), they explain that people with social anxiety can see only their social anxiety (the figure) and are unable to locate the sacred (the ground).

The 8-week manualized group program, entitled "Sacred Moments: Social Anxiety in a Larger Context," drew on a variety of spiritual resources including prayer, meditation, ritual, spiritual support, and spiritual coping. Each session was designed to teach people with social anxiety how to perceive the sacred in a specific area of their lives: bodies, emotions, the present moment, the self, relationships with others, suffering, meaning in life, and times of celebration. For example, in the session devoted to relationships, participants shared a story in which they received a sacred gift from someone else. The gift could take the form of something as ordinary as a comforting touch, the smile of a stranger, a friendly remark, or words of kindness at the right time. However, participants often used the language of sacred qualities (e.g., "unforgettable," "extraordinary," "touching") to describe these gifts. Moreover, the participants often reacted to the gifts with sacred emotions, such as awe, wonder, gratitude, and feeling uplifted. Through this process, participants found that receiving sacred gifts is not at all unusual, once one becomes practiced in seeing through the cloud of social anxiety. Although Sacred Moments has not yet been formally evaluated, some of the participants noted that their perspective on life had changed as a result of the program; they were now able to "think bigger" and, in the process, they had found that social anxiety had become less central to their day-to-day lives (p. 237).

ADDRESSING SACRED CLASHES
WITH THE DEVIL AND WITHIN

Demonization

Many clients are reluctant to mention the devil in psychotherapy for fear of being misinterpreted or labeled "crazy." Yet 45% of people in the United

States report that they definitely believe in the devil, and another 20% state that they probably do (Davis, Smith, & Marsden, 2005). Clinicians who listen for demonic language as carefully as they listen for signs of the sacred may find that talk about the devil is not altogether rare in psychotherapy. However, it is important to recognize that the devil can be understood in different ways. While some clients objectify the devil as an actual presence that can be as real and as manifest in oneself or in others as God is, others see the devil as an abstract symbol of evil. Still others speak of qualities associated with the demonic, such as wickedness, maliciousness, and sinfulness. Earlier, I noted that there is nothing inherently problematic about various beliefs in the devil. They are, after all, an integral part of many religious traditions and provide a way to make sense of pain, suffering, and injustice. But problems occur when people feel they are engaged in a losing battle with the demonic, when they identify themselves or others exclusively with the devil, or when they deny their own darker side and project it onto other people. To determine whether beliefs in the devil are a sign of spiritual dis-integration, clinicians should treat the mention of the demonic in therapy as a "red flag," an indicator of potential trouble that calls for further discussion.

Clinicians may find themselves uncomfortable with this discussion, particularly if they believe that the notion of the devil is absurd or abhorrent. They may feel tempted to challenge their clients immediately and forcefully (e.g., "You are not evil," "Your child is not demonic"). But interventions of this kind are likely to be rejected, for they ignore the reality of the demonic to the client. By accepting, learning about, and working with the client's view of the world, the therapist is in a better position to facilitate change when needed among those who demonize themselves or others.

Demonization of Self

Demonization is most often encountered in therapy among clients who perceive themselves to be battling with their own demons or who fear that they are becoming evil. Three clinical approaches are helpful in work with these clients. First, the client can be helped to place the demonic or the sense of evil in a larger spiritual context. To many people, the devil represents a threat to everything they hold sacred. Those who perceive themselves to be at spiritual risk may go to great lengths to protect themselves, and, in the process of avoiding the demonic, they may lose touch with their spiritual core. Recall the case of Crystal, the mother of three young children who developed a series of compulsions to ward off the possibility that she would be possessed by the devil. As I noted earlier, when asked to describe what she would be like if the devil claimed her, Crystal spoke of her fear that she would abandon her children. Abandonment was what Crystal herself had experienced as a child at the hands of her mother. Our conversa-

tion led Crystal to the realization that her greatest fear was not of possession by the devil but of possession by her mother. Placing a more human
face on Crystal's greatest fear helped reduce her feelings of terror and impo-
tence. In further sessions, I helped Crystal come to terms with her ambiva-
lent feelings toward her mother. Just as importantly, we explored Crystal's
own sense of sacredness in life. It was clear that she saw her children and
her role as mother as sacred gifts. She had, in fact, devoted her life to caring
for others and doing all she could not to follow in her mother's footsteps.
Through our conversations, Crystal was able to put her fears of the
demonic in a larger perspective. She began to see that her concerns about
possession were only one part of her life, and a small part at that, in comparison to what she held sacred. With time, Crystal came to a new conclusion: evil forces had never taken hold of her and, because of her spiritual
commitments, were unlikely to ever possess her. These insights were accompanied by dramatic reductions in Crystal's levels of anxiety, obsessiveness,
and compulsiveness.

Therapists can also draw on a variety of spiritual resources, such as
prayer and purification rituals, to help empower their clients in what they
perceive to be a battle with the demonic. In a qualitative study of Puerto
Rican migrants in the United States, Jacobson (2003) provides numerous illustrations of the value of prayer to people in the midst of their demonic
struggles. One devout, Evangelical, 35-year-old migrant described an experience in which he felt that he was being suffocated by the devil:

> RUBEN E.: I was sleeping this one night on my stomach for whatever reason.
> And it felt like an evil presence putting my head into the pillow.
>
> J.J.: Pushing you down?
>
> R.E.: Uhuh, and I was suffocating in the pillow and in my dream . . . but it was
> so real, that it was happening.
>
> J.J.: Like you were awake?
>
> R.E.: Yea. So at that moment, all I said in my dream, in conscious[ness],'cause
> I felt it happening, I said the name of Jesus seven times. Actually it was the
> seventh time I said Jesus' name, and the presence just lifted up off of me.
>
> J.J.: And then you woke up?
>
> R.E.: Then I woke up, and [he sighs deeply in relief]. (p. 24)

Because most therapists lack the formal power and legitimacy of religious traditions, collaboration with clergy is especially important in challenging the negative spiritual forces clients feel are at work in their lives.
For example, Greenberg and Witztum (2001) present the case of Ezra, a
24-year-old ultra-Orthodox Jewish student in Israel, who came to therapy
plagued with guilt for neglecting his father on the night he died. Ezra's con-

dition had deteriorated to the point that he was drinking so much that he was sleeping in his own vomit. Ezra had also begun to hear the voice of what he believed to be a punishing angel that ordered him to chastise himself by fasting, wearing torn clothing, and abstaining from sexual relations. Attempts by the therapists to encourage Ezra to take better care of himself were met by his reports of orders from the punishing angel to engage in more extreme ascetic practices. To neutralize the effect of the punitive angel, the therapists enlisted the help of Ezra's brother, who was a rabbi, and convened a lay Jewish court to place the angel on ritual trial. In the courtroom, Ezra was instructed to "talk to the angel. Tell him how much you have suffered, and ask him whether he thinks the time has come for him to forgive you. Tell him you would like to befriend him" (p. 282). The rabbi brother took the trial one step further and ordered the angel to "cease afflicting Ezra, never to return, 'neither for good or bad, not even to teach him mystical secrets' " (p. 282). Following the trial, Ezra's behavior and mood improved. Although he reported that he continued to receive visits from his angel, the angel had become supportive and encouraging rather than punitive.

Finally, without contradicting the client's beliefs about the devil, the therapist may encourage the client to consider alternate explanations for his or her problems. In fact, many clients attribute their problems to multiple causes. Explanations involving the devil can sit side by side with other explanations. In a recent survey of Pentecostal perspectives on the causes and cures of depression, Trice and Bjorck (2006) found that, even though many Pentecostals attributed depression to demonic oppression or spiritual failures, they also endorsed a variety of other explanations, such as social-relational problems (e.g., loneliness, poor relations with parents), financial problems, loss of control (e.g., a terminal illness), death, victimization (childhood abuse), and biological factors (e.g., heredity, chemical imbalance). These findings suggest that many religious clients, including those who are more conservative, will be open to exploring alternative explanations for their problems as long as their spiritual beliefs and practices are treated respectfully. Beliefs about the demonic are no exception to this rule.

There are times, however, when the clinician may need to take active steps to protect clients from beliefs and practices that turn self-destructive. Griffith and Griffith (2002) describe the case of a young woman with bipolar disorder who had been admitted to the hospital to remove a brain tumor. In preparation for her surgery, she injured her eye. Without treatment she could have lost sight in the eye, but she refused medical assistance, saying, "I don't care. I've got two eyes" (p. 244). When her doctors refused to release her from the hospital, she tried to escape and began to claw at her eye, quoting from the Bible: "If your eye offends you, pluck it out" (p. 244). Later she stated that "Satan was residing in her eye"

(p. 245). Her psychiatrist concluded that "psychosis was driving her religious zeal" and took legal steps to administer antipsychotic medications against her will. The medications were effective. The patient received treatment for her eye and later apologized to her psychiatrist "for making your life hell" (p. 245).

Demonization of Others

Blatant demonization of other people is not a common presenting problem in psychotherapy. Obviously, clients who demonize others to avoid facing their own darker side do not believe they themselves need help: the problem lies in someone else. It is rare, then, for a clinician to encounter clients who complain because they have projected the demonic onto others. However, clinicians may occasionally come across these individuals indirectly through therapeutic work with family members who have born the brunt of the demonization, such as an abused spouse or a child with a disability. Enlisting the demonizing individual in the therapeutic process is likely to be a major challenge in its own right. Not until a family protection agency or the victim of the demonization insists on therapy will the person who demonizes others enter counseling, and even then, probably unwillingly. Once the demonizer is in therapy, the clinical challenge is to shift the client's focus from the demonized other to the client's own personal demons, demons that may take many forms, such as alcohol and drugs, shame, rage, lust, or self-righteousness. In this vein, Rollo May (1970) advised clients to take the demonic into the self rather than to project or to deny it: "You take in the daimonic which would possess *you* if you didn't. The one way to get over daimonic possession is to possess *it*, by frankly confronting it, coming to terms with it, integrating it into the self-system" (p. 201). Of course, this is easier said than done, and perhaps for this reason we find few "success stories" in the clinical literature when it comes to the treatment of those who demonize others. Protecting the target of blatant demonization may be the only therapeutic recourse.

It is more common to see demonization in subtler form, as one element in a larger pattern of externalization of responsibility and scapegoating. Therapists can uncover this kind of demonization by listening carefully for demonic qualities in the clients' descriptions of people who are causing them trouble in their lives. "Wicked," "cruel," "malicious," "hateful," "mean-spirited," and "evil" are a few of the terms that hint at demonization. Keep in mind that this type of language, strong as it is, may be very appropriate when applied to people who knowingly, willingly, and consistently violate and damage others. But relatively few people fall into this category (Baumeister, 1997). Demonic language has several drawbacks: it freezes people into static traits, thereby reducing the likelihood of change; it tends to neglect the presence of balancing virtues in those who have been demonized; it diminishes the role of other factors that may contribute to undesirable behavior, such as biological, environmental, and interpersonal forces, including the actions of the person who is doing the demonizing; and because the demonic is seen as a threat to the sacred, it can lead to extremely powerful negative responses that only perpetuate the cycle of conflict.

In its subtler forms, the demonization of others can be addressed by making it more explicit. Clients may be quite surprised and disturbed to hear that they seem to be viewing and treating a family member, coworker, or acquaintance as if he or she was demonic. By naming the demonic, the therapist brings it to the surface and allows the client to take a step back from the problem, examine it, and explore more fully whether the person who is being demonized actually embodies the qualities of the devil. And, in this process, the therapist can offer different ways for the client to understand the actions of the other person, not necessarily to diminish the offensiveness of the behavior, but to place it in a broader, less malevolent context.

Internal Sacred Conflicts

Earlier, I noted that people encounter many new and different ways to understand and experience the sacred over the course of their development. New understandings do not fully replace old ones. Like the layers of an onion, very different images of the sacred can nestle comfortably next to each other. Internal or external changes, however, can lead to friction and strain in the individual's concept of the sacred. If left unresolved, these internal sacred struggles can become chronic and inflamed, eventually impacting other areas of life. Several steps can be helpful in working with clients who find themselves caught up in their own sacred wars.

First, make the internal struggle explicit. Just as clients may be unaware of their false gods, they may be unaware of their conflicting thoughts and feelings about the sacred. Clients may feel anger toward the God they thought they had fully disavowed, disappointment in the trusted sacred figure who let them down, fearful of the higher power they believed to be all loving, or abandoned by the God they assumed would always be there for them. Whatever its nature, giving a name to the conflicting images and experiences of the sacred brings what may be a hidden struggle to the surface. While this process may increase the client's distress, the discomfort can spur the client to explore his or her conflicts in what is now a clearer light.

Second, normalize internal sacred conflicts. Because internal conflicts can be a source of embarrassment, shame, and fear, therapists have to normalize these struggles to encourage further spiritual dialogue with their clients. One way to legitimize spiritual struggles is to provide illustrations of exemplary figures from the clients' own tradition who also struggled, such as Jesus, Buddha, Moses, or Muhammad. In Chapter 13, we saw that the biblical story of Job could serve as a model for people having difficulty tolerating terrible emotional pain. But the story can be understood at a number of levels. It can also be helpful to Jews and Christians who struggle with religious doubts (Schimmel, 1987). Job, a man of faith, becomes skeptical after his life is thrown into chaos by the loss of his health, his sons, and his worldly possessions. His struggle, however, is as much within himself as it is with God, for Job never disavows God's existence. He simply cannot reconcile the God he thought he knew with the God who allows him to suffer. God does not provide Job with an easy answer, but he does accept Job's questions and doubts, and Job is ultimately rewarded with a reaffirmation of his faith. For clients facing their own internal sacred conflicts, the story of Job suggests that doubt has an important place in the search for the sacred. In fact, doubt may well be a prerequisite for growth rather than an impediment to development.

To legitimize spiritual conflicts, therapists need to address the potential fears of their clients that their struggles will lead to punishment by God or rejection by their religious congregation. Efforts to enlarge the client's understanding of the sacred can be helpful in this situation. A collaborative relationship with sympathetic clergy can also play a valuable role in allaying the client's fears of religious criticism. In this vein, George Zornow (2001), a Lutheran pastor, developed a program entitled "Crying Out to God" that encourages participants to express whatever feelings they are experiencing about God to God. God, Zornow insists, is large enough and compassionate enough to accept any and all feelings the individual may have. Just as importantly, Zornow destigmatizes the topic, modeling openness and acceptance of spiritual conflicts and struggles, by expressing struggles of his own.

Third, bring the client's conflicting thoughts and feelings about the sacred into conversation with each other. Ana-Maria Rizzuto (1989) describes a case in which she did just that, almost literally. The case involved a parish priest who suffered from insomnia and hands that trembled so badly he could not distribute communion. Rizzuto noticed a sharp change in his demeanor when he talked about theological matters and when he spoke of his insomnia: "When he talked about the God of theology he was pleasant looking . . . he was expansive, he was gracious but when he was talking about the God of his prayers, of his insomnia, of his forgetting to consecrate, he was tense, frowning, scared" (p. 4). Rizzuto proceeded to name the conflict: "Listen father," she said, "you are a polytheist, you have two Gods" (p. 4). She then encouraged him to wrestle with his two Gods:

"Ask the God of theology in what ways He was different from the God of his prayers" (p. 4). The results, she reports, were impressive: "It was like curing someone of neurosis" (p. 4).

Finally, help the client accept some degree of internal conflict. Though we may aspire to a fully integrated life, few people achieve it on a consistent basis because inconsistencies, contradictions, and paradox are so much a part of human experience. This point certainly holds true for the spiritual dimension. Fortunately, we do not have to be perfectly integrated to live worthwhile lives. Clients can be encouraged to tolerate a level of internal sacred conflict. Kornfield (1993) has written a meditation to help people achieve greater peace within themselves, not by fighting to eliminate their inner struggles, but by accepting these struggles as part of who they are:

> Sit comfortably for a few minutes, letting your body be at rest. Let your breathing be easy and natural. Bring your attention into the present, sit quietly, and notice whatever sensations are present in your body. . . .
> Then cast your attention over all the battles that still exist in your life. Sense them inside yourself. . . . If you have been fighting inner wars with your feelings . . . sense the struggle you have been waging. Notice the struggles in your thoughts as well. Be aware of how you have carried on the inner battles. Notice the inner armies, the inner dictators, the inner fortifications. Be aware of all that you have fought within yourself. . . .
> Gently, with openness, allow each of these experiences to be present. Simply notice each of them in turn with interest and kind attention. In each area of struggle, let your body, heart, and soul be soft. Open to whatever you experience without fighting. Let it be present just as it is. Let go of the battle. Breathe quietly and let yourself be at rest. Invite all parts of yourself to join you at the peace table in your heart. (p. 30)

CONCLUSIONS

What is the hardest thing about being a therapist?, a graduate student once asked me. Encouraging people to give up old destinations and seek out new ones, I replied. People are incredibly tenacious in the pursuit of their aspirations. Whether their aspirations are constructive or destructive is immaterial to this point. People can cling tightly to the basest of goals just as they do to the noblest. When clinicians are faced with this kind of tenacity, their task of encouraging basic change in clients' strivings is exceptionally challenging. The challenge is even greater when it comes to clients' spiritual strivings, for we are talking about sacred matters here and, as we have seen, clients are especially protective of whatever they hold sacred. Nevertheless, the search for the sacred is not set in stone. Even in the spiritual realm, change is possible. In this chapter, I have presented a number of clinical ways to address problems of spiritual destinations. Work in this area is admittedly new, but clinicians have begun to make promising strides in their efforts to assist clients with the most fundamental of transformations. In the next chapter, we shift our attention to ways clinicians can help clients address problems of spiritual pathways.

15

Addressing Problems
of Spiritual Pathways

People experience spiritual problems not only in their choices of sacred destinations, but also in the pathways they take to reach these ends. In
this chapter, I consider how clinicians can respond to several problems of
spiritual pathways. Again, this review is selective. I focus on the ways
therapists can address three important and interrelated problems in the
pathways their clients take to the sacred: problems of breadth and depth,
problems of continuity and change, and problems of fit.

ADDRESSING PROBLEMS OF BREADTH AND DEPTH

Earlier, I noted that many people lack breadth and depth in their spiritual
pathways. The problem may have several causes: unfamiliarity with the full
resources of a religious tradition; a cafeteria-style approach to spirituality
that results in a hodgepodge of beliefs, practices, relationships, emotions,
and experiences; or a passive approach to spiritual learning in which the individual fails to internalize and adapt these teachings to his or her own life.
Whatever its roots, this kind of spirituality is short of power. People who
are missing breadth and depth in their spiritual pathways are not well
equipped to handle the full range of life problems. Not only that, a lack of
spiritual breadth and depth can create problems in and of itself. Therapists
can play a significant role in helping clients broaden and deepen their spirituality.

Broadening Spiritual Pathways

Many clients come to therapy with narrow spiritual orientations. Those who grew up within a religious tradition may have selectively abstracted particular beliefs and practices from the tradition on the basis of their religious education or their personal needs and preferences. Unfortunately, this process can leave them with incomplete, distorted, or imbalanced forms of spirituality (DiGiuseppe, Robin, & Dryden, 1990). And yet religious traditions are generally broad enough to encompass counterbalancing tendencies (Schreurs, 2002). They have a place for human choice as well as determinism, optimism as well as pessimism, freedom as well as bondage, concern for others as well as concern for self, forgiveness and compassion as well as sin and punishment, and positive as well as negative emotions. By drawing on the variegated pathways that define each religious tradition, therapists can help clients broaden and balance narrow their approaches to spirituality.

For example, Schreurs (2002) describes how she encouraged one client to find room for compassion, forgiveness, and positive emotions in her theology. The client, a 40-year-old woman who was a member of a small Protestant church, had lost her child in a car accident. She believed that her child's death had been inflicted on her by God as a punishment for her unfaithfulness to her husband. On the face of it, this problem might be simply understood in terms of the client's guilt at violating one of the Ten Commandments or her vision of a one-dimensional God who could only judge and punish. But Schreurs suggests that the problem goes beyond religious guilt and a small god to reflect a narrow and distorted theological understanding in which "the spiritual metaphor of trial and courtroom has become isolated from its biblical context of the spiritual journey" (101).

Instead of attempting to dismiss this woman's sense of guilt and punishment, Schreurs reframed it by suggesting that her client's self-inflicted estrangement from God is the real punishment, one that must be looked at from a wider perspective. Schreurs links the life of her client to a "master narrative of liberation" by drawing on stories from the Hebrew Bible and the New Testament of exemplary figures who also experienced a period of exile in the desert yet continued to seek God. Though they too occasionally strayed from the path, they were met with compassion, forgiveness, and love when they chose to return. By situating her client's experience in this larger religious narrative, Schreurs broadened and balanced her restricted theological understanding.

In contrast to Schreurs, who focuses on helping her client find a theological place for compassion and forgiveness, Bruce Narramore (1994) illustrates ways to help clients integrate negative emotions into their spiritual thinking. He describes how some clients cite Scripture to avoid addressing painful thoughts and feelings. For example, one of his clients proclaimed,

"The Bible says we should think on things that are lovely and pure. I don't think we should be trying to think about these upsetting things" (p. 256). In response, Narramore pointed to the broader context of this biblical verse:

> It's interesting that you quote Paul's statement about thinking on things that are lovely and pure. Do you remember what Paul says in the first part of that verse? If the patient says, "No, not exactly," I remind him that the verse beings with "Whatever is true . . . " (Phil. 4:8). . . . I know it would seem nice if we could only talk about the positive, but Paul starts off by telling us that we should think about whatever is true. Some true things are very painful and not very lovely, and it is scary to think about them. (p. 256)

Clients who have associated spirituality solely with traditional religious belief and practice can also be encouraged by their therapists to explore other times and places in which they have experienced the sacred, and urged to integrate these experiences more fully into their lives. I have sprinkled this book with numerous examples of people who discovered nontraditional pathways to the sacred, such as music, art, photography, conversation, quilting, and flying (see Chapters 3, 12, and 13). In their process of discovery, these individuals were able to move from spiritual fragmentation to a more inclusive spirituality that held broader implications for their lives.

Deepening Spiritual Pathways

People can involve themselves in a full range of spiritual thoughts, practices, emotions, relations, and experiences and yet still find that something is missing. The spiritual approach may be too thin and too simple to offer much more than the comfort of familiarity. Depth as well as breadth are prerequisites for spiritual integration. Without depth, spiritual pathways lack the profundity to lend life meaning and power. Therapists can encourage clients to explore their spirituality more deeply. Consider three examples that involve deepening rituals, deepening prayer, and deepening beliefs.

When they are repeated mechanically, rituals often become stagnant, unable to infuse life with a sense of sacredness. Family therapists Imber-Black and Roberts (1992) illustrate a number of ways to deepen the meaning of rituals. For instance, they describe one family that came to dread Christmas following the death of a family member, Jim, 6 years earlier. Since that time, the family had celebrated the holiday without any mention of Jim. Even so, his specter "hung over the holiday" and the family could take no pleasure in the ritual (p. 54). Eventually, two members of the family, Joel and Sophie, decided to take the risk of changing the way the family celebrated Christmas. Assembling photographs, letters he had written, and various other mementos, they created an album that honored Jim's life. During the exchange of gifts, Joel and Sophie presented their gift of the album to the entire family. One member left the room angrily, but returned to join the rest of the family who "poured over the album," reminiscing about Jim for the first time since he had died (p. 54). Joel's mother laughingly recalled how Jim had once opened his Christmas presents 2 days before the holiday, only to be caught in the act of trying to rewrap them. By acknowledging the powerful transformation that had taken place in their family and integrating this new reality into their holiday, the family gave Christmas a deeper and richer meaning. Imber-Black and Roberts concluded that "the family reclaimed the right to celebrate" (p. 54).

Therapists can also assist clients in developing greater openness and intimacy in their communications with God, just as they would help their clients build deeper relations with figures in their social network. Like ritual, prayer can become pro forma for many people, consisting of rote recitations that hold little connection to the client's deepest feelings or relationship with the sacred. The challenge in these cases is to encourage a shift from a spiritual monologue to a spiritual dialogue (Griffith & Griffith, 2002); that is, a shift from not only speaking to God, but also imagining or awaiting God's response.

Decker (2001) provides an example of this process in his clinical work with Emma, a young Pentecostal woman who had suffered the fourth in a series of unsuccessful pregnancies. Making matters even worse, she was required to carry the unborn child a little longer before the pregnancy could be terminated. In therapy, Decker tried to help Emma work through her terrible anger and grief not only toward other people in her life, but also toward God. His conversations with Emma, however, proved inadequate to the task. Emma's feelings were so overwhelming that she was unable to express herself. Ultimately, Decker asked Emma to put all of her feelings about God down on paper. Decker then reviewed Emma's prayer, identifying what she felt, what she told God, and what she perceived to be God's response. This process of "praying through" encouraged what Emma experienced as a deeper two-way communication with God, which in turn facilitated her ability to find meaning in her losses and emotional recovery.

As with ritual and prayer, people can hold spiritual beliefs that lack depth and meaning. During their early religious education, many people memorize the catechisms, codes, and commandments of their particular religious tradition, but fail to learn about the extensive theologies and commentaries that richly elaborate on these basic conventions (Pargament, 1997). Without further education, they are left with a shorthand set of rules to live by, such as "Honor thy mother and father," "Love thine enemies," and "Submit to God's will." Though there is great wisdom in many general religious aphorisms, they are only abbreviated guidelines for living and cannot prepare people to handle more complex problems. How does the commandment "Honor thy mother and father" apply to parents who have been abusive? How does the injunction "Love thine enemies" play itself out when the individual is faced with ruthless adversaries dedicated to the destruction of everything he or she holds dear? How does the directive "Submit to God's will" apply to the woman who discovers a lump in her breast? Simplistic spiritual understandings of complex issues can have devastating consequences.

Therapists can help clients develop deeper, more differentiated spiritual perspectives that increase their ability to deal with life's challenges. For example, abused clients who believe they must put anger and resentment behind them can be encouraged to distinguish forgiveness from forgetting, condoning, legal pardon, or reconciliation (Rye et al., 2005). Clients who believe that all anger is sinful can be encouraged to discriminate constructive "righteous" anger from destructive anger (Bassett, Hill, Hart, Mathewson, & Perry, 1992). And clients who believe that they are obliged to defer the responsibility for their lives to God can be asked to reflect on what God expects them to do to uphold their end of their relationship with the divine.

I must reemphasize my point that therapists need spiritual breadth and depth of their own if they are to help clients broaden and deepen their spirituality. To put it another way, it takes spiritual literacy on the part of therapists to help their clients develop a more integrated spirituality. It also takes therapeutic skill. The role of the therapist in this process of spiritual broadening and deepening is not to criticize, condemn, or proselytize. Debates about the truth of religious claims, I believe, should always be avoided, for the clinician has no privileged insight when it comes to matters of ultimate truth. Logical argument and challenge are also not the interventions of first choice, since clients themselves prefer less confrontational methods of treatment (McCullough & Worthington, 1995). The clinical rule of thumb "Start with the least intrusive approach to change" applies especially well to the spiritual domain. The therapist's job is to create an environment in which the client can safely explore all topics, including spiritual ones. Asking reflective questions, probing spiritual sensitive spots, raising alternative counterbalancing perspectives, suggesting new readings on the topic, and experimenting with change are some of the clinical methods that can help extend and deepen a client's spiritual pathways.

But these methods will be effective only with clients who have some degree of spiritual flexibility. Not all clients do. Some dig in their heels and resist any change. In these cases, the therapist may need to take a more challenging stance. We turn our attention now to the problem of spiritual continuity and change, focusing on one problem in particular: spiritual inflexibility.

ADDRESSING THE PROBLEM
OF SPIRITUAL INFLEXIBILITY

"Spiritual inflexibility" refers to an unwillingness to change that is based on spiritual reasons. I need to stress that the problem here is not an *inability* to change, it is an *unwillingness* to change. Spiritual inflexibility manifests itself through intolerance of ambiguity, differences, or novelty. In her novel *The Last Report on the Miracles at Little No Horse,* Louise Erdrich (2001) captures the difference between spiritual rigidity and spiritual flexibility in a debate between two priests:

> FATHER JUDE: Black is black and white is white.
>
> FATHER DAMIEN: The mixture is gray.
>
> FATHER JUDE: There are not gray areas in my philosophy.
>
> FATHER DAMIEN: I have never seen the truth without crossing my eyes. (p. 135)

Father Jude is speaking the language of spiritual rigidity. He sees life through the lens of stark polarities and clear-cut choices between white and black, good and bad, true and false. Refusing to consider alternative routes to the sacred, he sticks to the same spiritual pathway, even though it may lead him to a dead end. What is true, he insists, remains true across time, for all people, and all situations. In contrast, Father Damien speaks the language of spiritual flexibility. He does not reject notions of good and bad, black and white, or true and false, but instead views them from a more differentiated, shifting, binocular perspective. He insists on grays in the world and openness to surprise in the search for truth.

Dogmatism, perfectionism, and authoritarianism may all be signs of spiritual inflexibility. Spiritual rigidity can also reveal itself through resistance to change in psychotherapy. Clients present a variety of spiritual rationales for terminating counseling, such as "I shouldn't need therapy; I'm a failure for coming here because God should be enough for me," "I've decided to stop worrying about all of my problems and let God take care of them for me," and "The people in my church don't think I should be talking to you." In addition, spiritual reasons can be offered for beliefs and attitudes that block progress in therapy—for example, the client refuses to talk about painful feelings toward family members because she believes God wants her to be loving and forgiving of others.

"He was a simple man who died of complications." As this epitaph (from an anonymous soul) suggests, people who are unwilling to adjust to the world around them encounter serious trouble when the world calls for change. Because the capacity to adapt is a prerequisite for growth, rigidity leaves people vulnerable to the internal and external changes that are part of the normal course of development (Pargament, 1997). Spiritual inflexibility in particular creates problems at several levels. On a psychological level, people who refuse to modify their spiritual pathways are prone to anger, anxiety, guilt, and depression when they are unable to reach their spiritual destinations. On a social level, spiritually intolerant people often experience conflict with family members who do not conform to their spiritual worldview. Conflicts with people who fall entirely outside the individual's spiritual boundaries may be even more intense. On a spiritual level, inflexible people may continue to seek out the small gods of their childhoods through narrow spiritual pathways ill suited to the demands of adult life. And, as I noted above, spiritual rigidity can lead to early termination or difficult impasses in therapy. For these reasons, spiritual inflexibility often needs to be addressed directly in psychotherapy. Several methods can be helpful in this process.

Allaying Underlying Fears

Fear lies at the root of spiritual inflexibility. The fear is, in part, psychological. It is a fear of uncertainty, confusion, and aimlessness. Rigid spiritual frameworks offer a response to these fears. They provide people with a clear-cut sense of meaning and direction in a confusing and rapidly changing world filled with diverse individuals and lifestyles. Armed with unquestioning devotion to a fixed spiritual way of life, people don't have to struggle with definitions of who they are and who they are not or of how life should and should not be lived. The answers are simple, clear, and permanent. Rigid spiritual frameworks can protect people from other forms of psychological pain as well: the anxiety triggered by difficult life decisions, the fear of social abandonment and isolation, the experience of intensely painful emotions. Thus, even though the price for spiritual inflexibility can be steep, it does serve a key psychological purpose.

But it would be a mistake to interpret spiritual rigidity purely in psychological terms, for spiritual inflexibility also serves an important spiritual purpose. Think of it as a way, albeit an extreme way, of preserving and protecting the sacred, as an expression of the natural human tendency to conserve what matters most. Many people strongly resist change in the spiritual domain because the stakes are so high; the idea of spiritual change carries with it the possibility of profound loss.

In working with the spiritually rigid client, the therapist is unlikely to be successful if he or she fails to recognize that spiritual change can pose both psychological and spiritual menace to the person. Both the change and the relationship with the therapist may be rejected if the client perceives that they endanger his or her deepest values. After all, who is likely to win the battle when the client feels that he or she must choose between the therapist and God?

For this reason, therapists must approach the problem of spiritual rigidity very carefully. Both the spiritual and the psychological fears underlying the client's inflexibility have to be allayed. Though therapists may be tempted to jump quickly to underlying psychological fears, they should not bypass the client's spiritual concerns. Remember that the spiritual dimension is significant in its own right and, in some cases, may hold the most basic of all fears. Therapists therefore must demonstrate their own sensitivity and respect for sacred matters as a prelude to any conversation about spiritual change. It must be clear to clients that the goal of this dialogue is not to diminish or eliminate cherished beliefs and practices, but instead to enrich the place of the sacred in their lives. Psychologically, the therapist must also convey an appreciation for the client's need for answers to difficult questions and structure in living. It is important to reassure clients that discussions about change are not designed to throw their entire world into chaos, but rather to enable them to respond more effectively to the twists and turns that are a part of everyone's life. The critical message is that spiritual flexibility complements rather than opposes the need for stability and structure. Zerubavel (1991) aptly summarizes the goal: "Flexibility need not entail giving up structure altogether. It does imply, however, dynamic, elastic mental structures. Such structures would allow us to break away from the mental cages into which we so often lock ourselves, yet avoid chaos. With them, we can be creative as well as secure" (p. 122).

Drawing on Spiritual Resources to Encourage Flexibility

Change is a vital part of every religious tradition. The religions of the world acknowledge and celebrate the turns of seasons in nature and human life, marking these transitions with myths and rituals. The world's religions also contain models of change. Every religion recounts the dramatic stories of exemplary figures—for example, Abraham, Moses, Buddha, Jesus, and Muhammad—who undertake spiritual journeys in which they leave the safety of home, undergo a series of trials and tribulations, and emerge strengthened and steeled, with a powerful message to be shared with others. Neither is it hard to find modern-day exemplars of people who have completed their own remarkable spiritual journeys, such as Pope John Paul, Mahatma Gandhi, Nelson Mandela, Martin Luther King Jr., and Mother Teresa. None of these figures, past or present, remained fixed in place. They demonstrated a willingness to enter alien lands, accepting the risk and uncertainty that accompanied their journeys into unfamiliar territory. Even God has been described as responsive and flexible in many faiths. In the Hebrew Bible, for instance, God changes his mind several times in response to the pleas of his people. One way to facilitate spiritual flexibility is to frame the lives of religiously oriented clients in the context of their ever-changing, growing religious traditions. Like the exemplary figures of their religions, they are living out spiritual dramas of their own. They too have a story to tell, a story still in progress, one they can have a hand in shaping.

Therapists can draw on several other spiritual resources to promote greater flexibility in their clients. In their work with clients who resist change because they feel their involvement in therapy represents a betrayal of their church or religious teachings, therapists should be able to call on clergy from a variety of religious traditions who value psychotherapy and are willing to collaborate in treatment by reassuring clients that psychotherapy is not antithetical to religious commitment or by more direct participation in the counseling process. I have also found it helpful to reframe the counseling process in spiritual terms for clients who make hard-and-fast distinctions between psychotherapeutic and spiritual approaches to change. Psychotherapy, I suggest, may also be a part of the client's spiritual journey, and presents an important opportunity for spiritual growth.

Therapists can also encourage critical spiritual thinking to reduce inflexibility. Ano (2005) has developed a number of techniques to facilitate this process. Though his work focused on Christians struggling with perfectionism, his recommendations could be extended to other traditions. First, he stresses the importance of examining sacred literature in its context. Single verses from Scripture can paint a misleading picture when they are removed from their larger background. For example, he notes that at one point in the New Testament Jesus said, "If anyone comes to me and does not hate his father and mother . . . he cannot be my disciple" (Luke 14:26). Yet people familiar with the New Testament as a whole recognize that Jesus is not encouraging people to hate their families. Second, Ano recommends that people study Scriptures themselves. Much of religious learning, he notes, comes secondhand through parents, clergy, or religious educators. Yet if people are to reach their own conclusions about matters of faith and belief, they must come face to face with sacred literature. Third, when questions about spiritual meaning arise, Ano recommends seeking out respected spiritual leaders and teachers for their opinions and feedback.

Bibliotherapy is another potent resource for clients who have difficulty viewing spiritual beliefs and practices from several vantage points. Therapists who are well acquainted with spiritual literature can recommend books from their clients' own traditions that help them open their eyes to multiple levels of meaning in religious texts and teachings, the possibility that truth can be found within each of these levels, and the realization that mystery will always be a part of the spiritual domain (Doehring, 2006). For example, Christian theologian Michael Joseph Brown (2000) has written a very "user-friendly" book that contains 28 "Rules of Thumb" for interpreting biblical texts. Some of the rules encourage an active process of grappling with the material (e.g., "Rule of Thumb 5: When reading a text, don't ask and it won't tell"; p. 57). Others point to multiple levels of meaning (e.g., "Rule of Thumb 14: If the story sounds simple, then you can bet that the meaning isn't"; p. 81). Some offer the reminder to be open to paradox ("Rule of Thumb 10: The Bible means what it says and says what it means. Except when it doesn't"; p. 66). And others challenge the reader to be open to change (e.g., "Rule of Thumb 27: If your faith can't stand a little shaking, perhaps there wasn't much of a foundation there in the first place"; p. 141). Building on readings such as this one, therapists can help their clients to find new meanings in the spiritual stories, phrases, and terms that have kept them frozen in place in the past.

Therapists can also encourage clients to seek out spiritual support to help them face the fears that underlie their reluctance to change, be it the fear of intimacy, the fear of isolation, the fear of painful emotions, the fear of failure, or the fear of the loss of the sacred. Clients can write their own prayers, or they can find established prayers and meditations from traditional or nontraditional sacred literatures that have been specifically designed to support people struggling with change. For instance, consider the Serenity Prayer: "God grant me the serenity to accept the things I cannot change; courage to change the things I can; and wisdom to know the difference." In just a few brief lines, this prayer encourages people to be discerning about whether change is appropriate, accepting when change is not possible, and courageous when change is called for.

Although these approaches to facilitating change may seem relatively mild and nonintrusive, there is some level of challenge to the status quo inherent in each of them. But this challenge is cushioned by couching the encouragement to change within a familiar and stable religious context. The underlying message the therapist needs to convey is that, although life does insist on change, some things endure. Even in the midst of transformation, the client can be reassured, the sacred remains a constant.

Challenging Spiritual Inflexibility

In some cases, clients need more of a push. Nothing less than a direct challenge is likely to increase the client's spiritual flexibility. At this point, many therapists cringe. They are reluctant to act so assertively in counseling for fear of interfering with their clients' fundamental right to live life however they choose. These fears may be especially strong in the spiritual domain. After all, who has the right to question or challenge a client's spiritual beliefs and practices? These are legitimate concerns.

Nevertheless, keep in mind two points. First, there is an important difference between challenge and coercion. Challenge is built into virtually every psychotherapy, be it the challenge of sharing any and all thoughts in psychodynamic therapy, the challenge to irrational thoughts in rational-emotive therapy, or the challenge of facing painful issues with a spouse in couple therapy. Even the most basic of therapeutic skills—reflective listening, empathy, positive regard—can be disorienting to the client. The challenge for therapists from every perspective is to find a means of confronting their clients noncoercively, in ways that are respectful of their autonomy and ultimate responsibility for their own lives. Second, keep in mind that spiritual problems can have serious consequences, especially when the client adheres rigidly to degrading, extremist, or narrow beliefs and practices that are poorly suited to life's demands. When held inflexibly, the belief that God alone solves all problems may lead to refusals of life-giving medical treatment. The belief that God expects perfection of people may result in crushing guilt, shame, and compulsive striving. The belief that wives are religiously-obligated to submit to their husbands can keep women in abusive marriages. As with other forms of treatment, there are times when challenge is a necessary element of spiritually integrated therapy.

Several therapists have illustrated how they challenge inflexibly held spiritual beliefs (Eriksen et al., 2002; Narramore, 1994; Nielsen et al., 2001; Rayburn, 1985). A number of examples are presented in Table 15.1. Even though these illustrations all come from work with Christian clients, remember that spiritual rigidity is found in people from every religious tradition as well as among people who reject traditional teachings. Nielsen et al. (2001) have elaborated in great detail on various types of spiritual challenge. Consider three forms here. Pragmatic challenges push the client toward greater flexibility by pointing to the destructive consequences of his or her beliefs. Thus, the client who believes she is a worthless sinner can be asked, "What does it do for you or for God when you down-rate yourself?" (Nielsen et al., 2001, p. 133). Pointing to spiritual inconsistencies is another form of challenge that encourages flexibility by highlighting the gap between clients' beliefs and sacred teachings. In response to the Christian who maintains that suffering is a sign of spiritual purity, the therapist might ask, "Why did Jesus spend so much time healing people of various afflictions if suffering were so beneficial?" (Nielsen et al., 2001, p. 171). Offering alternative scriptural citations—that is, suggesting that there are different ways to interpret the most important lessons of a religious tradition—is a third form of challenge to spiritual rigidity. So the Christian who concludes that the Bible insists on perfection can be reminded that the New Testament also contains verses that maintain everyone is a sinner and no one can be perfect (e.g., "If we say we have no sin, we deceive ourselves and the truth is not in us"; 1 John 1:8) (Rayburn, 1985). Although clients may find these challenges to their rigidity provocative, clients will also find it difficult to dismiss such challenges out of hand because it is the client's interpretation of religious teachings that is being questioned, not the ultimate truth of these teachings. Most importantly, each of these challenges is com-

TABLE 15.1. Illustrative Challenges to Rigidly Held Spiritual Beliefs

Rigidly held spiritual belief	Illustrative challenge
I am a worthless sinner.	What does it do for you or for God when you down-rate yourself? Does it help you help others or pray or go to church or repent? Does it do any good for His works?[a] (p. 133)
Suffering is a sign of spiritual purity.	Why did Jesus spend so much time healing people of various afflictions (physical and emotional) if suffering were so beneficial?[a] (p. 171)
The Bible says I have to be perfect.	Only the divine has absolute perfection and so Matthew 5:48 ("You, therefore must be perfect, as your heavenly Father is perfect") is complemented by I John 1:8 ("If we say we have no sin, we deceive ourselves and the truth is not in us").[b] (pp. 39–40)
The Bible says that women should obey their husbands.	Yes, but what are your thoughts about some other verses, like Ephesians 5:21, "Be subject to one another out of reverence for Christ," and Ephesians 5:25, "Husbands love your wives, as Christ loved the church and gave himself up for her."[a] (p. 195)
I shouldn't need anyone but God.	But you know, when God saw that Adam was alone, He didn't tell Adam, "What's the matter with you Adam? You have me. That should be enough." He created Eve. God apparently made us so that we need each other.[c] (p. 253)
I don't have to take care of myself because I know that God will take care of me.	It sounds like God is holding up His end of the relationship with you. What are you doing to hold up your end of the relationship?
It is sinful for me to focus on myself.	In fact, Matthew 22:30 says "You shall love your neighbor as yourself" not instead of yourself.[d] (p. 55)

Note. Adapted from [a]Nielsen, Johnson, and Ellis (2001); [b]Rayburn (1985); [c]Narramore (1994); [d]Eriksen, Marston, and Korte (2002).

municated in a way that conveys the therapist's respect for sacred texts and spiritual commitment.

Brief Words on Humor

One more way to challenge spiritual inflexibility deserves consideration: the use of humor. By "humor," I do not mean making fun of clients, their situation, or their faith. Ridicule is probably the quickest way to destroy a therapeutic relationship. Like a bad comedian on stage, therapists who misuse humor will quickly get the hook. But humor, at its best, helps people recognize that there are many ways to look at themselves. Several years ago, a couple in the midst of a marital breakup brought their 6-year-old daughter into therapy because they were concerned about the effects of their marital problems on their little girl. The tension was thick in the room, but before we went very far, the little girl scanned my office, looked to her parents, and then asked, "Is this where diverse people go?" The mother was as puzzled as I was, and immediately asked her daughter, "What do you mean?" The daughter responded, "You know. Is this where people like you and Dad go to—people going through a diverse?" Both parents began to laugh and the tension in the room dissipated (at least for a while). Things were certainly bad in the family but, the humor suggested, not critical; there might be other ways to experience the situation. In Peter Berger's (1997) words, there was something "redeeming" about the laughter. According to Berger, "The comic conjures up a separate world, different from the world of ordinary reality, operating by different rules. It is also a world in which the limitations of the human condition are miraculously overcome. The experience of the comic is, finally, a promise of redemption" (p. x).

Properly used, humor can unthaw clients who seem to be spiritually frozen in place. For example, I have told a few of my intransigent Jewish clients (who know that I too am Jewish) this story from Berger (1997): "Under some tyrannical regime or other three Jews are about to be shot. The officer in charge of the execution offers them a last cigarette. The first accepts, so does the second. The third refuses. Whereupon the second turns to him and says, 'Moishe, don't make trouble' " (p. 92). How silly it is, this story suggests, to stick to old habits when the realities of life have changed. Of course, the joke would be less effective (and perhaps even offensive) if told by a therapist who was not Jewish. For Jewish clients and therapists, however, this kind of story joins them together in a long and well-recognized history of self-deprecating humor.

Humor in which therapists make light of themselves can be especially useful in challenging client's spiritual resistances. For instance, when faced with a religious client who questions whether God would want him or her to see a therapist, Eriksen et al. (2002) suggest the following response: "If God used an ass [to speak to Balaam in the Bible], do you think God might be able to use me to help you?" (p. 58).

There is something elusive about humor. It is not clear, at least not to me, what makes a story or a little joke funny. But good humor does create possibilities for change in seemingly intractable situations, including spiritual ones. My client Krista suffered from sporadic episodes of deep and disabling depression. Krista was a devout Roman Catholic whose faith had been a tremendous consolation to her throughout her life. She took particular comfort from attending mass. Even in the worst of her depressive periods, Krista forced herself to get out of bed in the morning, go to mass, and take communion. During her good periods, however, she was very troubled by fears that she would become totally disabled by her depression. Most of all, Krista was worried that she would be unable to attend mass. I could offer my client no guarantees. She had a strong family history of depression and her depressed periods were, in fact, becoming more frequent, in spite of psychotherapy and medication. One day as I was listening to Krista tearfully describe her spiritual fears, I spontaneously commented, "It sounds to me like you're afraid of becoming a 'massket case.' " Krista caught the pun right away, stopped crying, and started to laugh. This pun wouldn't win any awards for humor, but it did prove helpful to Krista in this session and subsequent ones. Her discovery that she could laugh about her worries opened up new possibilities for her. It challenged the notion that there was only one way to approach her greatest fears, and it offered the possibility of change, the hope that even the most painful of life situations can be transcended.

Without some degree of spiritual flexibility clients cannot adapt to changing times and circumstances, cannot grow in their understanding of the sacred, and cannot broaden and deepen their spiritual pathways. Helping clients loosen their "spiritual straightjackets" is a key element in spiritually integrated psychotherapy. Most of the examples I have presented in this section have focused on individuals. Yet spiritual rigidity can also manifest itself in problems between people. We turn our attention now to some of the ways therapists can address problems of fit, focusing particularly on problems of spiritual fit between the individual and the larger social system.

ADDRESSING PROBLEMS OF FIT

Mental health professionals tend to see psychological problems from an individualistic perspective. Like medical illnesses, psychological problems are said to lie within the person. Earlier, however, I noted that some spiritual problems are better understood as lying in the relationship between clients and their life situations or between clients and their larger social context. These are problems of fit and they call for a different set of spiritual solutions. Below I consider some of these strategies for enhancing fit, paying special attention to the problems of tension between the individual and the social system.

When Spiritual Conflicts Mask Other Conflicts

Several years ago, I saw a couple in therapy that was engaging in spiritual warfare. Ilya, an immigrant from Armenia, had been raised in the Russian

Orthodox Church. As an adolescent, he lost interest in the church and all things religious. In his mid-20s, he met Ellen, a Jewish woman. The only child of parents who had survived the Holocaust, Ellen felt a strong commitment to passing on her heritage to her children. Prior to their marriage, Ilya and Ellen had spoken in great detail about religious matters. Because he attached little importance to religion, Ilya had willingly agreed to raise the children as Jewish, attend milestone religious events with the family in the synagogue, and be buried next to his wife in a Jewish cemetery. What brought the family into therapy was Ilya's sudden decision to change the terms of this arrangement. He decided that he now wanted his children to be raised in the religious tradition of their father. They had spent several years in Hebrew school and he felt it only fair that they begin attending Sunday school at the local Russian Orthodox church. Ellen's reaction was immediate and furious. How dare he violate the contract that was the very foundation of their marriage? Hadn't she made it clear to him before they were married that she would not raise the children outside the Jewish tradition? Ilya responded by increasing his demands. No longer would he attend his wife's synagogue, a place in which he had never felt welcome, and no longer could he imagine himself being buried in a cemetery surrounded by an alien people. All of this information spilled out within the first half hour of the first session of therapy. Both partners were so upset they could barely contain themselves. Clearly, the issue was too hot to touch this early in treatment. I said as much to the couple and shifted the focus to other topics.

Over the next few sessions, I learned that Ilya had recently suffered a series of life-changing losses: the death of a parent in Armenia, demotion from his upper-level managerial position, and a back injury. While his fortunes were declining, Ellen's seemed to be thriving. She had switched from her role as stay-at-home mom to marketing executive and was advancing rapidly in her company. But caught up in the excitement of her own transition, Ellen was unaware of Ilya's terrible feelings arising from his loss of the roles and responsibilities—son, breadwinner, strong husband—that had given his life meaning and purpose.

Where did Ilya's sudden religious change of heart fit in here? It was not precipitated by a powerful spiritual experience. Ilya had little interest in returning to the Russian Orthodox Church for himself. Neither did he show any interest in pursuing other spiritual paths. Instead, by renegotiating the religious rules of the family, Ilya hoped to create a new identity for himself and a new place for himself in the family. It soon became clear to me that the spiritual battle between the spouses was masking Ilya's personal conflicts and a growing distance that had been unfolding in their marriage. In this case, I sidestepped the obvious spiritual conflict of the couple to address what turned out to be more fundamental individual and marital tensions. In the process, the spiritual conflict receded in intensity and importance.

Sidestepping spiritual conflicts is not always appropriate, however. When is it inappropriate? Spiritual conflicts should be addressed head-on when clients reject the therapist's attempt to shift the focus away from spiritual topics, when the spiritual issue reemerges after other issues have been resolved, when the spiritual conflict is judged to be a significant concern in and of itself, and when the spiritual conflict has to be addressed before other problems can be resolved. Butler and Harper (1994) illustrate this latter point in their work with religious couples. Not uncommonly, they found, these couples diffuse the tension in their marriages by "triangling" sacred objects into their relationship. Triangling can take several guises. Each spouse may argue that God is on his or her side. Both partners may project the strain in their marriage onto sacred objects, such as a specific church neither can stand, self-righteous religious hypocrites, or a God they feel let them down. Or one or both partners may seek out intimacy with God as a surrogate for closeness with their spouse. Complicating matters further, both spouses may vie to create a spiritual coalition with the therapist against their partner (Rotz, Russell, & Wright, 1993), with devastating results for treatment. Though these spiritual conflicts often grow out of deeper tensions and frustrations in the marriage, they cannot be sidestepped. The therapist must help the couple find a more constructive place for the sacred in their relationship before addressing other problems.

Addressing Problems of Individual–Systems Fit

There are several ways that therapists can help clients resolve problems of conflicts between themselves and their social systems: by making the spiritual conflict explicit, building greater spiritual discernment, encouraging sanctification of the relationship, promoting spiritual tolerance, and exploring new spiritual niches.

Making the Spiritual Conflict Explicit

Seemingly insignificant conflicts can have deep spiritual significance. Unaware of the spiritual dimension of their conflict, clients may find themselves stuck in what may appear to be a relatively minor disagreement. For instance, Roger was a 45-year-old man who came to my office for help in maintaining his sobriety. Earlier in his life, Roger had been the CEO of an international company. By all external criteria, he was highly successful. He made a great deal of money, was admired by family and friends, and traveled and vacationed extensively. The only problem was that he hated his job. Roger had gone into business under pressure from his family, although his real loves were art and literature. Ironically, in spite of the fact that he hated everything about his job, Roger was good at his work, and he quickly ascended the career ladder. In the process, he also began to drink heavily. Eventually, the drinking took its toll, and Roger lost his job, his marriage, and his savings. When I saw Roger, he was living in an efficiency apartment, attending AA, and trying to find a new direction for his life.

Our conversation ranged over many topics, but one issue arose repeatedly: the conflict he was having with his girlfriend over his hobby, pottery. Roger had taken several courses in pottery and ceramics and had apprenticed himself to a seasoned potter. Roger's idea of heaven was an afternoon spent sitting in front of his potter's wheel at the local art museum learning the craft. Roger's girlfriend felt otherwise. All of this energy devoted to pottery, she insisted, was wasted because it took him away from what should be his most important task: finding a real job that produced a decent income. Roger couldn't understand why they continued to argue over something as trivial as his hobby. He himself recognized that he needed to find a job to support himself, but for some reason he kept digging in his heels whenever the topic of pottery came up.

Perhaps, I suggested, the conflict was not so trivial after all. Something about pottery seemed to move Roger deeply. At the potter's wheel, Roger experienced spiritual emotions—peace, fulfillment, even transcendence— that he had never found elsewhere. And yet his girlfriend wanted him to put this "hobby" aside in favor of more "adult" pursuits. Thinking back to the tug-of-war he had faced with his parents as a younger man, Roger realized that once again he was facing conflict between what he wanted for himself and what others wanted for him. There was, he recognized, nothing trivial about it. I encouraged Roger to talk to his girlfriend about the spiritual meaning that pottery held for him. He did, and their conversation shifted from bickering about Roger's "hobby" to enlightening dialogue about their spiritual strivings. By making the spiritual dimension of their conflict more explicit, Roger and his girlfriend were able to move to a clearer resolution of their problems.

Building Greater Spiritual Discernment

As we have seen, part of the power of spirituality lies in its diversity. Spiritual beliefs and practices come in a variety of shapes and sizes. Within the spiritual domain, people can find resources to help them deal with a wide range of situations and contexts. Problems arise, though, when people fail to apply their spiritual resources judiciously. In these instances, therapists can try to encourage greater discernment on the part of their clients. In building spiritual discernment, the therapist does not challenge any particular belief or practice of the client; the challenge instead is to the appropriateness of the belief or practice to the situation or context. For example, John, a 30-year-old man, was referred to me by his supervisor because he had been causing some problems on the job. Over the previous few months, he had begun to sing religious hymns, sway in apparent ecstasy as he worked on a machine press, and talk to coworkers about religious matters on lunch breaks. The supervisor was concerned that John was having a mental breakdown. On top of that, John's coworkers were complaining about his "weirdness." I found no signs of a thought disorder or other serious mental illness in John. I did learn that he had had a recent born-again experience and felt a strong desire to share the good news with everyone he encountered. Perhaps John's behavior would have been less problematic in another setting, but he was working in a factory with young, blue-collar coworkers who had little patience for his religious enthusiasm. Making matters worse, John was naïve about the impact he was having on his coworkers. I made no attempt to temper his religious enthusiasm. Instead, I tried to help him discern when, where, and how he might express his newfound fervor. This worked out well for John and his company. He continued to sing religious hymns at work, but quietly to himself, stopped swaying at the machine press, and limited his religious conversations to a more receptive audience of family, friends, and church members.

Promoting Spiritual Tolerance

Differences in the spiritual arena can be very hard to resolve without some degree of spiritual forbearance. Group therapy is a particularly appropriate context for facilitating spiritual tolerance. Nancy Kehoe (1998) is an expert in this area. For many years, she has been leading religious issues therapy groups for people from varied religious backgrounds with serious mental illness. These groups are designed to help clients explore any and all feelings about their religious beliefs, practices, and backgrounds, or lack of religiousness. The group has little external structure and few rules, with the exception of one. Kehoe insists on spiritual tolerance: "The basic ground rule and fundamental value of the group is that each person and his or her beliefs are to be respected. The group is not a prayer group, nor is it a Bible study group; no one is allowed to proselytize" (pp. 47–48). By insisting on this rule, Kehoe instills a norm for spiritual tolerance that allows group participants to explore diverse attitudes and approaches to spirituality in a safe environment. This is not to say that the group does not experience conflicts. Kehoe presents the following exchange that occurred after the group leader proposed an interdenominational Passover seder to celebrate the universal yearning for freedom:

> EVE: That makes me so angry. That means that Christians are appropriating a significant Jewish holiday . . .
>
> RICHARD: Being Jewish in this culture means that you are devaluated. This is a good example of how Jews feel oppressed.

JOHN: [The leader] is only showing us that there was a historical connection. Jesus was Jewish and so he was celebrating a seder.

CLAIRE: : I am not going to participate in the seder. I don't like this discussion.

TOM: I believe in every word that the Bible says, and I have always believed that the Jews killed Jesus.

PETER: This is an example of why there are holy wars. Each religion wants to dominate the others and say it is the best.

EVE: Well, if we have a seder, I'm not coming.

TOM: I'm not, either.

LEADER: There have been many strong feelings expressed today and I think that it will be important for us to continue this discussion next week. (pp. 51–52)

What is extraordinary about this exchange is the willingness of the participants to share such powerful feelings so openly, including challenges to the group leader. The next week, the therapist and group members continued to discuss their strong feelings with no ill effects. "No one in the program became more delusional," Kehoe writes. "No one left the group or the program precipitously. No one's beliefs were shattered because of the discussion. In fact, members became more aware of common ground with other beliefs and increased their level of tolerance. Everyone in the program participated in the Passover seder that year" (pp. 52–53).

Spiritual tolerance can also be encouraged in the context of family therapy. Family therapists have long been committed to enhancing the psychological autonomy of individual family members. In much the same way, therapists can encourage the spiritual autonomy of their clients. For example, Griffith (1986) described his work with Penny S. and her mother, Mrs. S. Throughout her adolescence, Penny had grappled with drug abuse, truancy, and violent conflicts with her parents over the rules of the family. At the age of 20, she was hospitalized following a suicide attempt and diagnosed with borderline personality disorder and major depression. Two years earlier, Penny had converted to a strict fundamentalist Christian church. Mrs. S. had also become increasingly religious during Penny's adolescence in an effort to gain more control over her daughter. Having experienced a terrible childhood of her own, Mrs. S. saw herself in Penny and desperately tried to solve her daughter's problems for her. In spite of the tremendous abuse she had suffered at Penny's hands, Mrs. S. devoted her life to her daughter and felt compelled to make every possible sacrifice for her. She pointed to God's unending love as the model for this sacrificial relationship. Yet Mrs. S admitted that she may have been overly dominating.

Griffith tried to create more distance, psychologically and spiritually, between Mrs. S and Penny. Citing the biblical parable of the prodigal son in which the father had no choice but to let his youngest son leave home and squander his inheritance in a foreign land, Griffith concluded with the statement, "Sometimes to love means to let go" (p. 612). Griffith encouraged Mrs. S. to recognize the limitations of her control rather than try to solve Penny's problems by relying on her own resources. The therapist suggested that Mrs. S., like the good father in the parable, should trust in God to care for her daughter. In essence, Griffith was asking Mrs. S. to shift from a self-directing to a deferring style of spiritual coping in an effort to create greater tolerance of what seemed to be spiritually intolerable. Mrs. S. was responsive to this advice. She began to give up the role of rescuer, accept her powerlessness with Penny, and refocus on developing her own relationship with God. Penny, in turn, moved away from home, started college part-time, and took the first steps to creating a more autonomous spirituality.

Encouraging Sanctification of the Relationship

Differences over spiritual matters can threaten many personal values: security, identity, comfort, meaning, and the individual's relationship with God. In response to these perceived threats, people may retreat into their own space, lash out against others, or seek spiritual allies to side with them in their battle. Each of these mechanisms is self-protective in nature, but each is also capable of inflicting a great deal of damage on intimate relationships.

   Therapists can help counteract this problem by shifting the client's focus from self-protection to the sacred connection between the couple. The "love intervention" described in Chapter 13 is one way to facilitate this shift. Butler and Harper (1994) present another in their work with a husband and wife both engaged in attempts to enlist God on their side of the marital conflict. In one session, the wife produced a written record from her purse that showed that she prayed more frequently than her husband. The husband responded with a speech of his own in which he described "God's unconditional love for him and God's disgust for vain and repetitious prayers" (p. 282). After observing this pattern of escalating religious conflict several times, the therapist intervened by raising several provocative questions that were designed to remove God from the marital tug-of-war, placing Him instead on the side of the marriage itself. "How could God side with either of them against the other without violating the sanctity of their marriage? It would be almost as if God had chosen to have an affair with one or both of them. How could a God who is interested in encouraging loving marriages be so disrespectful of the boundary of their own marriage?" (p. 282). This kind of intervention encourages couples to look beyond their own immediate needs to the sacred value of their relationship. By reminding the couple of the sanctity of their marriage, the therapist creates new possibilities for giving and sacrifice by each partner, based not on coercion, fear, or the expectation of something in return, but on the desire to contribute to a larger sacred connection.

Exploring New Spiritual Niches

Not all differences between an individual and a system are reconcilable, even after the differences are made explicit, even after tolerance is encouraged, even after the sacred nature of the relationship is emphasized. People may remain spiritually at odds with their partners, families, religious institutions, organizations, or communities that are unsupportive or destructive. Just as therapists encourage clients to explore new jobs when they cannot resolve conflicts at work, therapists can encourage clients to explore new spiritual niches for themselves when old settings no longer meet their needs.

One option is to help clients find a niche for themselves in their existing spiritual homes. Megachurches, for instance, provide their members with multiple social and educational offerings. Clients unhappy with one aspect of church life might find another more comfortable setting under the same roof. Smaller congregations can pose a stiffer challenge. There, clients may need to do some minor or major remodeling to create a new niche for themselves. As with all change, this process can lead to organizational resistance. In these instances, therapists can anticipate the resistance with their clients and support them through the course of change. For instance, a number of years ago, I worked with Peter, a 55-year-old man suffering from depression associated with a progressive neurological illness. The illness had been accompanied by many losses in Peter's life. Spiritual losses were among the most significant. Over the years, Peter had been a linchpin of his church, serving in numerous roles including president and deacon. Particularly painful to Peter was the loss of his ability to participate fully in the life of the church. Wheelchair-bound, Peter could no longer attend the Bible study and social events that were held in the basement of the church. Ironically, the sign above the doorway at the bottom of the narrow stairs read, "Everyone is welcome here." I encouraged Peter to approach the other leaders of the church about the possibility of creating a wheelchair-accessible entrance into the basement. Although several leaders were sympathetic, they balked at the expense. Peter persisted, however, and eventually the church agreed to construct a new entrance. In the process, Peter's depression lifted, not only because of the spiritual support he gained from his renewed involvement in the religious life of the church, but from his vigorous efforts to create a place for all people in the congregation, disabled as well as healthy.

A second option is to help clients find new spiritual homes. For example, people struggling with alcoholism can find a number of AA meetings to choose from in virtually every city. Like religious congregations, each meeting has its own distinctive personality. Thus, clients who are uncomfortable in one setting can often find themselves perfectly at home in another. Similarly, a quick tour of almost any community in the United States will show that there is no shortage of religious congregations from which to choose. Large, small, formal, informal, homogenous, diverse—these congregations have distinctive climates that appeal in their own unique ways to different potential members. I often encourage clients who are unable to find or create a comfortable niche for themselves in their congregations to "shop around." It is important to remember, however, that congregations are more than social institutions. They are spiritual institutions, purveyors of ultimate truths. Thus, the decision to change congregations should not be made casually; instead, it should be carefully considered, particularly when the client may be shopping around for congregations from other denominations.

A final option is to encourage clients to build their own spiritual homes. Creating brand-new settings can be a daunting task, but it is not impossible. New congregations and spiritual associations of one kind or another are constantly under construction. Clients unable to fit within existing contexts may be exhilarated by the chance to build a new spiritual home, be it a new Bible study group, a new church, or a new social ministry to serve homeless people. Similarly, therapists can empower clients to create fundamental spiritual change in the larger social system. Ali et al. (2004) present a nice clinical illustration. Mona, a 21-year-old Muslim American college student, came to therapy complaining of diffuse physical symptoms, such as headaches, body aches, and fatigue, that could be not attributed to a medical cause. Initially, the therapist, a male, had difficulty forming a relationship with Mona. Unaware of the prohibition against physical contact between women and male strangers in Islam, he tried to shake her hand in the first session, an invitation she declined. The therapist also found himself frustrated by Mona's lack of self-disclosure. Fortunately, the therapist recognized that part of the difficulty he was experiencing might reflect his own stereotypical beliefs regarding Muslim Americans. Through supervision and consultation with Muslim colleagues, he familiarized himself with Palestinian Muslims and became more sensitive to the impact of his own behavior on the therapeutic relationship. Mona responded positively to the signs of growing cultural awareness on the part of her therapist. She began to disclose more about herself and the conflicts she was experiencing as a Muslim with her parents, the college environment, and life in an Islamophobic society. Again, the therapist was able to respond sensitively. He provided Mona with additional information on the prevalence of anti-Muslim discrimination in the United States that reassured her that she was not the only one experiencing religious conflicts. Soon, Mona began to bring questions about her own religious identity to therapy. Should she continue to wear her headscarf? Should she continue with her daily prayers? The therapist gave Mona a safe space to discuss the pros and cons of these choices, in part by making clear his own appreciation for the potential value of religion without attempting to impose this value on her. Eventually, she decided to reaffirm her faith. Mona became actively involved in educational programs on campus to combat religious hate acts. Thus, through the process of therapy, Mona was empowered to seek fundamental religious change in her environment.

CONCLUSIONS

No topic is off-limits in psychotherapy. Spiritually integrated psychotherapy brings an often neglected topic—the sacred—to the foreground of the clinical conversation. In this dialogue, spirituality may surface as an unplumbed but vital resource for change. On the other hand, spirituality may be revealed as a significant problem in itself. There is no guarantee that an individual's spiritual approach will remain unchanged through psychotherapy. As Grosch (1985) writes, "The self-discovery is devious and may lead to the unmasking of, and disenchantment with, what one thought was genuine. It might be that the patient needed to discover what little faith he or she really had" (p. 126). Remember, however, that the goal of spiritually integrated psychotherapy is not the elimination of spirituality, but the enrichment and integration of spirituality in the client's life.

Over the course of the last four chapters, I described a variety of ways clinicians can draw upon spiritual and psychological resources to address spiritual and psychological problems. We have seen that spiritually integrated therapy is multimodal, encompassing a broad spectrum of clinical methods that can be applied through almost any system of therapy to individuals, couples, families, and groups confronted with the full range of human problems. Even though this review of methods has been illustrative rather than comprehensive, I hope it has made the point that spiritually integrated therapy adds another critical dimension to psychotherapy. Nevertheless, this approach is only just beginning to emerge as a new orientation to treatment. Many important clinical questions remain unanswered. For instance, what is the best way to work with problems of spiritual extremism? How should clinicians approach clients who are spiritually hypocritical? What about clients who jump from one spiritual fad to another? How might therapists help clients engaged in a spiritual quest form deeper and more lasting spiritual commitments? Clearly, there is more work to be done, including more clinically relevant research. In the concluding chapter, we turn our attention to the future of spiritually integrated psychotherapy and some of the ways it might be advanced.

Part IV

CONCLUSIONS

16

Steps toward a More Spiritually Integrated Psychotherapy

Thirty years ago, I gave my first colloquium to a department of psychology. I spoke about religion and mental health. I don't remember much about the talk, but I do recall an incident afterward. The chairman of the department came up to me, leaned over the podium, and whispered, "I'm Catholic." Fortunately, I was trained as a clinical psychologist so I knew how to respond. "Oh," I said quietly. After pausing for a moment, I asked, "Why are we whispering?" In a voice still hushed, the chairman said, "Religion . . . you know, it's not something we talk about around here." This was not an uncommon reaction 30 years ago.

This picture has begun to change, however (see Weaver et al., 2006). Even in the 5 years it has taken me to write this book, there has been a sharp increase in open conversation on the topic of spirituality by scientists and practitioners. How do we account for this change? Perhaps it reflects a sense that, in spite of the advances that have been made in the field, there has been something missing from the ways we have tried to understand and help people. Perhaps it reflects a yearning for a psychology that touches the deeper levels of what it means to be human. Perhaps it also reflects the growing body of research that points unequivocally to spirituality as a potent predictor of health and well-being. And perhaps it reflects the growing realization that we can actually address the spiritual dimension in psychotherapy.

Whatever the reason, times have changed. Even so, this area of study and practice is far from well established. Spiritually integrated psychotherapy, in particular, is still in its early stages of development. Where do we go from here? In this final chapter, I conclude by discussing three steps that are critical to advancing spiritually integrated psychotherapy: demonstrating the effectiveness of spiritually integrated therapy, extending the reach of spiritually integrated approaches to change, and developing skills in this method of treatment.

DEMONSTRATING THE EFFECTIVENESS OF SPIRITUALLY INTEGRATED PSYCHOTHERAPY

Spiritually integrated psychotherapy will not gain widespread use and acceptance until it has been proven to be effective. That is as it should be. Deep personal spiritual convictions or faith in the value of spiritually oriented treatment are no substitute for scientific support. As with any form of psychotherapy, spiritually integrated therapy should lead to meaningful change if it is indeed worthwhile. Researchers and therapists have begun to evaluate the impact of spiritually integrated treatments and, as we have seen in some of their findings reviewed in this book, the results have been promising. Nevertheless, this research is only a start; several critical questions remain about the effectiveness of spiritually integrated therapy.

Can Spiritually Integrated Psychotherapy Be Manualized?

Before any kind of treatment can be formally evaluated, it must be clearly articulated so practitioners can be trained in the method, so the method itself can be implemented with a reasonable degree of standardization, and so others can replicate the findings of evaluative studies. Treatment manuals are the critical vehicle for defining and evaluating new methods of psychotherapy. Nevertheless, many therapists shudder at the idea of treatment manuals. The very word "manual" can bring to mind therapies as dry, regimented, and lifeless as the instructions for assembling a bicycle. The chills that run down the spine may be especially intense for therapists interested in spirituality, a dimension of life so rich, varied, and dynamic that it would seem virtually "unmanualizable" without trivializing or distorting it beyond recognition. And yet, in spite of these concerns, therapists and researchers have begun to manualize spiritually integrated psychotherapies, with some success. In Table 16.1, I have summarized the manualized spiritually integrated treatments that I was able to locate in the literature.[1]

These treatments are far from trivial. Spiritually integrated therapies

---

[1]Although a few spiritually integrated treatments have been described as "manualized" in the literature, I included only those therapies for which I was able to find a published or unpublished treatment manual.

TABLE 16.1. Manualized Spiritually Integrated Psychotherapies

Program	Researchers	Target	Goal	Spiritual resources
From Vice to Virtue	Ano (2005)	Four-session Christian-based group for people struggling with vices and imperfections	To cultivate the development of virtues and resistance to vices	Diverse spiritual coping methods (e.g., spiritual support, spiritual visualization, purification), prayer, use of Scriptures
Spiritual Self-Schema (3-S) Therapy	Avants & Margolin (2003)	8-week group nonsectarian intervention for addiction and HIV risk behavior	To replace the "addict self-schema" with a "spiritual self-schema"	Meditation, prayers and affirmations, spiritual reframing, training in spiritual virtues
Re-Creating Your Life	Cole & Pargament (1998)	Six-session group nondenominational intervention for the medically ill	To enhance overall adjustment and facilitate sense of control, meaning, identity, and intimacy	Diverse spiritual coping methods (e.g., spiritual support, surrender), meditation, spiritual visualization
Sacred Moments	McCorkle, Bohn, Hughes, & Kim (2005)	10-session group nondenominational intervention for social anxiety disorder	To help people place social anxiety into a larger spiritual perspective	Sanctification, meditation, ritual, spiritual support
Solace for the Soul	Murray-Swank (2003)	Eight-session theistic intervention for female survivors of sexual abuse	To help people address and resolve spiritual struggles	Diverse spiritual coping methods (e.g., revisioning God, spiritual support, spiritual reframing), prayer, spiritual visualization, meditation, affirmations, spiritual journaling
Lighting the Way	Pargament, McCarthy, et al. (2004)	Eight-session theistic intervention for women with HIV/AIDS	To address spiritual struggles and facilitate wholeness and healing	Diverse spiritual coping methods (e.g., spiritual support, spiritual reframing, revisioning God, spiritual surrender), sanctification, spiritual journaling, meditation, prayer, ritual, forgiveness

(continued)

TABLE 16.1. (*continued*)

Program	Researchers	Target	Goal	Spiritual resources
Spiritual Renewal	Richards, Hardman, & Berrett (2000)	10-week theistic group intervention for people with eating disorders	To help people with eating disorders grow spiritually and achieve greater spiritual harmony	Address false gods, spiritual support, identify spiritual strivings, spiritual surrender, forgiveness, gratitude, spiritual reframing
Coping with Divorce	Rye & Pargament (2003)	Eight-session Christian-based forgiveness group for divorced men and women	To help people become more forgiving of their ex-spouses	Prayer, purification rituals, spiritual surrender, spiritual reframing, spiritual modeling, meditation, use of Scripture
Becoming a More Forgiving Christian	Worthington (2004)	Six-session Christian-based intervention for community members who experienced transgressions by others	To help people become more forgiving toward those who have hurt them	Use of Jesus Christ as model of forgiveness, prayer, meditation, encouraging spiritual virtues (e.g., empathy, gratitude)

have been designed to meet the needs of people facing a wide range of serious problems. For example, one program, Solace for the Soul, is designed for women who have been sexually abused (Murray-Swank, 2003; see Chapters 11 and 14). Another manualized treatment, Spiritual Self-Schema (3-S) Therapy, is aimed at people dealing with drug addiction and HIV risk behavior (see Avants & Margolin, 2003; Chapter 14). Still another program, Sacred Moments, is tailored to help people with social anxiety disorder (McCorkle et al., 2005; see Chapter 14). A few programs have been developed to help individuals move toward greater forgiveness of others (Worthington, 2004). Other programs, such as Re-Creating Your Life, are designed for people struggling with serious medical illness (Cole & Pargament, 1998).

Manualized treatments address weighty psychological, social, and spiritual issues. Consider two examples. Table 16.2 describes the goals of each session of "Lighting the Way," an eight-session, manualized, group treatment for women who have been infected with HIV/AIDS (Pargament, McCarthy, et al., 2004). Lighting the Way addresses questions of deepest concern: Does a diagnosis of HIV/AIDS mean that the individual is fundamentally contaminated? Is intimacy still possible after HIV/AIDS? How can the person move beyond shame and guilt? How can the individual come to

TABLE 16.2. Session-by-Session Goals of Lighting the Way

- *Session 1: Wholeness and Healing.* Define healing; encourage the view of healing as a process; identify barriers and resources toward feeling healed.

- *Session 2: Body and Spirit.* Identify how body and spirit interact with one another; identify eternal things about the self that cannot be touched by the disease; identify how to recognize when the spirit is hungry and how to sustain it.

- *Session 3: Isolation and Intimacy.* Normalize the experiences of isolation and concerns with intimacy and explore the possible impact on coping; discuss experiences of isolation and concerns about intimacy; explore the disconnection from God and other people that can result from living with HIV/AIDS.

- *Session 4: Letting Go of Anger.* Discuss different ways of experiencing and expressing anger; discuss the effects of anger; identify objects of anger; discuss and normalize anger at God; introduce the possibility of letting go of destructive anger.

- *Session 5: Shame and Guilt.* Normalize the experience of shame and guilt and the potential impact of shame and guilt on healing; identify messages, spiritual and otherwise, of shame that people hear from others, messages of guilt people tell themselves, and messages of God that counter these shame and guilt messages; encourage self-love and self-forgiveness as healing alternatives to shame and guilt.

- *Session 6: Control versus Active Surrender.* Embrace the paradoxical nature of surrender; identify things that are under personal control and things that are beyond personal control; identify barriers that make letting go difficult; learn how to surrender to God and begin the process of letting go.

- *Session 7: Hopes and Dreams.* Identify dreams before HIV; discuss dreams that have been lost; identify dreams that are still possible; discuss the differences between false dreams and possible dreams; identify new dreams to pursue and how to redefine God's purpose in life.

- *Session 8: A Review of the Journey.* Review the process of healing; discuss the goals that group members have attained and those they feel they have yet to achieve; review the main points of each session; say good-bye.

Note. Drawn from Pargament, McCarthy, et al. (2004).

terms with uncontrollable aspects of life? What hopes and dreams are still possible?

Table 16.3 describes the focus of each session of "Spiritual Renewal," a 10-session, manualized, theistic treatment for women with eating disorders (Richards et al., 2000). Here too therapists encourage clients to face profound issues, including the faith the individual has misplaced in food and other addictions; the loss of a sense of divine worth and mission in life; anger and bitterness toward God, others, and oneself; and the lack of balance and harmony in life. Spiritual Renewal confronts these deep-seated problems.

There are points of commonality among the manualized treatments. They deal with significant human problems and deep-rooted psychological, social, and spiritual concerns. They also draw upon various combinations of powerful spiritual resources that include meditation, prayer, spiritual

TABLE 16.3. Session-by-Session Goals of Spiritual Renewal

- *Session 1: The Healing Power of Faith and Spirituality.* Identify eating disorders as a form of misplaced faith in the effort to find fulfillment in life; encourage placing faith in a more constructive, benevolent source of significance.

- *Session 2: Understanding and Accepting the Human Predicament.* Recognize that life is hard and raise the possibility of heroism in response to adversity; distinguish what has worked from what has failed in coping; commit to more effective ways of coping in the future.

- *Session 3: Affirming Your Divine Worth.* Recognize the inherent self-worth of the individual; distinguish self-worth based on appearance, achievement, and approval from self-worth based on spiritual beliefs and love; distinguish times in life when people experienced self-worth from times when they felt worthless.

- *Session 4: Discovering Your Personal Life Purpose and Mission.* Identify a guiding vision in life; encourage a plan and commitment to realizing this vision.

- *Session 5: Accepting Responsibility.* Identify barriers to taking responsibility (e.g., perfectionism, shame, disgust); recognize the dangers of overresponsibility, and encourage spiritual responsibility for what can be controlled.

- *Session 6: Forgiveness and Saying Goodbye to the Old.* Encourage forgiveness of oneself, others, and God: identify barriers to forgiveness; shift role of prosecutor, judge, and jury from self to God.

- *Session 7: Embracing Congruence and Balance.* Define importance of living a balanced life, including balance between process and outcome, between behavior and intentions, and between public and private behavior.

- *Session 8: Understanding and Growing in Divine Love.* Distinguish what love is from what love is not; encourage acts of kindness and compassion toward others; consider looking to God as a partner in love.

- *Session 9: Belonging and Gratitude.* Identify importance of feeling a sense of belonging with others and God; cultivate gratitude for the good things of life.

- *Session 10: Embracing Spiritual Harmony.* Stress importance of spiritual harmony; encourage being in tune with one's heart and expressing one's heart to others; identity spiritual practices to nurture spiritual harmony.

Note. Drawn from Richards, Hardman, and Berrett (2007).

coping methods, rituals, visualizations, journaling, and sanctification. In spite of their similarities, existing manualized treatments have different points of emphasis. For example, Sacred Moments encourages people with social anxiety to view their problem and life more generally through the larger lens of the sacred (McCorkle et al., 2005). The goal of the therapy is not to talk people out of their anxiety, but rather to help people see their anxiety within the context of a greater field of forces. Rituals, meditation, and exercises to promote sanctification are used to encourage participants to make and sustain this perceptual shift. In contrast, helping people visualize a compassionate, supportive God plays a more central role in other manualized interventions, such as Solace for the Soul for abused women (Murray-Swank, 2003) and Re-Creating Your Life for people with serious medical illness (Cole & Pargament, 1998). Meditation is key to some interventions (e.g., Spiritual Self-Schema Therapy; Avants & Margolin, 2003), prayer and Scripture to others (e.g., From Vice to Virtue; Ano, 2005), and spiritual methods of coping to still others (e.g., Lighting the Way; Pargament, McCarthy, et al., 2004). In short, although manualized spiritually integrated treatments are similar in some respects, they are distinctive in other ways; there is no single spiritually integrated therapy.

Manualized spiritual interventions provide guidelines and standards for treatment. Even so, they can be sensitive to individual differences. Most of these therapies acknowledge the varied ways people understand and relate to the sacred. Individuals are encouraged to draw on their own distinctive spiritual perspectives in the process of treatment. Although some manualized treatments are designed exclusively for Christians (e.g., Ano, 2005; Worthington, 2004), others are nondenominational and can be applied to people from diverse religious and spiritual backgrounds (e.g., Cole & Pargament, 1998; McCorkle et al. 2005).

Certainly, manualized treatments have their limitations. They are brief and can leave clients feeling the need for additional help. In my experience, this is the most common complaint about manualized spiritually integrated therapy. Clients generally enjoy the chance to explore the spiritual side of their lives and are often reluctant to stop once they get started. All in all, however, I believe that it is possible to manualize spiritually integrated psychotherapy in systematic yet sensitive ways that retain rather than distort much of the distinctive character of spirituality. The key question that follows is whether these interventions are effective. Evaluations of the effectiveness of manualized and other types of spiritually integrated interventions are not plentiful, but initial results have been encouraging.

Does Spiritually Integrated Psychotherapy Work?

On the face of it, the question "Does spiritually integrated psychotherapy work?" seems pretty straightforward. All we have to do is determine whether clients who receive this type of treatment, in fact, improve. A number of evaluative studies have shown that people who receive some form of spiritually integrated therapy do indeed make positive changes in their health and well-being. Consider a few examples. Tarakeshwar, Pearce, and Sikkema (2005) tested an eight-session spiritual coping group intervention for 13 men and women with HIV. Similar to Lighting the Way, the intervention focused on helping participants draw more fully on their spiritual resources and address their spiritual struggles. Over the course of the intervention, participants showed significant reductions in depression and spiritual struggles, and significant increases in positive religious coping. Similarly, Richards, Owen, and Stein (1993) designed and tested an 8-week group treatment for Mormon undergraduates dealing with perfectionism. The program integrated Mormon teachings with cognitive-behavioral methods. From pre- to posttreatment, the researchers found significant declines in perfectionism and depression, and significant improvements in self-esteem, religious well-being, and existential well-being.

Promising as studies such as these are, they do not provide strong evidence in support of the effectiveness of spiritually integrated therapy. After all, it is well known that people with serious problems often change by drawing on their own personal and social resources without the help of psychotherapy. Perhaps many of the clients in these studies would have changed had they not been in treatment. Stronger evidence would come from studies that compare clients in spiritually integrated therapy to clients who are not receiving psychotherapy. A few of these comparative studies have been conducted. They have shown that spiritually integrated therapy results in more positive changes than those reported by people who do not receive psychotherapy (e.g., Pechour & Edwards, 1984; Propst, 1980).

These studies suggest that spiritually integrated therapy is more effective than no therapeutic help. But before we get too excited about these results, it is important to remember that a number of therapeutic approaches have proven to be more effective than no treatment at all. The issue many therapists are interested in is how spiritually integrated therapy compares to other forms of treatment.

Is Spiritually Integrated Psychotherapy More Effective Than Other Treatments?

A growing body of research has compared spiritually integrated psychotherapy to other types of treatment, with encouraging results. A few studies have found no difference in the effectiveness of "religion-accommodative" cognitive-behavioral treatments and standard cognitive-behavioral therapies for Christian clients with depression (e.g., Johnson & Ridley, 1992; Johnson, DeVries, Ridley, Pettorini, & Peterson, 1994).

A number of studies, however, offer a different picture (e.g., Propst, 1980; Propst, Ostrom, Watkins, Dean, & Mashburn, 1992; Smith, Bartz, & Richards, in press). Here are some examples:

1. Amy Wachholtz (2005) found that spiritual meditation was superior to secular meditation and progressive relaxation for college students with vascular headaches.
2. R. D'Souza and colleagues presented preliminary evidence that indicated that "spiritually augmented cognitive behaviour therapy" appeared to be more effective than supportive case management in samples of depressed patients (D'Souza, Rich, Diamond, Godfery, & Gleeson, 2002) and

patients with schizophrenia (D'Souza, Rich, Diamond, & Godfery, 2002) in Australia.

3. Azhar and colleagues compared a religiously based psychotherapy to supportive psychotherapy plus medication in the treatment of Muslim patients from Malaysia diagnosed with generalized anxiety disorder (Azhar, Varma, & Dharap, 1994), dysthymic disorder (Azhar et al., 1995a), and major depression (Azhar & Varma, 1995b). The religiously based therapy consisted of encouraging readings from the Koran, prayers of relaxation, and religious discussions in treatment. Patients with major depression were rated as less depressed than the comparison group at both 1-month and 6-month follow-ups. The anxious and dysthymic patients were rated less anxious and depressed, respectively, than those in the supportive therapy condition 1 month after treatment; however, these findings were not maintained at the 6-month follow-up.

4. Lampton and colleagues compared the effects of a Christian-oriented forgiveness workshop (Worthington, 2004) to an assessment-only comparison condition in a sample of students who were interested in becoming more forgiving (Lampton, Oliver, Worthington, & Berry, 2005). Although the researchers hypothesized that the workshop would be more helpful than the assessment-only condition, they also predicted that participation in the assessment-alone condition would promote some change by encouraging positive reflections about forgiveness. In support of these predictions, participants in the assessment-only condition did show significant increases over time in positive thoughts, feelings, and behavior toward forgiveness of a specific transgression, but participants in the workshop reported even greater changes in the direction of positive responses of forgiveness and less of a tendency to avoid transgressors.

5. Richards, Berrett, Hardman, and Eggett (2006) studied 122 women with eating disorders in an inpatient setting. They compared the effectiveness of three treatments: a spirituality group that read a spiritual workbook and then discussed the readings during a weekly meeting; a cognitive group that read a cognitive-behavioral self-help workbook and then discussed the readings at a weekly meeting; and an emotional support group that discussed a variety of nonspiritually related topics (e.g., self-esteem, nutrition) at weekly meetings. All three groups reported positive changes over the course of treatment. However, in comparison to the other two groups, the spiritual group showed significantly greater improvement in eating attitudes and spiritual well-being, and significantly greater declines in symptom distress, relationship distress, and social role conflict.

How do we make sense of these findings? Some studies show no difference between spiritually integrated psychotherapy and other treatments. In contrast, another set of studies shows that spiritually integrated psychotherapy is modestly more effective than comparative treatments. Overall, the weight of the current evidence suggests that spiritually integrated therapy has distinctive therapeutic benefits (see Smith, Bartz, & Richards, in press). Nevertheless, it is too early to arrive at definitive conclusions on the question of the relative efficacy of spiritually integrated therapy.

Two points are important to keep in mind as we await the results of new evaluative studies. First, comparisons of spiritually integrated therapy with "secular" treatments may be a bit misleading, for it may be impossible to fully separate the spiritual component out of even presumably secular therapies. Recall the studies led by Mark Rye that compared religious forgiveness groups with secular forgiveness groups (Rye & Pargament, 2002; Rye et al., 2005). The secular and religious forgiveness groups grew out of the same model of forgiveness, a model loosely based on Worthington's (1998) forgiveness program. The only difference between the two groups was that spiritual resources were explicitly interwoven into the religious groups, while no mention of religion or spirituality was made in the secular groups (see Table 16.4). Both groups proved to be equally effective in promoting forgiveness of romantic partners (Rye & Pargament, 2002) and former spouses (Rye et al., 2005). However, when asked about the resources that helped them forgive, *members of the secular groups* indicated that two of the three most common resources they used were spiritual in nature (e.g., "I asked God for help and/or support as I was trying to forgive"). Thus, in spite of our efforts to compare the effects of secular and religious approaches to forgiveness, we were unable to implement and evaluate a fully secular forgiveness group. To label an approach to treatment as "secular" may thus be a misnomer, for the spiritual dimension continues to operate in the background. It may be more appropriate to frame these evaluative studies as comparisons between "explicitly spiritual" versus "not explicitly spiritual" groups.

Second, even if it is true that spiritually integrated therapies are not generally more effective than other types of treatment, it is equally true that other types of treatment are not generally more effective than spiritually integrated therapies (McCullough, 1998). Given that many clients prefer spiritually sensitive counselors and counseling (see Worthington, Kurusu, McCullough, & Sandage, 1996), spiritually integrated therapy is likely to remain a treatment of choice for a significant number of people. This latter point leads to another, more complex question.

Does Spiritually Integrated Psychotherapy Work Better in Some Instances than Others?

Psychotherapy researchers generally answer the question, Does psychotherapy work?, with the frustrating but accurate answer, "It depends." Years of evaluation research have suggested that general questions about the efficacy of therapy should be replaced with more specific questions of the kind

TABLE 16.4. Comparing Content of Secular and Religious Forgiveness Groups for Divorced Men and Women in Rye et al. (2005)

Sessions	Content	Secular group	Religious group (added components)
1–3	Processing and Coping with Negative Feelings	1. Attend to ways in which ex-spouse hurt you 2. Identify helpful and harmful consequences of anger and hostility 3. Identify how divorce has affected the way you see yourself	1. Visualize divine presence at your side, giving you the courage to face your pain 2. Identify how your anger affects your relationship with God 3. Consider how your view of yourself fits with the way God sees you
4–5	Learning about Forgiveness	1. Identify useful strategies for coping 2. Discuss the benefits of forgiveness 3. Identify obstacles to forgiveness 4. Discuss the fundamental attribution error (i.e., tendency to judge others more harshly than oneself)	1. Identify different types of spiritual coping strategies 2. Discuss the spiritual benefits of forgiveness 3. Think about forgiveness as a leap of faith 4. Consider how the fundamental attribution error relates to the Christian view of compassion
6–8	Moving Closer to Forgiveness	1. Seek support for forgiveness 2. Find models of forgiveness 3. Consider ways you have wronged others 4. Continue to hold on to forgiveness and redefine relation with ex-spouse	1. Seek spiritual support for forgiveness 2. Read the story of the prodigal son as a model of forgiveness 3. Draw on spiritual support when reminded of your own transgressions 4. Identify spiritual resources (e.g., prayers, daily affirmations) to deal with recurring resentment

raised by Paul (1967): "What treatment, by whom, is most effective for this individual with that specific problem, and under which set of circumstances?" (p. 111). Evaluations of spiritually integrated psychotherapy may require a similar level of specificity. For instance, the value of spiritually integrated psychotherapy may depend on the type of client in treatment. It seems only logical that this kind of therapy would be of particular value to more spiritually oriented clients. However, only a few studies have looked at this issue. In one recent investigation of 271 clients who visited Christian counseling centers or a secular agency, Wade, Worthington, and Vogel (2007) found that when religious interventions were used, clients who were more religiously committed reported greater closeness to their therapists and greater change in the presenting problem than clients who were less religiously committed. However, other studies have yielded mixed results on the benefits of matching spiritual treatments to spiritual clients (Worthington & Sandage, 2002). In this book, I have suggested that spiritually integrated therapy could be quite relevant to ostensibly nonspiritual clients who may be unaware of the role that spirituality plays in their lives. Conversely, the spiritual dimension is not necessarily relevant to the issues that bring even the most spiritually oriented client to therapy. Thus, the value of spiritually integrated therapy may depend as much on the particular problems the client is confronting as on the client's degree of personal spirituality.

Illustrative of this point, Brenda Cole evaluated the impact of Re-Creating Your Life, a six-session group intervention for people dealing with medical illnesses that addressed spiritual resources and struggles tied to four existential themes: meaning, control, relationships, and identity (Cole & Pargament, 1998). In a pilot evaluation of Re-Creating Your Life, Cole focused on 16 women with cancer. Nine of the women participated in Re-Creating Your Life and seven were in a nontreatment control condition. Over the course of the 6 weeks, pain severity and depression increased significantly for the women in the nontreatment control condition, while they remained relatively stable for women in the spiritually focused intervention (Cole, 2005). Encouraged by these findings, Cole (1999) evaluated Re-Creating Your Life in a sample of patients with syncope, a cardiac abnormality in which individuals experience episodes of dizziness or full loss of consciousness. Twenty-six people were randomly assigned to Re-Creating Your Life or a cognitive-behavioral comparison condition. Twelve people participated in the non-treatment control condition. In contrast to the findings in the oncology sample, the patients in the cognitive behavioral condition showed a significant reduction in state anxiety over the course of treatment, while the patients in Re-Creating Your Life remained stable, and the patients in the nontreatment control condition increased in anxiety.

In an effort to make sense of the different results, Cole conducted some additional analyses and found that, unlike the women with cancer who reported a great deal of depression and distress, the syncope patients were not experiencing high levels of depression or anxiety. Their level of well-being may have reflected the fact that their disease had been successfully treated through pacemakers or defibrillators. In contrast to the women with cancer, the patients with syncope were living relatively normal lives, with little immediate threat to their health and well-being. Cole (1999) tentatively concluded that the spiritual coping intervention might be better suited to people in low-control and high-stress situations. Her findings suggest that, as with other forms of psychological change, spiritual interventions may need to be tailored to meet the needs of particular people faced with particular problems,

The value of spiritually integrated psychotherapy may depend not only on the type of client and problem, but also on the type of therapist. Although it could be argued that spiritually oriented therapists should be more effective delivering spiritually integrated therapy than their less spiritually minded counterparts, some evidence suggests otherwise. In one of the most rigorous evaluative studies of spiritually integrated therapy, Rebecca Propst and her colleagues (1992) compared religious and nonreligious therapists providing 18 sessions of religious and nonreligious cognitive behavioral therapy (CBT) to depressed clients from the community. In addition, the participants in these four groups were compared to clients who received pastoral counseling from religious counselors and a waiting list control. Clients in both the religious CBT and pastoral counseling conditions showed more improvements in depression and social adjustment than clients in the nonreligious CBT and waiting list conditions. Surprisingly, though, nonreligious therapists outperformed the religious therapists in the religious CBT condition. These findings need to be replicated. However, at the very least, they suggest that nonreligious therapists can be effective in delivering spiritually integrated psychotherapy. These findings are also consistent with a point that I stressed earlier in the book: personal religiousness or spirituality does not necessarily equip a therapist to conduct spiritually integrated psychotherapy. Even more important are the therapist's openness, sensitivity, and willingness to learn about the part that spirituality plays in the life of the client. This attitude can be found in both spiritual and nonspiritual therapists. It can also be missing in both spiritual and nonspiritual therapists.

Finally, the efficacy of spiritually integrated therapy may depend on the type of spiritually integrated therapy. Remember that spiritual resources and problems come in many shapes and sizes. To speak of the value of a spiritually integrated psychotherapy without specifying the kind of spiritually integrated psychotherapy conveys as much information as speaking about the value of medical treatment without any further elaboration. As yet, however, researchers have not compared the relative efficacy of different types of spiritually integrated therapy, with a few exceptions (see Smith, Bartz, & Richards, in press). Comparisons of this kind require careful attention to the critical ingredients of spiritually integrated therapy and systematic presentations of these critical ingredients in the form of treatment manuals.

Studies on the effectiveness of spiritually integrated psychotherapy are encouraging, but it is too soon to draw firm conclusions. Questions continue to outnumber answers about this new approach to treatment. This will likely be true for some time to come. What kind of research is needed? Larger scale clinical trials of spiritually integrated treatments are necessary. In this research, it will be particularly important to delineate the critical ingredients of spiritually integrated treatments more sharply. It will also be important to extend evaluative studies of this therapy beyond those raised in largely Christian contexts to people who come from other religious traditions. In addition, virtually no research has been conducted as yet on the efficacy of integrating spirituality into marital and family therapy; this is, as Worthington and his colleagues (1996) put it, "a wasteland" (p. 477). Qualitative analyses of clients' perceptions of spiritually integrated therapy and its impact on their lives would also enrich the findings from quantitative studies. Finally, researchers should be sure to evaluate the impact of spiritually integrated therapy not only on measures of psychological, social, and physical well-being, but also on measures of spiritual well-being, including indices of spiritual virtues, growth, and integration.

DEVELOPING SKILLS IN SPIRITUALLY INTEGRATED PSYCHOTHERAPY

In the first chapter, I introduced Alice, my client who suffered from bipolar illness. Even though spirituality had helped to sustain her throughout her life, she had never mentioned this resource to any of her therapists. When I asked her why, she replied, "They already think I'm crazy." Alice was not unusual in her reluctance to broach the topic in psychotherapy. MacMinn and Foskett (2004) cite other examples in their study of mental health service users in England. One person said, "You have to be very cautious about what you say because being not main stream, a little off track, you have to be very careful you're not condemned for what you believe by the professionals" (p. 27).

A few studies suggest that these perceptions are not off-base. For example, one study pointed to a bias among mental health professionals against less familiar religious traditions. O'Connor and Vandenberg (2005) developed vignettes that accurately described several of the beliefs and practices of Roman Catholics, Mormons, and members of the Nation of Islam. They then asked 110 mental health practitioners to rate the "psychotic pathology" of these vignettes. The members of the less familiar religious traditions (Mormonism and Nation of Islam) were rated as more pathological than the Roman Catholics. These differences held even when the beliefs and practices in all three sets of vignettes were described as harmful. Along similar lines, McVittie and Tiliopoulos (in press) found that practicing therapists tended to underestimate the significance of religious beliefs, to stereotype religious clients as intransigent, and to marginalize and exclude the religious dimension in the context of therapy.

Perhaps it should not come as a great surprise that therapists respond to spiritual issues with their own personal biases and stereotypes. After all, as I noted earlier, only a small proportion of therapists have had any formal training in the area of religion and spirituality (Brawer et al., 2002; Schulte et al., 2002). But bias and stereotypes about spirituality are only one type of problem often manifested by clinicians without training in this type of psychotherapy (see Table 16.5). I have touched on others throughout this book. For example, many clinicians suffer from a kind of spiritual myopia; they have difficulty seeing the spiritual dimension of problems and solutions and instead look beyond spirituality to presumably more basic, biopsychosocial processes. Other clinicians may be able to see the spiritual dimension, but are timid about addressing it in psychotherapy. They may believe that the topic is "too sensitive," or they may confuse the value of separation of church and state in the United States with the separation of spirituality and psychology in therapy. Clinicians who are more spiritual themselves are vulnerable to the problems of spiritual overenthusiasm (i.e., seeing spirituality as the root of all problems and source of all solutions) and spiritual cockiness (i.e., overestimating one's own competence based on one's own personal spirituality). Finally, beginning students often find it difficult to tolerate the ambiguity and uncertainty that arise when a spiritual issue is broached in psychotherapy. "Just tell me what to do," is the frequent plea. Yet simple solutions are not appropriate to the kinds of complex problems students are likely to encounter in spiritually integrated psychotherapy. Training is clearly needed if practitioners are to treat the spiritual dimension in psychotherapy with more wisdom, skill, and sensitivity. What should this training look like? I believe it should have both formal and informal components.

Formal Training

I have stressed in this book that personal religiousness and spirituality in themselves do not prepare someone to do spiritually integrated psychotherapy.

TABLE 16.5. Problems Clinicians Often Bring to Training in Spiritually Integrated Psychotherapy

- *Spiritual bias*: the tendency to hold stereotyped views of religion and spirituality
- *Spiritual myopia*: difficulty seeing the spiritual dimension of problems and solutions; the tendency to see spirituality from a global, undifferentiated perspective
- *Spiritual timidity*: the fear of addressing spirituality in therapy based on the belief that spirituality should be separated from treatment
- *Spiritual overenthusiasm*: the tendency to see spirituality as the root of all problems or the source of all solutions
- *Spiritual cockiness*: overestimations of the therapist's own level of competence in spiritually integrated psychotherapy based on his or her personal spirituality
- *Intolerance of ambiguity*: the desire for definitive, simple solutions to complex problems

The most critical ingredient of this approach to treatment is an *understanding* of religiousness and spirituality. To build that kind of understanding, formal training is needed. Several psychologists have already begun to envision this kind of education (Richards & Bergin, 2005; Shafranske & Maloney, 1996). Drawing on this work, I offer six recommendations for formal training:

1. A graduate seminar in the psychology of religion and spirituality that introduces students to the rich classic and contemporary literature, both theoretical and empirical, on these topics.
2. A course in comparative religion that provides students with background on the diversity of religious traditions, beliefs, and practices in the world.
3. A course in spiritually integrated psychotherapy that offers students ways to understand, evaluate, and address spirituality as both a source of problems and a source of solutions in psychotherapy.
4. Integration of spiritual issues in other graduate classes, including psychopathology, assessment, various forms of psychotherapy, supervision, and consultation.
5. Spiritually sensitive supervision of clinical cases.
6. Continuing education on spirituality that updates clinicians on recent developments and advances in this rapidly growing area of study and practice.

Informal Learning

Personal piety and spiritual devotion may enrich therapists personally, but they do not equip them to become effective in conducting spiritually integrated psychotherapy. Furthermore, important as it is, expertise in spiritually integrated therapy requires more than formal training and academic knowledge. Whether or not they are deeply involved in spirituality themselves, therapists should have an integrated perspective on spirituality. What goes into this perspective? I can think of several things: an appreciation for the depth, richness. and diversity of spirituality; an awareness of the role of spirituality in the lives of clients, therapists, and the process of therapy: and a willingness on the part of therapists to share themselves authentically in treatment. This kind of integration grows as much out of personal experience as it does from formal training, experiences with traditional and nontraditional forms of spirituality, and experiences that promote spiritual self-awareness.

I would guess that, despite the exceptional diversity of spirituality in the United States, relatively few therapists have attended the regular worship services of religious groups other than their own. Most therapists have not explored the sacred literature from the world's great religious traditions. Few have sat down with religious leaders and members of diverse groups and spoken with them about the part that the church, synagogue, mosque, or temple plays in their lives. And it is the unusual therapist who has witnessed rituals and spiritual coping methods enacted by members of other traditions. Lacking these kinds of direct experiences, therapists are often left instead with spiritual stereotypes and misinformation. Fortunately, these stereotypes can be corrected. What it takes is the courage to leave the safety of familiar religious settings (or clinical offices), venture into new, unfamiliar religious homes, and express a sincere interest in learning about the spiritual lives of their inhabitants. Fears of suspicious or hostile reactions, I have found, are overblown. In my own experience, the leaders and members of virtually every tradition are more than happy to teach interested newcomers about their faith. Visits of this kind can also lead to long-term relationships that prove to be helpful to both the practitioner and the spiritual community. For example, over the years, through my own visits with diverse congregations, I have developed relations with a group of clergy who have served as invaluable sources of spiritual knowledge, consultation, and collaboration in my clinical work.

Spiritual self-awareness is also an essential component of spiritually integrated psychotherapy. I have stressed that, for better or worse, the therapists' own attitudes and approaches to the sacred, and to religion more generally, will have an impact on their work with clients. Self-awareness is the most effective antidote to the dangers of spiritual imposition on clients. Toward this end, I encourage therapists to write their own spiritual autobiographies, including a spiritual genogram of their own history (Frame, 2001). In these autobiographies, clinicians should ask themselves many of the same spiritual questions that they are likely to pose to their clients in the process of spiritual assessment (see Table 16.6). In grappling with these issues, therapists will have to do a great deal of soul-searching. But I highly recommend the spiritual autobiography as a tool, for in the process of getting to know themselves better spiritually, therapists will become better equipped to help their clients address spiritual issues of their own.

Small Steps

The idea of developing greater competence in spiritually integrated psychotherapy may seem overwhelming to therapists who are already overtaxed with the demands of learning about new therapies, keeping up with developments in medications, and dealing with the burdens of managed care. Some practitioners may choose to pursue spiritually integrated therapy as an area of clinical specialization. Let me stress, however, that specialized expertise is not a prerequisite to addressing spirituality in psychotherapy.

TABLE 16.6. Questions to Guide the Spiritual Autobiography

• What are my deepest values and what do I strive for in my life?

• What do I hold sacred?

• How did I discover the sacred?

• How has my larger family and institutional religious context shaped my attitudes toward spirituality and religion?

• How have I tried to develop and sustain myself spiritually over the years?

• What kinds of struggles have I encountered in the process of developing and conserving my spirituality?

• What kinds of spiritual transformations have I experienced, if any?

• Where do I currently stand in the search for the sacred?

• What are the areas of spiritual integration and dis-integration in my life?

• In what ways has my spirituality affected my life? In what ways has it not affected my life?

• What are my areas of spiritual strength and vulnerability in working with clients?

• Are there clients from particular spiritual or religious backgrounds whom I may not be able to help?

Feel free to start small. When a client raises a religious or spiritual issue, try asking a follow-up question and listening carefully to the client's response. When a client expresses powerful emotions about a spiritual experience, positive or negative, reflect on the feeling and watch what happens. When a client struggles to put spiritual sentiments into words, avoid the temptation to change the subject and observe the results when you give the client a chance to sort it out. My guess is that you will find yourself engaged in a meaningful spiritual conversation with the client, you will get to know the client at a deeper level, and you will learn more about the power of spirituality in the client's life. By starting small, you may find yourself captivated rather than burdened by the idea of learning more about spiritually integrated psychotherapy.

EXTENDING THE REACH OF SPIRITUALLY INTEGRATED PSYCHOTHERAPY

Although this book has focused on spirituality and psychotherapy, the effort to understand and address the sacred has implications for other forms of helping as well. Innovative activities are now underway that attempt to integrate spiritual resources into settings ranging from correctional institutions to the workplace (e.g., Bormann et al., 2006). Below I briefly illustrate a few of the ways practitioners interested in spiritually integrated change could extend their reach beyond the psychotherapy office.

Spiritually Integrated Change in Medical Institutions

Medical institutions have taken promising steps toward greater integration of spiritual resources into health care. For instance, over the past decade, a number of medical schools have introduced spirituality into the curriculum of first-year medical students. Spiritual resources have also been interwoven into holistic health care programs for patient populations, with good results (e.g., Kennedy, Abbott, & Rosenberg, 2002). In addition, health professionals have begun to work with various religious communities to develop spiritually based interventions for patients and their families. For instance, Nancy Dann, a minister, and Wilson Mertens, a physician, created an interdenominational event entitled "A Sacred Gathering for Those Touched by Cancer" (Dann & Mertens, 2004). The program consisted of three services in which the attendees were presented with music, Scripture, and prayer specifically designed to address the spiritual and emotional issues most salient to cancer: surrendering fear, instilling hope, finding peace, experiencing God's love, and creating community. Ninety percent of the 200 participants who completed surveys indicated that the services were "very helpful." Finally, a few practitioners and researchers have tried to integrate spirituality directly into the physicians' interactions with patients.

The work of Jean Kristeller and her colleagues is particularly noteworthy in this regard (Kristeller, Rhodes, Cripe, & Sheets, 2005). These researchers trained four oncologists to open the door to a spiritual conversation with 118 patients through brief, semistructured questions. The topic of spirituality was introduced using the following statement: "When dealing with a serious illness, many people draw on religious or spiritual beliefs to help cope. It would be helpful to me to know how you feel about this" (p. 18). Based on their patients' responses, the oncologists adjusted their own response accordingly. If the patient responded positively to the question, the physician asked, "What have you found most helpful about your beliefs since your illness?" (p. 18). If the patient responded neutrally to the initial question, the oncologist asked, "How might you draw on your faith or spiritual beliefs to help you?" (p. 18). If the patient reacted with signs of spiritual distress or struggle, the oncologist said, "Many people feel that way . . . what might help you come to terms with this?" (p. 18). And if the patient responded defensively, the oncologist responded, "It sounds like you're uncomfortable I brought this up. What I'm really interested in is how you are coping . . . can you tell me about that?" (p. 18). The goal of this process was to support and affirm the patients' spirituality, encourage the use of spiritual resources, and link patients in spiritual distress to other resources, such as the hospital chaplain.

This was a brief intervention, a necessity given the heavy demands on the oncologists' time. On average, the spiritual conversations lasted only 6 minutes. The oncologists in the program rated themselves as "quite" or "very" comfortable in 85% of the spiritual conversations with their patients. The large majority of the patients in the study were also comfortable with the intervention. Three weeks after the intervention, patients in the program reported significantly greater reductions in depression, better quality of life, and a stronger sense of caring from their physician than control patients. Kristeller and her colleagues concluded that spiritual resources and concerns could be addressed in a sensitive, efficient, and effective way within the framework of regular clinical practice.

Spiritually Integrated Change in Religious Institutions

Religious institutions have a long and deep tradition of involvement in efforts to facilitate their members' spiritual well-being, defined broadly to encompass the psychological, social, and physical spheres of life. Thus, pastoral and lay counseling programs and religiously based social services are commonplace throughout the United States. These services, studies suggest, can be quite effective (e.g., Baker, 2000; Benes, Walsh, McMinn, Dominguez, & Aikins, 2000; Toh & Tan, 1997). Congregations have also been used successfully as sites for preventive screening and health promotion programs for groups that have been disconnected from traditional health services (e.g., Maton & Wells, 1995; Resnicow et al., 2001). Furthermore, some religious institutions are developing programs to meet the spiritual needs of members who are dealing with specific traumas and challenges, such as divorce and sexual abuse (e.g., Guido, 2004; Hopkins, 1991; Murray, 2002). For example, in response to the needs of sexual abuse survivors in the Roman Catholic Church, Guido (2004) recommends "healing remembrance" activities that acknowledge—to the survivors, family and friends, the larger church, and God—the reality of the sexual abuse and the complicity of those who were involved. Healing remembrance activities include periodic masses for survivors and their families, homilies and prayers that speak directly of sexual abuse in the church, and "a renewed theology of redemption" that faces squarely the causes and consequences of clergy sexual abuse (p. 31).

Even though psychologists and other mental health professionals and researchers have worked together with religious institutions to develop and evaluate some of these spiritually integrated programs, this kind of collaboration remains the exception rather than the rule. There are plenty of exciting opportunities for cross-disciplinary exchange (see Pargament & Maton, 2000). However, mental health practitioners willing to venture out of their own professional homes must remember that religious institutions are not mental health centers. They have a distinctive mission: to help their members know God. Collaboration, at its best, grows out of the shared commitment of religious and mental health communities to well-being, and a mutual respect for the distinctive resources each partner brings to the helping process (Kloos & Moore, 2000; Tyler et al., 1983). Practitioners in particular are likely to find that they have as much to learn from religious communities as they have to offer to them.

Education and Prevention

Important as psychotherapy is, it has one major disadvantage. It takes place *after* problems have developed. Education and prevention in the area of spirituality *before* problems arise therefore make good sense. What might education and prevention look like in the spiritual realm? Consider three examples (see Pargament, Maton, & Hess, 1992, for a more extensive review).

Spiritual Education in Middle School

Earlier, I noted that religious education often ends just when it should be beginning. Many young adolescents complete their religious training just at the time in their lives when they are starting to realize their capacity for abstract reasoning, a prerequisite for grappling with the symbols, paradoxes, and complexities of religious traditions and spirituality more generally. While they will continue to grow intellectually, physically, socially, and psychologically, many adolescents will be stunted in their spiritual development, left to deal with the greatest challenges of adult life with the spirituality of 13-year-olds. Those who continue in some form of religious education may find that these programs fail to integrate spirituality with the special worries, concerns, and challenges of adolescence. As a result, spirituality and religion become disconnected from everyday life.

For example, a few years ago, my colleagues and I interviewed a group of middle-school students at a Jewish day school about the role of Judaism in their lives. The results were surprising and disconcerting. While all of the students voiced pride in being Jewish, most were unable to articulate how Judaism played a part of their daily lives. Judaism, for the majority, had to do with going to synagogue on weekends, ritual practices (e.g., fasting on Yom Kippur), and family get-togethers on Jewish holidays. Virtually nothing was said of Jewish values, ethics, and models that might guide the students through the ups and down of adolescence.

In response to these interviews, my colleagues and I developed a 12-week program entitled "Mi Ahni," Hebrew for "Who am I." Three weeks were devoted to four values that are esteemed within Judaism, though certainly not unique to this religion:

1. Learning, the value of knowledge and the hard work required to get it.
2. Honesty, the value of being open and truthful with oneself, with others, and with God.

3. Teshuva (repentance), the value of maintaining relationships with others and with God.
4. Tikkum Olam, the value of being a good person and "repairing the world."

Drawing on biblical and modern Jewish stories, commentaries on the Bible, role playing of problem situations commonly faced by adolescents, and discussion and debate among the students, the sessions brought Judaism down to earth and face to face with the concrete problems and dilemmas commonly faced by these adolescents. Students were presented with hard questions in Mi Ahni: To live life as a Jew, what do you do when a popular classmate invites you to a party that conflicts with a prior engagement with a less popular classmate? As a Jew, what should you do when your parents are driving you crazy? How should you handle it when your baseball team has scheduled a game on a Jewish holiday? The leaders of the group did not answer the questions for the students, but rather let the students move toward their own answers by personal soul-searching, discussion, and religious study.

Developing Mi Ahni wasn't easy. It took three revisions before we felt that we finally got it right. But the last version of the program proved to be successful. Over the course of the program, students demonstrated more ability to integrate Jewish beliefs, practices, and values in the way they handled concrete problems, and they showed significant increases in their Jewish identity. Helping the students develop a more integrated spirituality was a goal of Mi Ahni in and of itself. In addition, we hope that, with greater spiritual integration, the students became better equipped to deal with the full range of problems they are likely to encounter in coming years.

Spiritual Education in College

Spiritual education should not be restricted to adolescence or any other time of life. There is, after all, a great deal to learn about spirituality: the processes of discovery, conservation, and transformation of the sacred; spiritual struggles as a natural part of life; spiritual integration and disintegration; and spiritual tools for change. If we think about spiritual education as a lifelong process, then we can look for opportune times and places for further spiritual development.

College is one such ideal time. In contrast to the commonly accepted view that students generally put their spirituality on hold when they enter college, studies suggest that the college years are a period of spiritual struggle for many students. In a recent pioneering survey of over 100,000 entering college students at more than 200 diverse colleges and universities in the United States, over half of the students revealed that they at least occasionally "felt distant from God," "questioned their religious beliefs," and disagreed with their families about religious issues. Almost half of the students also reported that they "felt angry with God" at least occasionally (Astin et al., 2005). Moreover, the findings from the survey indicated that many students look to college as a place to develop personally and spiritually as well as intellectually. About two-thirds of the students considered it "essential" or "very important" that college enhance their self-understanding, develop their personal values, and encourage their emotional development. Almost half of the student sample said that it was "essential" or "very important" that college encourage their personal expression of spirituality. Unfortunately, however, colleges do not appear to be very supportive of their students' spiritual quests. According to a survey of third-year undergraduates, most students say that their professors never encourage discussion of spiritual or religious topics, and almost half voiced dissatisfaction with the degree to which college provides them with "opportunities for religious/spiritual reflection" (Astin et al., 2005).

With a bit of energy and imagination, colleges could respond more fully to the spiritual yearnings of students. More explicit attention to spiritual matters could be woven into the college experience, from residential life to the academic curriculum, including the hard sciences, social sciences, and arts and humanities. There are faculty and administrators who believe that spiritual conversation has no place on a freethinking college campus (paralleling the concerns of some therapists about discussing spirituality in psychotherapy). It is important to stress, however, that spiritual education does not refer to attempts to proselytize students to adopt one spiritual perspective or another. Instead, spiritual education is all about creating opportunities for students to study, engage with, debate, and discuss spiritual values, issues, and concerns. This kind of spiritual education would only foster the larger mission of higher education.

Spirituality as a Resource for the Prevention of Marital Problems

Couples about to enter marriage are another group that is ripe for spiritual education. Why? First, there is a clear need for help. Studies indicate that almost one in two marriages today will end in divorce. Second, spirituality is a potential resource for many of these couples. The vast majority of married couples in the United States report some religious affiliation (Glenn, 1982). Higher levels of religious and spiritual involvement have also been consistently linked to a lower risk of divorce and higher levels of marital commitment and satisfaction (Mahoney et al., 2001). Third, as we have noted, spirituality can be a source of conflict for couples (Mahoney, 2005).

Howard Markman and Scott Stanley pioneered a spiritually integrated program called "PREP" (Prevention and Relationship Enhancement Program) for couples to reduce the risk of marital distress and to improve marital life more generally. PREP grows out of Markman and Stanley's exten-

CONCLUSIONS

sive line of research that has pinpointed factors that distinguish stable and distressed married couples over time (e.g., Markman, 1981), and used these factors to develop a communication-oriented approach to prevent marital distress (Markman, Renick, Floyd, Stanley, & Clements, 1993).

Well aware of the commitment of religious traditions to strong marriages, Markman, Stanley, and their colleagues developed two spiritually integrated PREP programs, one tailored to Christians (Stanley, Trathen, McCain, & Bryan, 1998) and one tailored to Jews (Crohn, Markman, Blumberg, & Levine, 2001). Both programs address a common set of issues: communication, problem solving, commitment, acceptance, and forgiveness. However, each program also draws on the distinctive resources of the particular religious tradition.

The Christian PREP encourages couples to see their marriage through a sacred lens. "God's design for marriage," Stanley et al. (1998) note, "is that it be a covenant of spiritual unity in which the souls and hearts of both partners are joined before Him and with Him into a 'three-fold cord' providing direction and meaning in the bond of love" (p. 15). Broadening and deepening their relationship with Jesus Christ, the couple is taught, sets the stage for greater acceptance, commitment, and openness with each other. Spiritual intimacy is also encouraged by regular spiritual conversation, praying together, sharing spiritual struggles, and joint worship.

The Jewish PREP focuses on issues specific to Jewish couples (Crohn et al., 2001). For example, the authors note that as Jews have become more assimilated into U.S. culture, many have internalized the larger culture's negative stereotypes about Jews. These anti-Semitic stereotypes may manifest themselves through negative attitudes toward oneself and/or the opposite sex that spill over into the marital relationship. Participants in PREP are guided in ways to identify and resolve any of their own ambivalence about being Jewish. The Jewish PREP also responds to the high rate of interfaith marriage among Jews by raising and addressing the challenges of reconciling different faith traditions in the creation of a new family.

Clinicians knowledgeable about spiritually integrated change have resources that could be of value in many helping capacities that go beyond psychotherapy, including prevention, consultation, education, and social change. In this section, I have merely scratched the surface of these possibilities. In future years, practitioners are likely to discover new opportunities for the integration of spirituality into efforts to improve the human condition.

NO NEED TO WHISPER

Throughout this book, I have encouraged clinicians to take a closer look at the spiritual dimension of life. In the process, I hope it has become clear that there is no longer any need to whisper about spirituality in psychotherapy—not to our clients, not to other therapists, and not to ourselves. Let me highlight four reasons why it makes good sense to give spirituality a greater voice in psychotherapy.

• *Reason 1*: Spirituality is a natural and normal part of life. In the past, many therapists whispered about spirituality or avoided the topic entirely because they didn't know what to say. It is true that there are special challenges in trying to make sense of this elusive process. Yet spirituality does not fall outside the realm of human knowledge and comprehension. We can develop a better understanding of spirituality just as we can learn more about other dimensions of life: biological, psychological, and social. This understanding must go beyond simple stereotypes if we are to do justice to the richness and complexity of spirituality. In developing this understanding, we must also avoid the temptation to view spirituality as illusory, as a set of beliefs and practices ostensibly devoted to the sacred, but in reality designed to satisfy more basic needs. Spiritually integrated therapy rests on the fundamentally different premise that the yearning for the sacred is a primary, irreducible aspect of human nature. The sacred speaks to our deepest dreams and aspirations, the truths we hold to be timeless, our sense that there is something that lies beyond our everyday experience, and our most fundamental assumptions about why we are here, how we should live our lives, and what if anything we leave behind. Any psychology of human behavior remains incomplete without an appreciation for the motivation to know and connect to the sacred.

• *Reason 2*: Spirituality contributes to a more complete accounting of human strengths and weaknesses. Even though spirituality is a natural and normal part of life, it is not inherently good. Spirituality does speak to the best of human nature. As we have seen, a wide range of empirical studies and clinical reports point to the same conclusion: spirituality plays a positive role in the lives of many people. But we have also seen that the sacred quest can go awry in as many ways as a car can break down: people can define the sacred in narrow, constricting ways that squeeze the life out of themselves or others; they can elevate themselves to the position of gods; they can follow pathways that destroy the spiritual goals they are trying to achieve; they can freeze the search for the sacred into static, lifeless form: and so on. I have presented a way to distinguish spirituality at its best from spirituality at its worst through the notion of spiritual integration. But regardless of whether it is part of the problem or part of the solution, expressions of spirituality reflect a natural human desire: the desire to know something transcendent, something boundless, and something of ultimate value and truth.

• *Reason 3*: Spirituality is a therapeutic fact of life. The reality is we cannot divorce spirituality from the therapeutic process. The choices are to be more explicit about it, to tiptoe around it, or to reduce it to something else. I have argued for the former approach—to take spirituality seriously in its own right—because doing so makes for better treatment. Like it or not, spirituality is fully interwoven into human experience, including what takes place in the therapy room. The question, then, isn't *whether* to address spirituality in psychotherapy. Therapeutic neutrality toward spirituality is impossible. As with every other dimension of behavior, spirituality will be shaped one way or another by the therapy process. The real question is *how* we choose to address spirituality in psychotherapy.

• *Reason 4*: We are now in a position to move from theory to practice. I have not written a cookbook here. Because people see the sacred and approach it in so many diverse ways, there can be no single approach to dealing with spirituality in therapy, no single course of treatment. However, spirituality can be assessed as carefully, thoughtfully, and systematically as any other dimension of life. Questions about a client's spirituality are just as important as questions about his or her medical history, social relationships, and emotions. Therapists can encourage their clients to draw on their spiritual resources in therapy, just as they encourage them to access other resources, such as medical help, social support, physical exercise, and self-help books. Therapists can also address a variety of spiritual problems that may interfere with clients' health and well-being, just as they would attend to other problems that pose a barrier to change. Practitioners do their clients a great service when they understand and address spirituality as a significant issue in and of itself, a potential resource as well as a potential source of problems. In contrast, practitioners who overlook spirituality in treatment diminish their effectiveness as helpers, for they neglect the part of life that makes people most distinctively human.

In short, times have changed. Mental health professionals can now talk about spirituality openly and unapologetically. There is no need to whisper. We do, however, need to become more spiritually literate and articulate as individual clinicians and as a helping profession. There is more work to be done.

PUTTING THINGS TOGETHER

In the preface of this book, I said that I believe in a "unified field theory," a perspective that could link a way to understand spirituality, based on theory and research, with a way to address spirituality in our efforts to help people. We aren't there yet, but we are taking some promising steps in the direction of "putting things together" for our clients and for ourselves as therapists.

Of course, helping clients achieve greater spiritual integration in the course of psychotherapy is not a panacea; it does not lead to a life free of failure, longings, or pain. It means confronting challenges as best we can, while recognizing our limits as human beings. Attempts to eliminate all suffering, experience all there is to experience, or refuse to see that every choice comes with loss are bound to fail. Integration means a life that is constructed as much around defeat and hurt as around attainment and joy. This is certainly not a new idea, but spirituality at its best offers another perspective, a different way of viewing the world. Through the sacred lens, we see that pain and loss, while part of life, are only that. They are not the full story and they don't have the last word: in suffering, we can find meaning and purpose; in the confrontation with human limitations, we can discover new sources of strength and inspiration; in the most difficult of relationships, we can transcend self-preoccupation by attending to the pain of someone else. And, through the lens of the sacred, we can see ourselves in broader perspective, as small but significant parts of the larger stream that flows through and beyond our individual lives.

Spirituality at its best also offers a different way of viewing psychotherapy. Seen from the perspective of the sacred, the therapy office is more than a room; it becomes sacred space. The role of therapist is more than a job; it becomes a vocation. The relationship between client and therapist is more than a professional working alliance; it becomes imbued with sacred power. Furthermore, once sanctified, psychotherapy functions like other sacred objects: generating sacred emotions of awe, gratitude, humility, and trepidation; serving as a center of identity and self-definition for the therapist; and becoming a resource that supports the practitioner throughout his or her career (Brady, Guy, Poelstra, & Brokaw, 1999; Oman, Hedberg, Downs, & Parson, 2003). I like the way therapist Nancy Devor (2002) put it: "I am aware at times of the power I hold and how tender a plant, the human spirit. One should never enter the therapy room without humility. . . . I cannot imagine having the courage to do this work without faith" (p. 3). Thus, the integration of spirituality into psychotherapy adds a vital dimension to the way we understand our work. When we look at psychotherapy through the lens of the sacred, we transform the way we see our clients, ourselves, and the nature of change.

References

Abraído-Lanza, A. F., Vásquez E., & Echeverría, S. E. (2004). En las manos de Dios [in God's Hands]: Religious and other forms of coping among Latinos with arthritis. *Journal of Consulting and Clinical Psychology, 72,* 91–102.

Abramowitz, J. S., Huppert, J. D., Cohen, A. B., Tolin, D. F., & Cahill, S. P. (2002). Religious obsessions and compulsions in a non-clinical sample: The Penn Inventory of Scupulosity (PIOS). *Behaviour Research and Therapy, 40,* 825–838.

Abramowitz, L. (1993). Prayer as therapy among the frail Jewish elderly. *Journal of Gerontological Social Work, 19,* 69–75.

Ahmadi, F. (2006). *Culture, religion, and spirituality in coping: The example of cancer patients in Sweden.* Uppsala, Sweden: Uppsala University.

Ai, A. L., Peterson, C., & Huang, B. (2003). The effect of religious-spiritual coping on positive attitudes of adult Muslim refugees from Kosovo and Bosnia. *International Journal for the Psychology of Religion, 13,* 29–47.

Alexander, C. N., Rainforth, M. V., & Gelderloos, P. (1991). Transcendental meditation, self-actualization, and psychological health: A conceptual overview and statistical meta-analysis. *Journal of Social Behavior and Personality, 6,* 189–247.

Alferi, S. M., Culver, J. L., Carver, C. S., Arena, P. L., & Antoni, M. H. (1999). Religiosity, religious coping, and distress: A prospective study of Catholic and Evangelical Hispanic women in treatment for early-stage breast cancer. *Journal of Health Psychology, 4,* 343–356.

Ali, S. R., Liu, W. M., & Humedian, M. (2004). Islam 101: Understanding the religion and therapy implications. *Professional Psychology: Research and Practice, 35,* 635–642.

Allport, G. W. (1950). *The individual and his religion.* New York: Macmillan.

Altemeyer, B. (1988). *Enemies of freedom.* San Francisco: Jossey-Bass.

Anderson, H., & Foley, E. (1998). *Mighty stories, dangerous rituals: Weaving together the human and the divine.* San Francisco: Jossey-Bass.

347

Anderson, S. R., & Hopkins, P. (1991). *The feminine face of God: The unfolding of the sacred in women.* New York: Bantam Books.

Ano, G. A. (2005). *Spiritual struggles between vice and virtue: A brief psychospiritual intervention.* Unpublished doctoral dissertation, Bowling Green State University, Bowling Green, OH.

Ano, G. A., & Vasconcelles, E. B. (2005). Religious coping and psychological adjustment to stress: A meta-analysis. *Journal of Clinical Psychology, 61,* 1–20.

Aoki, W. T., Barsness, R., & Leong, S. B. (2001). Honor, wonder, awe and love: Sacred moments in relationship with clients. *Journal of Psychology and Christianity, 20,* 80–84.

Armstrong, K. (1993). *A history of God.* New York: Bantam Books.

Astin, A. W., Astin, H. S., Lindholm, J. A., Bryant, A. N., Calderone, S., & Szelenyi, K. (2005). *The spiritual life of college students: A national study of college students' search for meaning and purpose.* Los Angeles: Higher Education Research Institute.

Astin, J. A. (1997). Stress reduction through mindfulness meditation. *Psychotherapy and Psychosomatics, 66,* 97–106.

Atallah, S. F., El-Dosoky, A. R., Coker, E. M., Nabil, K. M., & El-Islam, M. F. (2001). A 22-year retrospective analysis of the changing frequency and patterns of religious symptoms among inpatients with psychotic illness in Egypt. *Social Psychiatry and Psychiatric Epidemiology, 36,* 407–415.

Austin, J. T., & Vancouver, J. B. (1996). Goal constructs in psychology: Structure, process, and content. *Psychological Bulletin, 120,* 338–375.

Avants, S. K., Beitel, M., & Margolin, A. (2005). Making the shift from "addict self" to "spiritual self": Results from a Stage I study of spiritual self-schema (3–S) therapy for the treatment of addiction and HIV risk behavior. *Mental Health, Religion, and Culture, 8,* 167–177.

Avants, S. K., & Margolin, A. (2003). *The Spiritual Self-Schema (3–S) Development Program.* Retrieved December 31, 2006, from http://www.3-s.us/3–S_manuals/ 3S_general.doc.

Azhar, M. Z., & Varma, S. L. (1995a). Religious psychotherapy as management of bereavement. *Acta Psychiatrica Scandinavica, 91,* 233–235.

Azhar, M. Z., & Varma, S. L. (1995b). Religious psychotherapy in depressive patients. *Psychotherapy and Psychosomatics, 63,* 165–173.

Azhar, M. Z., Varma, S. L., & Dharap, A. S. (1994). Religious psychotherapy in anxiety disorder patients. *Acta Psychiatrica Scandinavica, 90,* 1–3.

Baer, R. A. (2003). Mindfulness training as a clinical intervention: A conceptual and empirical review. *Clinical Psychology: Science and Practice, 10,* 125–143.

Baer, R. A., Smith, G. T., Hopkins, J., Krietemeyer, J., & Toney, L. (2006). Using self-report assessment methods to explore facets of mindfulness. *Assessment, 13,* 27–45.

Baider, L., & De-Nour, A. K. (1987). The meaning of a disease: An exploratory study of Moslem Arab women after a mastectomy. *Journal of Psychosocial Oncology, 4,* 1–13.

Bakan, D. (1966). *The duality of human existence: An essay on psychology and religion.* Chicago: Rand McNally.

Baker, D. C. (2000). The investigation of pastoral care interventions as a treatment for depression among continuing care retirement community residents. *Journal of Religious Gerontology, 12,* 63–85.

Baker, R., & Gorgas, J. (1990, July 19). Crash broke her back, but not her spirit. *News Journal* (Mansfield OH), p. 5A.

Baldwin, J. (1963). *The fire next time*. New York: Dial Press.

Barbour, J. G. (1974). *Myths, models, and paradigms: A comparative study in science and religion*. New York: Harper & Row.

Bassett, R. L., Hill, P. C., Hart, C., Mathewson, K., & Perry, K. (1992). Helping Christians reclaim some abandoned emotions: The ACE model of emotions. *Journal of Psychology and Theology, 21*, 165–173.

Batson, C. D., & Schoenrade, P. (1991). Measuring religion as quest: 1. Validity concerns. *Journal for the Scientific Study of Religion, 30*, 416–429.

Batson, C. D., Schoenrade, P., & Ventis, W. L. (1993). *Religion and the individual: A social-psychological perspective*. New York: Oxford University Press.

Baumeister, R. F. (1997). *Evil: Inside human violence and cruelty*. New York: Freeman.

Beck, C. (1989). *Everyday Zen: Love and work*. San Francisco: Harper.

Beit-Hallahmi, B. (1992). *Despair and deliverance: Private salvation in contemporary Israel*. Albany: State University of New York Press.

Bellah, R. N. (1970). Confessions of a former establishment fundamentalist. *Bulletin of the Council on the Study of Religion, 1*, 3–6.

Bellah, R. N., Madsen, R., Sullivan, W. M., Swidler, A., & Tipton, S. M. (1985). *Habits of the heart: Individualism and commitment in American life*. New York: Harper & Row.

Benes, K. M., Walsh, J. M., McMinn, M. R., Dominguez, A. W., & Aikins, D. C. (2000). Psychology and the church: An exemplar of psychologist–clergy collaboration. *Professional Psychology: Research and Practice, 31*, 515–520.

Benore, E. R., & Park, C. L. (2004). Death-specific religious beliefs and bereavement: Belief in an afterlife and continued attachment. *International Journal for the Psychology of Religion, 14*, 1–22.

Berger, P. L. (1969). *A rumor of angels: Modern society and the discovery of the supernatural*. Garden City, NY: Anchor Books.

Berger, P. L. (1997). *Redeeming laughter: The comic dimension of human experience*. New York: de Gruyter.

Bergin, A. E. (1985). Proposed values for guiding and evaluating counseling and psychotherapy. *Counseling and Values, 29*, 99–116.

Bergin, A. E. (1991). Values and religious issues in psychotherapy and mental health. *American Psychologist, 46*, 394–403.

Bergin, A. E., & Payne, I. R. (1991). Proposed agenda for a spiritual strategy in personality and psychotherapy. *Journal of Psychology and Christianity, 10*, 197–210.

Berkovits, E. (1979). *With God in hell: Judaism in the ghetto and deathcamps*. New York: Sanhedrin Press.

Bibby, R. W. (1987). *Fragmented gods: The poverty and potential of religion in Canada*. Toronto: Irwin.

Bickel, C. O., Ciarrocchi, J. W., Sheers, N. J., Estadt, B. K., Powell, D. A., & Pargament, K. I. (1998). Perceived stress, religious coping styles, and depressive affect. *Journal of Psychology and Christianity, 17*, 33–42.

bin Laden, O. (1998, February 23). [Text of fatwah urging jihad against Americans.] Retreived July 1, 2004, from http://.www.ict.org.il/articles/fatwah.htm.

Bjorck, J. P., & Thurman, J. W. (in press). Negative life events, patterns of positive and negative religious coping, and psychological functioning. *Journal for the Scientific Study of Religion.*

Blake, W. (1977). Auguries of innocence. In *The complete poems* (A. Ostriker, Ed.) (pp. 506–510). New York: Penguin Books.

Bobgan, M., & Bobgan, D. (1987). *Psychoheresy: The psychological seduction of Christianity.* San Francisco: East Gate.

Bormann, J. E., Oman, D., Kemppainen, J. K., Becker, S., Gershwin, M., & Kelly, A. (2006). Mantram repetition for stress management in veterans and employees: A critical incident study. *Journal of Advanced Nursing, 53,* 502–512.

Bowman, E. S. (2000). The assets and liabilities of conservative religious faith for persons with severe dissociative disorders. *Journal of Psychology and Christianity, 19,* 122–138.

Brady, J. L., Guy, J. D., Poelstra, P. L., & Brokaw, B. F. (1999). Vicarious traumatization, spirituality, and the treatment of sexual abuse survivors: A national survey of women psychotherapists. *Professional Psychology: Research and Practice, 30,* 386–393.

Brawer, P. A., Handal, P. J., Fabricatore, A. N., Roberts, R., & Wajda-Johnston, V. A. (2002). Training and education in religion/spirituality within APA-accredited clinical psychology programs. *Professional Psychology: Research and Practice, 33,* 203–206.

Brenner, E. E. (1985). *Winning by letting go: Control without compulsion, surrender without defeat.* San Diego, CA: Harcourt Brace Janovich.

Brenner, R. R. (1980). *The faith and doubt of Holocaust survivors.* New York: Free Press.

Brenner, R. R. (2007) *Jewish, Christian, Chewish, and Eschewish: Interfaith pathways for the new millennium.* Unpublished manuscript. Washington, DC.

Brotherson, S. E., & Soderquist, J. (2002). Coping with a child's death: Spiritual issues and therapeutic implications. *Journal of Family Psychotherapy, 13,* 53–86.

Brown, M. J. (2000). *What they don't tell you: A survivor's guide to biblical studies.* Louisville, KY: Westminster John Knox Press.

Brown, P. D. (2003). *Paths to prayer: Finding your own way to the presence of God.* San Francisco: Jossey-Bass.

Brown, R. P. (2003). Measuring individual differences in the tendency to forgive: Construct validity and links with depression. *Personality and Social Psychology Bulletin, 29,* 759–771.

Brown, S. L., Nesse, R. M., House, J. S., & Utz, R. L. (2004). Religion and emotional compensation: Results from a prospective study of widowhood. *Personality and Social Psychology Bulletin, 30,* 1165–1174.

Browning, D. S. (1987). *Religious thought and the modern psychologies.* Philadelphia: Fortress Press.

Buber, M. (1970). *I and thou.* New York: Scribner's.

Buechner, F. (1992). *Listening to your life: Daily meditations with Frederick Buechner.* New York: HarperCollins.

Bulman, R. J., & Wortman, C. B. (1977). Attributions of blame and coping in the "real world": Severe victims react to their lot. *Journal of Personality and Social Psychology, 35,* 351–363.

Burker, E. J., Evon, D. M., Sedway, J. A., & Egan, T. (2005). Religious and nonreligious coping in lung transplant candidates: Does adding God to the picture tell us more? *Journal of Behavioral Medicine, 28*, 513–526.

Burtt, E. A. (Ed.). (1982). *The teachings of the compassionate Buddha.* New York: Mentor Books.

Bushbaum, L. (1999). Quilting. In S. W. Alexander (Ed.), *Everyday spiritual practice: Simple pathways for enriching your life* (pp. 231–236). Boston: Skinner House Books.

Butler, M. H., & Harper, J. M. (1994). The divine triangle: God in the marital system of religious couples. *Family Process, 33*, 277–286.

Butler, M. H., Gardner, B. C., & Bird, M. H. (1998). Not just a time-out: Change dynamics of prayer for religious couples in conflict situations. *Family Process, 37*, 451–475.

Butter, E. A., & Pargament, K. I. (2003). Development of a model for clinical assessment of religious coping: Initial validation of the Process Evaluation Model. *Mental Health, Religion, and Culture, 6*, 175–194.

Castelli, J. (1994). (Ed.). *How I pray: People of different religions share with us that most sacred and intimate act of faith.* New York: Ballantine Books.

Cineplex Church. (2002, May 31). *Religion and Ethics Newsweekly.* Available online at http://www.pbs.org/wnet/religionandethics/week539/feature.html.

Clothey, F. W. (1981). Ritual, nature and theories. In K. Crim, R. A. Bullard, & L. D. Shinn (Eds.), *The perennial dictionary of world religions* (pp. 624–628). San Francisco: Harper & Row.

Cohen, A. B., & Rozin, P. (2001). Religion and the morality of mentality. *Journal of Personality and Social Psychology, 81*, 697–710.

Cole, B. S. (1999). *The integration of spirituality and psychotherapy for people who have confronted cancer.* Unpublished doctoral dissertation, Bowling Green State University, Bowling Green, OH.

Cole, B. S. (2005). Spiritually-focused psychotherapy for people diagnosed with cancer: A pilot outcome study. *Mental Health, Religion, and Culture, 8*, 217–226.

Cole, B. S., Hopkins, C., Steel, J. S., Carr, B. L. & Tisak, J. (in press). Assessing spiritual growth and spiritual decline following a diagnosis of cancer: Reliability and validity of the Spiritual Transformation Scale. *Psycho-Oncology.*

Cole, B. S., & Pargament, K. I. (1998). Re-creating your life: A spiritual/psychotherapeutic intervention for people diagnosed with cancer. *Psycho-Oncology, 8*, 395–407.

Cole, B. S., & Pargament, K. I. (1999). Spiritual surrender: A paradoxical path to control. In W. R. Miller (Ed.), *Integrating spirituality into treatment: Resources for practitioners* (pp. 179–198). Washington, DC: American Psychological Association.

Coleman, S. B., Kaplan, J. D., & Downing, R. W. (1986). Life cycle and loss: The spiritual vacuum of heroin addiction. *Family Process, 25*, 5–23.

Conway, K. (1985–1986). Coping with the stress of medical problems among black and white elderly. *International Journal of Aging and Human Development, 21*, 39–48.

Crohn, J., Markman, H. J., Blumberg, S. L., & Levine, J. R. (2001). *Beyond the chuppah: A Jewish guide to happy marriages.* San Francisco: Jossey-Bass.

352 References

Croog, S. H., & Levine, S. (1972). Religious identity and response to serious illness: A report on heart patients. *Social Science and Medicine, 6*, 17–32.

Csordas, T. J. (1983). The rhetoric of transformation in ritual healing. *Culture, Medicine, and Psychiatry, 7*, 333–375.

Csordas, T. J. (1994). *The sacred self: A cultural phenomenology of charismatic healing*. Berkeley, Los Angeles: University of California Press.

Dann, N. J., & Mertens, W. C. (2004). Taking a "leap of faith": Acceptance and value of a cancer program-sponsored spiritual event. *Cancer Nursing, 27*, 134–141.

Davis, C. G., Wortman, C. B., Lehman, D. R., & Silver, R. C. (2000). Searching for meaning in loss: Are clinical assumptions correct? *Death Studies, 24*, 497–540.

Davis, J. A., Smith, T. W., & Marsden, P. (2005). *General Social Surveys, 1972–2004: Cumulative files* (2nd ICPSR version). Chicago: NORC.

DeChant, D. (2003). The economy as religion: The dynamics of consumer culture. *Civic Arts Review, 16*, 1–6.

Decker, E. E. Jr. (2001). "Praying through": A Pentecostal approach to pastoral care. *Journal of Psychology and Christianity, 20*, 370–377.

Devor, N. G. (2002, October and November). Spirituality and psychotherapy: A multidisciplinary journey. In M. Jordan (Chair), *Spirituality and psychotherapy*. Symposium conducted at the Danielsen Institute at Boston University.

Dieter, M. E., Hoekema, A. A., Horton, S. M., McQuilken, J. R., & Walvoord, J. F. (1987). *Five views on sanctification*. Grand Rapids, MI: Academic Books.

DiGiuseppe, R. A., Robin, M. W., & Dryden, W. (1990). On the compatability of rational-emotive therapy and Judeo-Christian philosophy: A focus on clinical strategies. *Journal of Cognitive Psychotherapy: An International Quarterly, 4*, 355–368.

Doehring, C. (1993). *Internal desecration: Traumatization and representations of God*. Lanham, MD: University Press of America.

Doehring, C. (2004). Pastoral care of Bess in Breaking the Waves: A contextual practical theological approach. *Pastoral Sciences, 23*, 55–70.

Doehring, C. (2006). *The practice of pastoral care: A postmodern approach*. Louisville, KY: Westminster John Knox Press.

Doehring, C., Clarke, A., Pargament, K. I., Hayes, A., Hammer, D., Nikolas, M., & Hughes, P. (in press). Perceiving sacredness in life: Correlates and predictors. *Archives for the Psychology of Religion*.

Domback, M., & Karl, J. (1987). Spiritual issues in mental health care. *Journal of Religion and Health, 26*, 183–197.

Doyle, T. P. (2003). Roman Catholic clericalism, religious duress, and clergy sexual abuse. *Pastoral Psychology, 51*, 189–231.

D'Souza, R., Rich, D., Diamond, I., & Godfery, K. (2002). An open randomized control trial using a spiritually augmented cognitive behavioural therapy for demoralization and treatment adherence in patients with schizophrenia. *Proceedings of the 37th Royal Australian and New Zealand College of Psychiatrists and Congress, 36*(Suppl.), A9.

D'Souza, R., Rich, D., Diamond, I., Godfery, K., & Gleeson, D. (2002). An open randomized control trial of a spiritually augmented cognitive behaviour therapy in patients with depression and hopelessness. *Proceedings of the 37th Royal Australian and New Zealand College of Psychiatrists and Congress, 36*(Suppl.), A9.

Dupre, L. (1976). *Transcendent selfhood: The loss and rediscovery of the inner life.* New York: Seabury Press.

Dubus, A. (2001). Sacraments. In D. Henry (Ed.), *Sorrow's company: Writers on loss and grief* (pp. 156–165). Boston: Beacon Press.

Durkheim, E. (1965). The *elementary forms of the religious life.* New York: Free Press.

Eck, B. E. (1996). Integrating the integrators: An organizing framework for a multi-faceted process of integration. *Journal of Psychology and Christianity, 15,* 101–115.

Edmonds, S., & Hooker, K. (1992). Perceived changes in life meaning following bereavement. *Omega, 25,* 307–318.

Einstein, A. (1988). Science and religion are interdependent. In J. Rohr (Ed.), *Science and religion: Opposing viewpoints* (pp. 91–96). St. Paul, MN: Greenhaven Press.

Eliade, M. (1957). *The sacred and the profane: The nature of religion.* New York: Harvest Books.

Elkins, D. N. (1995). Psychotherapy and spirituality: Toward a theory of the soul. *Journal of Humanistic Psychology, 35,* 78–98.

Elkins, D. N. (1998). *Beyond religion: Eight alternative paths to the sacred.* Wheaton, IL: Quest Books.

Ellis, A. (1986). *The case against religion: A psychotherapist's view and the case against religiosity.* Austin, TX: American Atheist Press.

Ellis, A. (2000). Can rational emotive behavior therapy (REBT) be effectively used with people who have devout beliefs in God and religion? *Professional Psychology: Research and Practice, 31,* 29–33.

Ellison, C. W., & Smith, J. (1991). Toward an integrative measure of health and well-being. *Journal of Psychology and Theology, 19,* 35–48.

Emmons, R. A. (1999). *The psychology of ultimate concerns: Motivation and spirituality in personality.* New York: Guilford Press.

Emmons, R. A. (2000). Gratitude as a human strength: Appraising the evidence. *Journal of Social and Clinical Psychology, 19,* 56–69.

Emmons, R. A., Cheung, C., & Tehrani, K. (1998). Assessing spirituality through personal goals: Implications for research on religion and subjective well-being. *Social Indicators Research, 45,* 391–422.

Emmons, R. A., & Hill, J. (2001). *Words of gratitude for mind, body, and soul.* Philadelphia: Templeton Foundation Press.

Emmons, R. A., & McCullough, M. E. (2003). Counting blessings versus burdens: Experimental studies of gratitude and subjective well-being in daily life. *Journal of Personality and Social Psychology, 84,* 377–389.

Emrick, C. D. (1987). Alcoholics Anonymous: Affiliation processes and effectiveness as treatment. *Alcoholism: Clinical and Experimental Research, 11,* 416–423.

Erdrich, L. (2001). *The last report on the miracles at Little No Horse.* New York: Perennial Books.

Eriksen, K., Marston, G., & Korte, T. (2002). Working with God: Managing conservative Christian beliefs that may interfere with counseling. *Counseling and Values, 47,* 48–68.

Estleman, L. D. (2004). *Port Hazard.* New York: Forge Book.

Ethics of the Fathers (1995). Brooklyn, NY: Mesorah Publications.

Exline, J. J. (2002). Stumbling blocks on the religious road: Fractured relationships, nagging vices, and the inner struggle to believe. *Psychological Inquiry, 13*, 182–189.

Exline, J. J., & Martin, A. (2005). Anger toward God: A new frontier in forgiveness research. In E. L. Worthington (Ed.), *Handbook of forgiveness* (p. 73–88). New York: Routledge.

Exline J. J., & Rose, E. (2005). Religious and spiritual struggles. In R. F. Paloutzian & C. L. Park (Eds.), *Handbook of the psychology of religion and spirituality* (pp. 315–330). New York: Guilford Press.

Exline, J. J., Smyth, J. M., Gregory, J., Hockemeyer, J., & Tulloch, H. (2005). Religious framing by individuals with PTSD when writing about traumatic experiences. *International Journal for the Psychology of Religion, 15*, 17–33.

Exline, J. J., Yali, A. M., & Sanderson, W. C. (2000). Guilt, discord, and alienation: The role of religious strain in depression and suicidality. *Journal of Clinical Psychology, 56*, 1481–1496.

Fallot, T. (1998). Spiritual and religious dimensions of mental illness recovery narratives. *New Directions for Mental Health Services, 80*, 35–44.

Falsetti, S. A., Resick, P. A., & Davis, J. L. (2003). Changes in religious beliefs following trauma. *Journal of Traumatic Stress, 16*, 391–398.

Farber, B. A. (2006). *Self-disclosure in psychotherapy.* New York: Guilford Press.

Fishbein, M., & Ajzen, J. (1975). *Belief, attitude, intention, and behavior: An introduction to theory and research.* Reading, MA: Addison-Wesley.

Fitchett, G., Murphy, P., Kim J., Gibbons, J. L., Cameron, J., & Davis. J. A. (2004). Religious struggle: Prevalence, correlates and mental health risks in diabetic, congestive heart failure, and oncology patients. *International Journal of Psychiatry in Medicine, 34*, 179–196.

Fitchett, G., Rybarczyk, B. D., DeMarco, G. A., & Nicholas, J. J. (1999). The role of religion in medical rehabilitation outcomes: A longitudinal study. *Rehabilitation Psychology, 44*, 1–22.

Fitzpatrick, J. G. (1991). *Something more: Nurturing your child's spiritual growth.* New York: Penguin Books.

Flaherty, S. M. (1992). *Women, why do you weep?: Spirituality for survivors of childhood sexual abuse.* New York: Paulist Press.

Ford, D., & Nichols, C. W. (1987). A taxonomy of human goals and some possible applications. In M. E. Ford & D. H. Ford (Eds.), *Humans as self-constructing living systems: Putting the framework to work* (pp. 289–311). Hillsdale, NJ: Erlbaum.

Frame, M. W. (2001). The spiritual genogram in training and supervision. *Family Journal: Counseling and Therapy for Couples and Families, 9*, 109–115.

Freedman, S. R., & Enright, R. D. (1996). Forgiveness as an intervention goal with incest survivors. *Journal of Consulting and Clinical Psychology, 64*, 983–992.

Freud, S. (1961). *The future of an illusion.* New York: Norton. (Original work published 1927)

Freud, S. (1961). *Civilization and its discontents.* New York: Norton. (Original work published 1930)

Friedman, E. H. (1985). *Generation to generation: Family process in church and synagogue.* New York: Guilford Press.

Fromm, E. (1950). *Psychoanalysis and religion.* New Haven, CT: Yale University Press.

Gaer, J. (1958). *Wisdom of the living religions*. New York: Dodd, Mead.

Galanter, M. (1989). *Cults: Faith healing and coercion*. New York: Oxford University Press.

Gall, T. L. (2000). Integrating religious resources within a general model of stress and coping: Long-term adjustment to breast cancer. *Journal of Religion and Health, 39*, 167–182.

Gallup, G. Jr., & Lindsay, D. M. (1999). *Surveying the religious landscape: Trends in U. S. beliefs*. Harrisburg, PA: Morehouse.

Gandhi, M. K. (1962). *My God*. Ahmedabad, India: Navajivan.

Geertz, C. (1966). Religion as a cultural system. In M. Banton (Ed.), *Anthropological approaches to the study of religion* (pp. 1–46). London: Tavistock.

Geertz, C. (1968). *Islam observed: Religious developments in Morocco and Indonesia*. New Haven, CT: Yale University Press.

Genia, V. (1991). The Spiritual Experience Index: A measure of spiritual maturity. *Journal of Religion and Health, 30*, 337–346.

Germer, C. K., Siegel, R. D., & Fulton, P. R. (Eds.). (2005). *Mindfulness and psychotherapy*. New York: Guilford Press.

Glenn, N. D. (1982). Interreligious marriages in the United States: Patterns and recent trends. *Journal of Marriage and the Family, 44*, 555–566.

God's silence plagued soul of Mother Teresa. (2003, September). *Toledo Blade*, p. A6.

Goleman, D. (1977). *The varieties of the meditative experience*. New York: Dutton.

Gorsuch, R. L. (1968). The conceptualization of God as seen in adjective ratings. *Journal for the Scientific Study of Religion, 7*, 56–64.

Gorsuch, R. L., & Venable, G. D. (1983). Development of an "age universal" I-E scale. *Journal for the Scientific Study of Religion, 22*, 181–187.

Green, L. L., Fullilove, M. T., & Fullilove, R. E. (1998). Stories of spiritual awakening: The nature of spirituality in recovery. *Journal of Substance Abuse Treatment, 15*, 325–331.

Greenberg, D., & Witztum, E. (2001). *Sanity and sanctity: Mental health work among the ultra-orthodox in Jerusalem*. New Haven, CT: Yale University Press.

Greenberg, D., Witztum, E., & Pisante, J. (1987). Scrupulosity: Religious attitudes and clinical presentations. *British Journal of Medical Psychology, 60*, 29–37.

Greenberg, J., Porteus, J., Simon, L., Pyszczynski, T., & Solomon, S. (1995). Evidence of a terror management function of cultural icons: The effects of mortality salience on the inappropriate use of cherished cultural symbols. *Personality and Social Psychology Bulletin, 21*, 1221–1228.

Griffith, J. L. (1986). Employing the God–family relationship in therapy with religious families. *Family Process, 25*, 609–618.

Griffith, J. L., & Griffith, M. E. (2002). *Encountering the sacred in psychotherapy: How to talk with people about their spiritual lives*. New York: Guilford Press.

Grosch, W. N. (1985). The psychotherapist and religious commitment. In E. M. Stern (Ed.), *Psychotherapy and the religiously committed patient* (pp. 123–127). New York: Haworth Press.

Guidelines for Providers of Psychological Services to Ethnic, Linguistic, and Culturally Diverse Populations. (1993). *American Psychologist, 48*, 45–48.

Guido, J. J. (2004). Transforming memory. *Human Development, 25*, 26–31.

Haidt, J. (2003). Elevation and the positive psychology of morality. In C. L. M. Keyes

& J. Haidt (Eds.), *Flourishing: The positive person and the life well lived* (pp. 275–289). Washington, DC: American Psychological Association.

Haidt, J., & Keltner, D. (2003). Appreciation of beauty and excellence. In C. Peterson & M. E. P. Seligman (Eds.), *Character strengths and virtues* (pp. 537–551). Washington, DC: American Psychological Association.

Halberstam, D. (2001). *War in a time of peace.* New York: Scribner's.

Halevi, Y. K. (2001). *At the entrance to the Garden of Eden: A Jew's search for hope with Christians and Muslims in the Holy Land.* New York: Perennial Books.

Hall, T.A. (1995). Spiritual effects of childhood sexual abuse in adult Christian women. *Journal of Psychology and Theology, 23,* 129–134.

Hall, T. W., & Edwards, K. J. (1996). The initial development and factor analysis of the Spiritual Assessment Inventory. *Journal of Psychology and Theology, 24,* 233–246.

Hallinan, P. K. (1981). *I'm thankful each day.* Nashville, TN: Ideals Children's Books.

Hardy, A. (1979). *The spiritual nature of man: A study of contemporary religious experience.* Oxford, UK: Clarendon Press.

Harley, B., & Firebaugh, G. (1993). Americans' belief in an afterlife: Trends over the past two decades. *Journal for the Scientific Study of Religion, 32,* 269–278.

Hathaway, W. L. (2003). Clinically significant religious impairment. *Mental Health, Religion, and Culture, 6,* 113–129.

Hathaway, W. L. (2004). *Taking religion and spirituality seriously as a diversity domain.* Unpublished manuscript, Regent University, Virginia Beach, VA.

Hathaway, W. L., Douglas, D., & Grabowski, K. (2003). Faith Situations Questionnaire: Childhood normative data. *Journal of Psychology and Christianity, 22,* 141–154.

Hathaway, W. L., Scott, S. Y., & Garver, S. A. (2004). Assessing religious/spiritual functioning: A neglected domain in clinical practice. *Professional Psychology: Research and Practice, 35,* 97–104.

Havens, J. (1968). *Psychology and religion: A contemporary dialogue.* Princeton, NJ: Van Nostrand.

Hawkins, I. L., & Bullock, S. L. (1995). Informed consent and religious values: A neglected area of diversity. *Psychotherapy, 32,* 293–300.

Hays, J. C., Meador, K. G., Branch, P. S., & George, L. K. (2001). The Spiritual History Scale in four dimensions (SHS-4): Validity and reliability. *The Gerontologist, 41,* 239–249.

Hayes, S. C. (1984). Making sense of spirituality. *Behaviorism, 12,* 99–110.

Hayes, S. C. (2002). Acceptance, mindfulness, and science. *Clinical Psychology: Science and Practice, 9,* 101–106.

Hayes, S. C., Follette, V. M., & Linehan, M. M. (Eds.). (2005). *Mindfulness and acceptance: Expanding the cognitive-behavioral tradition.* New York: Guilford Press.

Hayes, S. C., Strosahl, K. D., & Wilson, K. G. (1999). *Acceptance and commitment therapy: An experiential approach to behavior change.* New York: Guilford Press.

Heiligman, R. M., Lee, L. R., & Kramer, D. (1983). Pain relief associated with a religious visitation: A case report. *Journal of Family Practice, 16,* 299–302.

Heilman, S. C., & Witztum, E. (2000). All in faith: Religion as idiom and means of coping with distress. *Mental Health, Religion, and Culture, 3,* 115–124.

Heller, D. (1986). *The children's God*. Chicago: University of Chicago Press.

Helminiak, D. A. (2005). *Meditation without myth*. New York: Cross.

Hendra, T. (2004). *Father Joe: The man who saved my soul*. New York: Random House.

Here I was sitting at the edge of eternity. (1989, August). *Life*, pp. 28–33, 38, 39.

Heschel, A. J. (1973). *A passion for truth*. New York: Farrar, Straus, & Giroux.

Heschel, A. J. (1986). *The wisdom of Heschel*. New York: Farrar, Straus, and Giroux.

Hill, P. C. (2001). Spiritual transformation: Forming the habitual center of personal energy. *Psychology of Religion Newsletter, 26*, 1–11.

Hill, P. C., & Hood, R. W., Jr. (Eds.). (1999). *Measures of religiosity*. Birmingham, AL: Religious Education Press.

Hill, P.C., & Pargament, K.I (2003). Advances in the conceptualization and measurement of religion and spirituality: Implications for physical and mental health research. *American Psychologist, 58*, 64–74.

Hillman, J. (1975). *Re-visioning psychology*. New York: Harper & Row.

Hite, Fr. Gregory (2005, August 14). I live alone. *Saint Joan of Arc Newsletter*, pp. 1–4.

Hodge, D. R. (2001). Spiritual assessment: A review of major qualitative methods and a new framework for assessing spirituality. *Social Work, 46*, 203–214.

Hoge, D. R. (1996). Religion in America: The demographics of belief and affiliation. In E. P. Shafranske (Ed.), *Religion and the clinical practice of psychology* (pp. 21–42). Washington, DC: American Psychological Associaition.

Hood, R. W. Jr. (1995). The facilitation of religious experience. In R. W. Hood Jr. (Ed.), *Handbook of religious experience* (pp. 569–597). Birmingham, AL: Religious Education Press.

Hood, R. W. Jr. (2003). The relationship between religion and spirituality. *Defining Religion: Investigating the Boundaries between Sacred and Secular Religion and the Social Order, 10*, 241–265.

Hood, R. W., Jr. (2005). Mystical, spiritual, and religious experiences. In R. F. Paloutzian & C. L. Park (Eds.), *Handbook of the psychology of religion and spirituality* (pp. 348–364). New York: Guilford Press.

Hopkins, N. M. (1991). Congregational intervention when the pastor has committed sexual misconduct. *Pastoral Psychology, 39*, 247–255.

Howe, I. (1976). *World of our fathers*. New York: Harcourt, Brace, Janovich.

Hughes, P. (2001). *Using theological perspectives in cross-disciplinary research and clinical practice to reclaim and redeem: A theological-clinical encounter*. Paper presented at the annual meeting of the American Psychological Association, Toronto, Canada.

Idler, E. L., Musick, M. A., Ellison, C. G., George, L. K., Krause, N., Ory, M. G., et al.. (2003). Measuring multiple dimensions of religion and spirituality for health research: Conceptual background and findings from the 1998 General Social Survey. *Research on Aging, 25*, 327–365.

Imber-Black, E., & Roberts, J. (1992). *Rituals for our times: Celebrating, healing, and changing our lives and our relationships*. New York: Harper Perennal Books.

Jacobs, J. L. (1992). Religious ritual and mental health. In J. F. Schumaker (Ed.), *Religion and mental health* (pp. 291–299). New York: Oxford University Press.

Jacobson, C. J., Jr. (2003). "Espiritus? No. Pero la maldad existe": Supernaturalism, religious change, and the problem of evil in Puerto Rican folk religion. *Ethics, 31*, 1–30.

James, W. (1936). *The varieties of religious experience: A study in human nature.* New York: Modern Library. (Original work published 1902)

James, W. (1975). *Pragmatism.* Cambridge, MA: Harvard University Press. (Original work published 1907)

Johnson, C. N., & Boyatzis, C. J. (2006). Cognitive-cultural foundations of spiritual development. In E. C. Roehlkepartain, P. E. King, L. Wagener, & P. L. Benson (Eds.), *The handbook of spiritual development in childhood and adolescence* (pp. 211–223). Thousand Oaks, CA: Sage.

Johnson, C. V., & Hayes, J. A. (2003). Troubled spirits: Prevalence and predictors of religious and spiritual concerns among university students and counseling center clients. *Journal of Counseling Psychology, 50,* 409–419.

Johnson, D. R., Feldman, S. C., Lubin, H., & Southwick, S. M. (1995). The therapeutic use of ritual and ceremony in the treatment of post-traumatic disorder. *Journal of Traumatic Stress, 8,* 283–298.

Johnson, P. E. (1959). *Psychology of religion.* Nashville, TN: Abingdon Press.

Johnson, W. B., DeVries, R., Ridley, C. R., Pettorini, D., & Peterson, D. R. (1994). The comparative efficacy of Christian and secular rational-emotive therapy with Christian clients. *Journal of Psychology and Theology, 22,* 130–140.

Johnson, W. B., & Ridley, C. R. (1992). Brief Christian and non-Christian rational-emotive therapy with depressed Christian clients: An exploratory study. *Counseling and Values, 36,* 220–229.

Jones, J. W. (1991). *Contemporary psychoanalysis and religion: Transference and transcendence.* New Haven, CT: Yale University Press.

Jones, J. W. (2002). *Terror and transformation: The ambiguity of religion in psychoanalytic perspective.* New York: Brunner-Routledge.

Jones, J. W. (2004). Religion, health, and the psychology of religion: How the research on religion and health helps us understand religion. *Journal of Religion and Health, 43,* 317–328.

Jones, S. L. (1994). A constructive relationship for religion with the science and profession of psychology: Perhaps the boldest model yet. *American Psychologist, 49,* 184–199.

Jordan, M. R. (1986). *Taking on the gods: The task of the pastoral counselor.* Nashville, TN: Abingdon Press.

Juergensmeyer, M. (2000). *Terror in the mind of God: The global rise of religious violence.* Berkeley and Los Angeles: University of California Press.

Jung, C. G. (1933). *Modern man in search of a soul.* New York: Harcourt, Brace, and Company.

Jung, C. G. (1938). *Psychology and religion.* New Haven, CT: Yale University Press.

Jung, C. G. (1964). After the catastrophe. In *Collected Works* (Vol. 10, pp. 194–217). New York: Pantheon Books. (Original work published 1945)

Kabat-Zinn, J. (2003). Mindfulness-based interventions in context: Past, present, and future. *Clinical Psychology: Science and Practice, 10,* 144–156.

Kahn, R. L., & Antonucci, T. C. (1980). Convoys over the life course: Attachment, roles, and social support. In P. B. Baltes & O. G. Brim (Eds.), *Life span development and behavior* (pp. 253–286). New York: Academic Press.

Kane, D., Cheston, S. E., & Greer, R. (1993). Perceptions of God by survivors of childhood sexual abuse: An exploratory study in an underresearched area. *Journal of Psychology and Theology, 21,* 228–237.

Kass, J. D. (1991). *Integrating spirituality into personality theory and counseling practice.* Paper presented at the annual meeting of the American Association for Counseling and Development, Reno, NE.

Keating, A. M., & Fretz, B. R. (1990). Christian anticipations about counselors in response to counselor descriptions. *Journal of Counseling Psychology, 36,* 292–296.

Kehoe, N. C. (1998). Religious-issues group therapy. *New Directions for Mental Health Services, 80,* 45–55.

Kennedy, J. F., Abbott, R. A., & Rosenberg, B. S. (2002). Changes in spirituality and well-being in a retreat program for cardiac patients. *Alternative Therapies, 8,* 64–73.

Keyes, R. (1995). *The wit and wisdom of Harry Truman.* New York: Gramercy Books.

Kimball, C. (2002). *When religion becomes evil.* San Francisco: Harper.

King, M. L. Jr. (1973). Unwise and untimely? In F. J. Streng & J. T. Allen (Eds.), *Ways of being religious: Readings for a new approach to religion* (pp. 197–202). Englewood Cliffs, NJ: Prentice-Hall.

Kirkpatrick, L. A., & Shaver, P. R. (1990). Attachment theory and religion: Childhood attachments, religious beliefs, and conversions. *Journal for the Scientific Study of Religion, 29,* 315–334.

Kirkpatrick, L. A., & Shaver, P. R. (1992). An attachment-theoretical approach to romantic love and religious belief. *Personality and Social Psychology Bulletin, 18,* 266–275.

Kirsch, I., & Lynn, S. J. (1999). Automaticity in clinical psychology. *American Psychologist, 54,* 504–515.

Kirvan, J. (1999). *God hunger: Discovering the mystic in all of us.* Notre Dame, IN: Sorin Books.

Kloos, B., & Moore, T. (2000). The prospect and purpose of locating community research and action in religious settings. *Journal of Community Psychology, 28,* 119–138.

Koenig, H. G., McCullough, M. E., & Larson, D. B. (2001). *Handbook of religion and health.* Oxford, UK: Oxford University Press.

Koenig, H. G., Pargament, K. I., & Nielsen, J. (1998). Religious coping and health status in medically ill hospitalized older adults. *Journal of Nervous and Mental Disease, 186,* 513–521.

Kohut, H. (1984). *How does analysis cure?* Chicago: University of Chicago Press.

Koltko, M. E. (1990). How religious beliefs affect psychotherapy: The example of Mormonism. *Psychotherapy, 27,* 132–141.

Kooistra, W. P. (1990). *The process of religious doubting in adolescents raised in religious environments.* Unpublished doctoral dissertation, Bowling Green State University, Bowling Green, OH.

Kooistra, W. P., & Pargament, K. I. (1999). Predictors of religious doubting among Roman Catholic and Dutch Reformed high school students. *Journal of Psychology and Theology, 27,* 33–42.

Kornfield, J. (1993). *A path with heart: A guide through the perils and promises of spiritual life.* New York: Bantam Books.

Krakauer, J. (2004). *Under the banner of heaven: A story of violent faith.* New York: Anchor Books.

Krause, N. (1998). Neighborhood deterioration, religious coping, and changes in health during late life. *The Gerontologist, 38,* 653–664.

Krause, N., Chatters, L. M., Metzer, T., & Morgan, D. L. (2000). Negative interaction in the church: Insights from focus groups with older adults. *Review of Religious Research, 41,* 510–533.

Krauss, P., & Goldfischer, M. (1988). *Why me?: Coping with grief, loss and change.* Toronto: Bantam Books.

Kristeller, J. L., Rhodes, M., Cripe, L. D., & Sheets, V. (2005). Oncologist Assisted Intervention Study (OASIS): Patient acceptability and initial evidence of effects. *International Journal for the Psychology of Religion, 35,* 329–347.

Kushner, H. (1981). *When bad things happen to good people.* New York: Schocken Books.

Kushner, H. (1989). *Who needs God?* New York: Summit Books.

LaMothe, R. (1998). Sacred objects as vital objects: Transitional objects reconsidered. *Journal of Psychology and Theology, 26,* 159–167.

Lampton, C., Oliver, G. J., Worthington, E. L. Jr., & Berry, J. W. (2005). Helping Christian college students become more forgiving: An intervention study to promote forgiveness as part of a program to shape Christian character. *Journal of Psychology and Theology, 33,* 278–290.

Last Words Browser. (2007). Online at www.alsirit.com/lastwords/

Lazar, S. W. (2005). Mindfulness research. In C. K. Germer, R. D. Siegel, & P. R. Fulton (Eds.), *Mindfulness and psychotherapy* (pp. 220–238). New York: Guilford Press.

Lewis, C. S. (1961). *A grief observed.* London: Faber & Faber.

Lewis, K. L., & Epperson, D. L. (1993). Values, pretherapy information and informed consent in Christian counseling. In E. L. Worthington Jr. (Ed.), *Psychotherapy and religious values* (pp. 85–103). Grand Rapids, MI: Baker Book House.

Lifton, R. J. (1973). The sense of immortality: On death and the continuity of life. *American Journal of Psychoanalysis, 33,* 3–15.

Lindgren, K. N., & Coursey, R. D. (1995). Spirituality and serious mental illness: A two-part study. *Psychosocial Rehabilitation Journal, 18,* 93–111.

Littlewood, R., & Lipsedge, M. (1989). *Aliens and alienists: Ethnic minorities and psychiatry.* London: Unwin Hyman.

Loewald, H. (1978). *Psychoanalysis and the history of the individual.* New Haven, CT: Yale University Press.

Loewenthal, K. M. (in press). *Religion, culture, and mental health.* Cambridge, UK: Cambridge University Press.

Loewenthal, K. M., Macleod, A. K., Goldblatt, V., Lubitsh, G., & Valentine, J. D. (2000). Comfort and joy?: Religion, cognition, and mood in Protestants and Jews under stress. *Cognition and Emotion, 14,* 355–374.

Lovinger, R. J. (1984). *Working with religious issues in therapy.* New York: Aronson.

Lovinger, R. J. (1996). Considering the religious dimension in assessment and treatment. In E. P. Shafranske (Ed.), *Religion and the clinical practice of psychology* (pp. 327–363). Washington, DC: American Psychological Association.

Lukoff, D., Lu, F., & Turner, R. (1992). Toward a more culturally sensitive DSM-IV: Psychoreligious and psychospiritual problems. *Journal of Nervous and Mental Disease, 180,* 673–682.

Lynn, E. C. (1999). The sacred moment. In S. W. Alexander (Ed.), *Everyday spiritual practice: Simple pathways for enriching your life* (pp. 61–65). Boston: Skinner House Books.

MacKnee, C. M. (2002). Profound sexual and spiritual encounters among practicing Christians: A phenomenological analysis. *Journal of Psychology and Theology, 30,* 234–244.

MacMin, L., & Foskett, J. (2004). "Don't be afraid to tell": The spiritual and religious experience of mental health service users in Somerset. *Mental Health, Religion, and Culture, 7,* 23–40.

Magee, J. J. (1994). Using themes from mystical traditions to enhance self-acceptance in life review groups. *Journal of Religious Gerontology, 9,* 63–72.

Magyar, G. M., Pargament, K. I., & Mahoney, A. (2000, August). *Violating the sacred: A study of desecration among college students.* Paper presented at the annual meeting of the American Psychological Association, Washington, DC.

Mahoney, A. (2005). Religion and conflict in marital and parent–child relationships. *Journal of Social Issues, 61,* 689–706.

Mahoney, A., Carels, R., Pargament, K. I., Wachholtz, A., Leeper, L. E., Kaplar, M., et al. (2005). The sanctification of the body and behavioral health patterns of college students. *International Journal for the Psychology of Religion, 15.* 221–238.

Mahoney, A., & Pargament, K. I. (2004). Sacred changes: Spiritual conversion and transformation. *Journal of Clinical Psychology: In Session, 60,* 481–492.

Mahoney, A., Pargament, K. I., Ano, G., Lynn, Q. Magyar, G., McCarghy, S., et al. (2002, August). *The devil made them do it: Demonization and desecration of the 9/11 terrorist attacks.* Paper presented at the annual meeting of the American Psychological Association, Chicago, IL.

Mahoney, A., Pargament, K. I., Cole, B., Jewell, T., Magyar-Russell, G., Tarakeshwar, N., et al. (2005). A higher purpose: The sanctification of strivings in a community sample. *International Journal for the Psychology of Religion, 15,* 239–262.

Mahoney, A., Pargament, K. I., Jewell, T., Swank, A. B., Scott, E., Emery, E., et al. (1999). Marriage and the spiritual realm: The role of proximal and distal religious constructs in marital functioning. *Journal of Family Psychology, 13,* 321–338.

Mahoney, A., Pargament, K. I., Murray-Swank, A., & Murray-Swank, N. (2003). Religion and the sanctification of family relationships. *Review of Religious Research, 44,* 220–236.

Mahoney, A., Pargament, K. I., Tarakeshwar, N., & Swank, A. B. (2001). Religion in the home in the 1980s and 90s: Meta-analyses and conceptual analyses of links between religion, marriage, and parenting. *Journal of Family Psychology, 15,* 559–596.

Mahoney, M. J. (2000). Core ordering and disordering processes: A constructive view of development. In R. A. Neimeyer & J. D. Raskin (Eds.), *Constructions of disorder: Meaning-making frameworks for psychotherapy* (pp. 43–62). Washington, DC: American Psychological Association.

Markman, H. J. (1981). Prediction of marital distress: A 5-year follow-up. *Journal of Consulting and Clinical Psychology, 49,* 760–762.

Markman, H. J., Renick, M. J., Floyd, F. J., Stanley, S. M., & Clements, M. (1993). Preventing marital distress through communication and conflict-management training: A four and five year follow-up. *Journal of Consulting and Clinical Psychology, 62,* 1–8.

Maslow, A. H. (1968). *Toward a psychology of being.* New York: Van Nostrand Reinhold.

Maton, K. I. (1989). The stress-buffering role of spiritual support: Cross-sectional and prospective investigations. *Journal for the Scientific Study of Religion, 28,* 310–323.

Maton, K. I., & Wells, E. A. (1995). Religion as a community resource for well-being: Prevention, healing, and empowerment pathways. *Journal of Social Issues, 51,* 177–193.

May, R. (1970). Psychotherapy and the daimonic. In J. Campbell (Ed.), *Myths, dreams, and religion* (pp. 196–210). New York: Dutton.

Mazumdar, S., & Mazumdar, S. (1993). Sacred space and place attachment. *Journal of Environmental Psychology, 13,* 231–242.

McCorkle, B. H., Bohn, C., Hughes, T., & Kim, D. (2005). "Sacred moments": Social anxiety in a larger perspective. *Mental Health, Religion, and Culture, 8,* 227–238.

McCullough, M. E. (1995). Prayer and health: Conceptual issues, research review, and research agenda. *Journal of Psychology and Theology, 23,* 15–29.

McCullough, M. E. (1998). Research on religion-accommodative counseling: Review and meta-analysis. *Journal of Counseling Psychology, 46,* 92–98.

McCullough, M. E., Emmons, R. A., & Tsang, J. (2002). The grateful disposition: A conceptual and empirical topography. *Journal of Personality and Social Psychology, 82,* 112–127.

McCullough, M. E., Hoyt, W. T., Larson, D. B., Koenig, H. G., & Thoresen, C. (2000). Religious involvement and mortality: A meta-analytic review. *Health Psychology, 19,* 211– 222.

McCullough, M. E., & Worthington, E. L. Jr. (1995). College students' perceptions of a psychotherapist's treatment of a religious issue: Partial replication and extension. *Journal of Counseling and Development, 73,* 626–634.

McCutcheon, L. E., Lange, R., & Houran, J. (2002). Conceptualization and measurement of celebrity worship. *British Journal of Psychology, 93,* 67–87.

McIntosh, D., Inglehart, M. R., & Pacini, R. (1990, May). *Flexible and central religious belief systems and adjustment to college.* Paper presented at the meeting of the Midwestern Psychological Association, Chicago, IL.

McIntosh, D. N., & Spilka, B. (1990). Religion and physical health: The role of personal faith and control. In M. L. Lynn & D. O. Moberg (Eds.), *Research in the social scientific study of religion* (Vol. 2, pp. 167–194). Greenwich, CT: JAI Press.

McReady, W. C. (1975). A survey of mystical experiences: A research note. In R. Woods (Ed.), *Heterodoxy/mystical experience: Religious dissent and the occult* (pp. 55–70). River Forest, IL: Listening Press.

McVittie, C., & Tiliopoulos, N. (in press). When 2–3% really matters: The (un)importance of religiosity in psychotherapy. *Journal of Social and Clinical Psychology.*

Memorandum on a mass murder. (1990, April 9). *Newsweek,* p. 25.

Merton, T. (1969). *Contemplative prayer.* New York: Herder & Herder.

Mickley, J., Pargament, K. I., Cowell, B., Belavich, T., Brant, C., & Hipp, K. (1998). God and the search for meaning among hospice caregivers. *Hospice Journal, 13,* 1–18.

Miethe, T. L. (1988). *The compact dictionary of doctrinal words.* Minneapolis, MN: Bethany House.

Miller, J., Fletcher, K., & Kabat-Zinn, J. (1995). Three-year follow-up and clinical implications of a mindfulness-based stress reduction intervention in the treatment of anxiety disorders. *General Hospital Psychiatry, 17,* 192–200.

Miller, L. (2005). Interpersonal psychotherapy from a spiritual perspective. In L. Sperry & E. P. Shafranske (Eds.), *Spiritually-oriented psychotherapy* (pp. 153–176). Washington, DC: American Psychological Association.

Miller, L., & Kelley, B. S. (2005). Relationships of religiosity and spirituality with mental health and psychopathology. In R. F. Paloutzian & C. L. Park (Eds.), *Handbook of the psychology of religion and spirituality* (pp. 460–478). New York: Guilford Press.

Miller, W. R., & C'de Baca, J. (2001). *Quantum change: When epiphanies and sudden insights transform ordinary lives.* New York: Guilford Press.

Moore, T. (1992). *Care of the soul.* New York: Harper Perennial Books.

Murray, K. A. (2002). Religion and divorce: Implications and strategies for counseling. *Family Journal: Counseling and Therapy for Couples and Families, 10,* 190–194.

Murray-Swank, A., Mahoney, A., & Pargament, K. I. (2006). Sanctification of parenting: Links to corporal punishment and parental warmth among Biblically conservative and liberal mothers. *International Journal for the Psychology of Religion, 16,* 271–387.

Murray-Swank, N. A. (2003). *Solace for the soul: An evaluation of a psychospiritual intervention for female survivors of sexual abuse.* Unpublished doctoral dissertation, Bowling Green State University, Bowling Green, OH.

Murray-Swank, N. A., & Pargament, K. I. (2005). God, where are you?: Evaluating a spiritually-integrated intervention for sexual abuse. *Mental Health, Religion, and Culture, 8,* 191–204.

Murray-Swank, N. A., Pargament, K. I., & Mahoney, A. (2005). At the crossroads of sexuality and spirituality: The sanctification of sex by college students. *International Journal for the Psychology of Religion, 15,* 199–220.

Narramore, B. (1994). Dealing with religious resistances in psychotherapy. *Journal of Psychology and Theology, 22,* 249–258.

Nash, R. (1990). Life's major spiritual issues: An emerging framework for spiritual assessment and diagnosis. *Caregiver Journal, 7,* 3–42.

Nelson, J. B. (2004). *Thirst: God and the alcoholic experience.* Louisville, KY: Westminster John Knox Press.

Neville, R. (1996). *The truth of broken symbols.* New York: State University of New York Press.

Nicholi, A. M. (1974). A new dimension of the youth culture. *American Journal of Psychiatry, 131,* 396–401.

Nielsen, S. L., Johnson, W. B., & Ellis, A. (2001). *Counseling and psychotherapy with religious persons: A rational emotive behavior therapy approach.* Mahway, NJ: Erlbaum.

Nosek, M. A. (1995). The defining light of Vedanta: Personal reflections on spirituality and disability. *Rehabilitation Education, 9,* 171–182.

O'Connor, S., & Vandenberg, B. (2005). Psychosis or faith?: Clinicians' assessment of religious beliefs. *Journal of Consulting and Clinical Psychology, 73,* 610–616.

Oden, T. C. (1983). *Pastoral theology: Essentials of ministry.* San Francisco: Harper & Row.

O'Hanlon, B. (1994). The third wave. *Family Therapy Networker, 18*(6), 18–29.

Oman, D., Hedberg, J., Downs, D., & Parsons, D. (2003). A transcultural spiritually-based program to enhance caregiving self-efficacy: A pilot study. *Complementary Health Practice Review, 8,* 201–224.

Otto, R. (1928). *The idea of the holy: An inquiry into the nonrational factor in the idea of the divine and its relation to the rational* (J. W. Harvey, Trans.). London: Oxford University Press. (Originally published 1917)

Paden, W. E. (1988). *Religious worlds: The comparative study of religion.* Boston: Beacon Press.

Palmer, P. J. (1998, September). The grace of great things: Reclaiming the sacred in knowing, teaching, and learning. *The Sun,* Baltimore, Maryland, pp. 24–28.

Paloutzian, R., & Ellison, C. W. (1982). Loneliness, spiritual well-being, and quality of life. In L. A. Peplau & D. Perlman (Eds.), *Loneliness: A sourcebook of current theory, research, and therapy* (pp. 224–237). New York: Wiley Interscience.

Paquette, J. M. (2005). Lutheran blessing for the divorced. *Beliefnet.com,* pp. 1–2. Accessed February 1, 2006 from www.beliefnet.com/story/75/story_75652.html

Pargament, K. I. (1997). *The psychology of religion and coping: Theory, research, practice.* New York: Guilford Press.

Pargament, K. I. (1999). The psychology of religion and spirituality?: Yes *and* no. *The International Journal for the Psychology of Religion, 9,* 3–16.

Pargament, K. I. (2002a). Is religion nothing but . . . ?: Explaining religion versus explaining religion away. *Psychological Inquiry, 13,* 239–244.

Pargament, K. I. (2002b). The bitter and the sweet: An evaluation of the costs and benefits of religiousness. *Psychological Inquiry, 13,* 168–181.

Pargament, K. I. (2006). The meaning of spiritual transformation. In J. D. Koss-Chioino & P. Hefner (Eds.), *Spiritual transformation and healing: Anthropological, theological, neuroscientific, and clinical perspectives* (pp. 10–24). Lanham, MD: AltaMira Press.

Pargament, K. I., Ensing, D. S., Falgout, K., Olsen, H., Reilly, B., Van Haitsma, K., et al. (1990). God help me (I): Religious coping efforts as predictors of the outcomes to significant negative life events. *American Journal of Community Psychology, 18,* 793–822.

Pargament, K. I., Kennell, J., Hathaway, W., Grevengoed, N., Newman, J., & Jones, W. (1988). Religion and the problem-solving process: Three styles of coping. *Journal for the Scientific Study of Religion, 27,* 90–104.

Pargament, K. I., Koenig, H. G., & Perez, L. (2000). The many methods of religious coping: Development and initial validation of the RCOPE. *Journal of Clinical Psychology, 56,* 519–543.

Pargament, K. I., Koenig, H. G., Tarakeshwar, N., & Hahn, J. (2001). Religious struggle as a predictor of mortality among medically ill elderly patients: A two-year longitudinal study. *Archives of Internal Medicine, 161,* 1881–1885.

Pargament, K. I., Koenig, H. G., Tarakeshwar, N., & Hahn, J. (2004). Religious coping methods as predictors of psychological, physical, and spiritual outcomes among medically ill elderly patients: A two-year longitudinal study. *Journal of Health Psychology, 9,* 713–730.

Pargament, K. I., Magyar, G. M., & Murray-Swank, N. (2005). The sacred and the search for the significance: Religion as a unique process. *Journal of Social Issues. 61,* 665–687.

Pargament, K. I., Magyar, G. M., Benore, E., & Mahoney, A. (2005). Sacrilege: A study of sacred loss and desecration and their implications for health and well-being in a community sample. *Journal for the Scientific Study of Religion, 44,* 59–78.

Pargament, K. I., & Mahoney, A. (2002). Spirituality: The discovery and conservation of the sacred. In C. R. Snyder & S. J. Lopez (Eds.), *Handbook of positive psychology* (pp. 646–659). New York: Oxford University Press.

Pargament, K. I., & Mahoney, A. (2005). Sacred matters: Sanctification as a vital topic for the psychology of religion. *International Journal for the Psychology of Religion, 15,* 179–198.

Pargament, K. I., & Maton, K. I. (2000). Religion in American life: A community psychology perspective. In J. Rappaport & E. Seidman (Eds.), *Handbook of community psychology* (pp. 495–522). New York: Kluwer Academic/Plenum Press.

Pargament, K. I., Maton, K. I., & Hess, R. E. (1992). (Eds.). *Religion and prevention in mental health: Research, vision, and action.* New York: Haworth Press.

Pargament, K. I., McCarthy, S., Shah, P., Ano, G., Tarakeshwar, N., Wachholtz, A. B., et al. (2004). Religion and HIV: A review of the literature and clinical implications. *Southern Medical Journal, 97,* 1201–1209.

Pargament, K. I., Murray-Swank, N., Magyar, G. M., & Ano, G. (2005). Spiritual struggle: A phenomenon of interest to psychology and religion. In W. R. Miller & H. Delaney (Eds.), *Judeo-Christian perspectives on psychology: Human nature, motivation, and change* (pp. 245–268). Washington, DC: American Psychological Association.

Pargament, K. I., Murray-Swank, N., & Mahoney, A. (in press). Problem and solution: The spiritual dimension of clergy sexual abuse and its impact on survivors. *Journal of Child Sexual Abuse.*

Pargament, K. I., & Park, C. (1995). Merely a defense?: The variety of religious means and ends. *Journal of Social Issues, 51,* 13–32.

Pargament, K. I., Smith, B. W., Koenig, H. G., & Perez, L. (1998). Patterns of positive and negative religious coping with major life stressors. *Journal for the Scientific Study of Religion, 37,* 710–724.

Pargament, K. I., Steele, R. E., & Tyler, F. B. (1979). Religious participation, religious motivation, and individual psychosocial competence. *Journal for the Scientific Study of Religion, 18,* 412–419.

Pargament, K. I., Trevino, K., Mahoney, A., & Silberman, I. (2007). They killed our Lord: The perception of Jews as desecrators of Christianity as a predictor of anti-Semitism. *Journal for the Scientific Study of Religion, 46,* 143–158.

Park, C. L. (2005). Religion and meaning. In R. F. Paloutzian & C. L. Park (Eds.), *Handbook of the psychology of religion and spirituality* (pp. 295–314). New York: Guilford Press.

Park, C. L., Cohen, L. H., & Herb, H. (1990). Intrinsic religiousness and religious coping as life stress moderators for Catholics versus Protestants. *Journal of Personality and Social Psychology, 54,* 551–577.

Parkin, D. (Ed.). (1985). *The anthropology of evil.* New York: Basil Blackwell.

Pattison, E. M. (1982). Management of religious issues in family therapy. *International Journal of Family Therapy, 4,* 140–163.

366 — References

Paul, G. L. (1967). Strategy of outcome research in psychotherapy. *Journal of Consulting Psychology, 31,* 109–118.

Pearce, M. J. (2005). A critical review of the forms and value of religious coping among informal caregivers. *Journal of Religion and Health, 44,* 81–118.

Pecheur, D. R., & Edwards, K. J. (1984). A comparison of secular and religious versions of cognitive therapy with depressed Christian college students. *Journal of Psychology and Theology, 12,* 45–54.

Peck, M. S. (1998). *People of the lie: The hope for healing human evil.* New York: Touchstone Books.

Pennebaker, J. (1997). *Opening up: The healing power of expression of emotions.* New York: Guilford Press.

Peradotto, J. (2006, Summer). Connecting mind, body, and spirit. *BP Magazine,* pp. 40–44.

Peterman, A. H., Fitchett, G., Brady, M., Hernandez, L, & Cella, D. (2002). Measuring spiritual well-being in people with cancer: The Functional Assessment of Chronic Illness Therapy-Spiritual Well-Being Scale (FACIT-Sp). *Annals of Behavioral Medicine, 24,* 49–58.

Peterson, C., & Seligman, M. E. P. (Eds.). (2004). *Character strengths and virtues: A handbook and classification.* New York: Oxford University Press.

Peterson, R. (1986). *Everyone is right: A new look at comparative religion and its relation to science.* Marina del Ray, CA: DeVorss.

Phillips, J. B. (1997). *Your God is too small.* New York: Touchstone Books.

Phillips, R. E. III, Lakin, R., & Pargament, K. I. (2002). The development of a psychospiritual intervention for people with serious mental illness. *Community Mental Health Journal, 38,* 487–495.

Phillips, R. E. III., & Stein, C. S. (in press). God's will, God's punishment, or God's limitations?: Religious coping strategies reported by young adults living with serious mental illness. *Journal of Clinical Psychology.*

Piaget, J. (1954). *The construction of reality in the child.* New York: Basic Books.

Piedmont, R. L. (1999). Does spirituality represent the sixth factor of personality?: Spiritual transcendence and the five-factor model. *Journal of Personality, 67,* 985–1013.

Pinker, S. (2002). *The blank slate: The modern denial of human nature.* New York: Viking.

Plato. (1951). *The symposium* (W. Hamilton, Trans.). Harmondsworth, UK: Penguin Books.

Poloma, M. M. (2003). *Main street mystics: The Toronto Blessing and reviving Pentacostalism.* Walnut Creek, CA: AltaMira Press.

Poloma, M. M., & Gallup, G. H. Jr. (1991). *Varieties of prayer: A survey report.* Philadelphia: Trinity Press International.

Pope, S. J. (2002). Relating self, others, and sacrifice in the ordering of love. In S. G. Post, L. G. Underwood, J. P. Schloss, & W. B. Hurlbut (Eds.), *Altruism and altruistic love: Science, philosophy, and religion in dialogue* (pp. 168–181). New York: Oxford University Press.

Porpora, D. V. (2001). *Landscapes of the soul: The loss of moral meaning in American life.* New York: Oxford University Press.

Post, S. G., Puchalski, C. M., & Larson, D. B. (2000). Physicians and patient spirituality: Professional boundaries, competency, and ethics. *Annals of Internal Medicine, 132,* 578–583.

Prabhu, R. K., & Rao, U. R. (Ed.). (1967). *The mind of Mahatma Gandhi.* Ahmedabad, India: Navajivan Publishing.

Prest, L. A., & Keller, J. F. (1993). Spirituality and family therapy: Spiritual beliefs, myths, and metaphors. *Journal of Marital and Family Therapy, 19,* 137–148.

Propst, L. R. (1980). The comparative efficacy of religious and nonreligious imagery for the treatment of mild depression in religious individuals. *Cognitive Therapy and Research, 4,* 167–178.

Propst, L. R. (1988). *Psychotherapy in a religious framework: Spirituality in the emotional healing process.* New York: Human Sciences Press.

Propst, L. R., Ostrom, R., Watkins, P., Dean, T., & Mashburn, D. (1992). Comparative efficacy of religious and nonreligious-behavioral therapy for the treatment of clinical depression in religious individuals. *Journal of Consulting and Clinical Psychology, 60,* 94–103.

Pruyser, P. W. (1968). *A dynamic psychology of religion.* New York: Harper & Row.

Pruyser, P. W. (1977). The seamy side of current religious beliefs. *Bulletin of the Menninger Clinic, 41,* 329–348.

Rajagopal, D., Mackenzie, E., Bailey, C., & Lavizzo-Mourey, R. (2002). The effectiveness of a spiritually-based intervention to alleviate subsyndromal anxiety and minor depression among older adults. *Journal of Religion and Health, 41,* 153–166.

Rayburn, C. A. (1985). The religious patient's initial encounter with psychotherapy. In E. M. Stern (Ed.), *Psychotherapy and the religiously committed patient* (pp. 35–45). New York: Haworth Press.

Resnicow, K., Jackson, A., Wong, T., De, A. K., McCarty, F., Dudley, W. N., et al. (2001). A motivational interviewing intervention to increase fruit and vegetable intake through black churches: Results for the Eat for Life trial. *American Journal of Public Health, 91,* 1686–1693.

Richards, P. S., & Bergin, A. E. (Eds.) (2000). *Handbook of psychotherapy and religious diversity.* Washington, DC: American Psychological Association.

Richards, P. S., & Bergin, A. E. (2005). *A spiritual strategy for counseling and psychotherapy.* Washington, DC: American Psychological Association.

Richards, P. S., Berrett, M. E., Hardman, R. K., & Eggett, D. L. (2006). Comparative efficacy of spirituality, cognitive, and emotional support groups for treating eating disorder inpatients. *Eating Disorders: Journal of Treatment and Prevention, 41,* 401–415.

Richards, P. S., Hardman, R. K., & Berrett, M. E. (2000). *Spiritual renewal: A journey of faith and healing.* Orem, UT: Center for Change.

Richards, P. S., Hardman, R. K., & Berrett, M. E. (2007). *Spiritual approaches in the treatment of women with eating disorders.* Washington, DC: American Psychological Association.

Richards, P. S., Owen, L., & Stein, S. (1993). A religiously oriented group counseling intervention for self-defeating perfectionism: A pilot study. *Counseling and Values, 37,* 96–104.

Richards, T. A., Acree, M., & Folkman, S. (1999). Spiritual aspects of loss among partners of men with AIDS: Postbereavement follow-up. *Death Studies, 23,* 105–127.

Rizzuto, A. M. (1979). *The birth of the living God: A psychoanalytic study.* Chicago: University of Chicago Press.

Rizzuto, A. M. (1989). Ana-Maria Rizzuto on God representation. *Psychologists Interested in Religious Issues Newsletter, 14,* 1–5.

Rizzuto, A. M. (1998). *Why did Freud reject God?: A psychodynamic interpretation.* New Haven, CT: Yale University Press.

Robinson, L. C. (1994). Religious orientation in enduring marriage: An exploratory study. *Review of Religious Research, 35,* 207–218.

Rogers, C. R. (1989). A newer psychotherapy 1942. In H. Kirschenbaum & V. Land Henderson (Eds.). *The Carl Rogers reader* (pp. 63–76). Boston: Houghton Mifflin.

Rolheiser, R. (1994). *The shattered lantern: Rediscovering God's presence in everyday life.* London: Hodder & Stoughton.

Roof, W. C. (1993). *A generation of seekers: The spiritual journeys of the baby boom generation.* San Francisco: Harper & Row.

Rose, E. M., Westefeld, J. S., & Ansley, T. N. (2001). Spiritual issues in counseling: Clients' beliefs and preferences. *Journal of Counseling Psychology, 48,* 61–71.

Rosenberg, M. (1962). The dissonant religious context and emotional disturbance. *American Journal of Sociology, 68,* 1–10.

Rosenberg, R. S. (2002). The religious dimensions of life. *America, 187,* 7–9.

Rosensaft, M. (2001). I was born in Bergen Belsen. In A. Berger & N. Berger (Eds.), *Second generation voices: Reflections by children of Holocaust survivors and perpetrators* (pp. 188–207). Syracuse, NY: Syracuse University Press.

Rotz, E., Russell, C. S., & Wright, D. W. (1993). The therapist who is perceived as "spiritually correct": Strategies for avoiding collusion with the "spiritually one-up" spouse. *Journal of Marital and Family Therapy, 19,* 369–375.

Rozin, P., & Royzman, E. B. (2001). Negativity bias, negativity dominance, and contagion. *Personality and Social Psychology Review, 5,* 296–320.

Rupp, J. (1997). *The cup of our live: A guide for spiritual growth.* Notre Dame, IN: Ave Maria Press.

Ryan, R. M., Rigby, S., & King, K. (1993). Two types of religious internalization and their relations to religious orientation and mental health. *Journal of Personality and Social Psychology, 65,* 586–596.

Rye, M., & Pargament, K. I. (2002). Forgiveness and romantic relationships in college: Can it heal the wounded heart? *Journal of Clinical Psychology, 58,* 419–441.

Rye, M., & Pargament, K. I. (2003). *Coping with divorce: A journey toward forgiveness.* Unpublished manual, University of Dayton, OH.

Rye, M., Pargament, K. I., Wei, P., Yingling, D. W., Shogren, K. A., & Ito, M. (2005). Can group interventions facilitate forgiveness of an ex-spouse?: A randomized clinical trial. *Journal of Consulting and Clinical Psychology, 73,* 880–892.

Schachter-Shalomi, Z., & Miller, R. S. (1995). *From age-ing to sage-ing: A profound new vision of growing older.* New York: Warner Books.

Scheepers, P., Gijsberts, M., & Hello, E. (2002). Religiosity and prejudice against ethnic minorities in Europe: Cross-national tests on a controversial relationship. *Review of Religious Research, 43,* 242–265.

Schimmel, S. (1987). Job and the psychology of suffering and doubt. *Journal of Psychology and Judaism, 11,* 239–249.

Schlauch, C. R. (1995). *Faithful companioning: How pastoral counseling heals.* Minneapolis, MN: Augsburg Fortress Press.

Schmidt, R., Sager, G. C., Carney, G. T., Jackson, J. J., Jr., Muller, A. C., & Zanca, K. J. (1999). *Patterns of religion.* Beltmont, CA: Wadsworth.

Schreurs, A. (2002). *Psychotherapy and spirituality: Integrating the spiritual dimension into therapeutic practice.* London: Kingsley.

Schuck, K. D., & Liddle, B. J. (2001). Religious conflicts experienced by lesbian, gay, and bisexual individuals. *Journal of Gay and Lesbian Psychotherapy, 5,* 63–82.

Schulte, D. L., Skinner, T. A., & Claiborn, C. D. (2002). Religious and spiritual issues in counseling psychology programs. *Counseling Psychologist, 30,* 118–134.

Schuster, M. A., Stein, B. D., Jaycox, L. H., Collins, R. L., Marshall, G. N., Elliott, M. N., et al. (2001). A national survey of stress reactions after the September 11, 2001, terrorist attacks. *New England Journal of Medicine, 345,* 1507–1512.

Segall, M., & Wykle, M. (1988–1989). The black family's experience with dementia. *Journal of Applied Social Sciences, 13,* 170–191.

Sered, S. S. (1989). The religion of relating: Kinship and spirituality among Middle Eastern Jewish women in Jerusalem. *Journal of Social and Personal Relationships, 6,* 309–325.

Shafranske, E. P. (2001). The religious dimension of patient care within rehabilitation medicine: The role of religious attitudes, beliefs, and personal and professional practices. In T. G. Plante & A. C. Sherman (Eds.), *Faith and health: Psychological perspectives* (pp. 311–338). New York: Guilford Press.

Shafranske, E. P., & Malony, H. N. (1990). Clinical psychologists' religious and spiritual orientation and their practice of psychotherapy. *Psychotherapy, 27,* 72–78.

Shafranske, E. P., & Malony, H. N. (1996). Religion and the clinical practice of psychology: A case for inclusion. In E. P. Shafranske (Ed.), *Religion and the clinical practice of psychology* (pp. 561–586). Washington, DC: American Psychological Association.

Shapiro, S. L., Schwartz, G. E., & Bonner, G. (1998). Effects of mindfulness-based stress reduction on medical and premedical students. *Journal of Behavioral Medicine, 21,* 581–599.

Siegel, K., & Schrimshaw, E. W. (2002). The perceived benefits of religious and spiritual coping among older adults living with HIV/AIDS. *Journal for the Scientific Study of Religion, 41,* 91–102.

Siegel, R. D. (2005). Psychophysiological disorders: Embracing pain. In C. K. Germer, R. D. Siegel, & P. R. Fulton (Eds.), *Mindfulness and psychotherapy* (pp. 173–196). New York: Guilford Press.

Silberman, I., Higgins, E. T., & Dweck, C. S. (2005). Religion and world change: Violence and terrorism versus peace. *Journal of Social Issues, 61,* 761–784.

Silver, S. M., & Wilson, J. P. (1988). Native American healing and purification rituals for war stress. In J. P. Wilson, Z. Harel, & B. Kahana (Eds.), *Human adaptation to extreme stress: From the Holocaust to Vietnam* (pp. 337–355). New York: Plenum Press.

Skinner, B. F. (1948). *Walden Two.* New York: Macmillan.

Skinner, B. F. (1971). *Beyond freedom and dignity.* New York: Knopf.

Smith, C., & Exline, J. J. (August, 2002). *Effects of homelessness on a person's perceived relationship with God.* Paper presented at the annual meeting of the American Psychological Association, Chicago, IL.

Smith, F. T., Hardman, R. K., Richards, P. S., & Fischer, L. (2003). Intrinsic religiosity and spiritual well-being as predictors of treatment outcome among women with eating disorders. *Eating Disorders: Journal of Treatment and Prevention, 11*, 15–26.

Smith, H. (1958). *The religions of man.* New York: Harper & Row.

Smith, J. E. (1968). *Experience and God.* New York: Oxford University Press.

Smith, M. (2004). A survivor's story. *Human Development, 25*, 5–10.

Smith, T. (1992). The polls: Poll trends. Religious beliefs and behaviors and the tele-vangelist scandals of 1987–1988. *Public Opinion Quarterly, 56*, 360–380.

Smith, T. B., Bartz, J. D., & Richards, P. S. (in press). Outcomes of religious and spiritual adaptations to psychotherapy: A meta-analytic review. *Psychotherapy Research.*

Smith, T. B., McCullough, M. E., & Poll, J. (2003). Religiousness and depression: Evidence for a main effect and the moderating influence of stressful life events. *Psychological Bulletin, 129*, 614–636.

Smith, W. C. (1962). *The meaning and end of religion.* Minneapolis, MN: Fortress Press.

Sormanti, M., & August, J. (1997). Parental bereavement: Spiritual connections with deceased children. *American Journal of Orthopsychiatry, 6*, 460–469.

Sperry, L. (2001). *Spirituality in clinical practice: Incorporating the spiritual dimension in psychotherapy and counseling.* Philadelphia: Brunner-Routledge.

Spilka, B. (1993, August). *Spirituality: Problems and directions in operationalizing a fuzzy concept.* Paper presented at the annual meeting of the American Psychological Association, Toronto, Canada.

Spilka, B., Armatas, P., & Nussbaum, J. (1964). The concept of God: A factor-analytic approach. *Review of Religious Research, 6*, 28–36.

Spilka, B., Hood, R. W. Jr., Hunsberger, B., & Gorsuch, R. (2003). *The psychology of religion: An empirical approach* (3rd ed.). New York: Guilford Press.

Stanley, S., Trathen, D., McCain, S., & Bryan, M. (1998). *A lasting promise: A Christian guide to fighting for your marriage.* San Francisco: Jossey-Bass.

Starbuck, E. E. (1899). *The psychology of religion.* New York: Scribner.

Steinberg, M. (1975). *Basic Judaism.* New York: Harcourt Brace Jovanovich.

Strunk, O. Jr. (1965). *Mature religion: A psychological study.* New York: Abingdon Press.

Suess, L., & Halpern, M. S. (1989). Obsessive–compulsive disorder: The religious perspective. In J. L. Rapaport (Ed.), *Obsessive–compulsive disorder in children and adolescents* (pp. 311–325). Washington, DC: American Psychiatric Press.

Swank, A. B. (1992). *Spiritual confession: A theoretical synthesis and experimental study.* Unpublished doctoral dissertation, Bowling Green State University, Bowling Green, OH.

Swinton, J. (2001). *Spirituality and mental health care: Rediscovering a "forgotten" dimension.* London: Kingsley.

Tan, S. Y. (1996). Religion in clinical practice: Implicit and explicit integration. In E. Shafranske (Ed.), *Religion and the clinical practice of psychology* (pp. 365–390). Washington, DC: American Psychological Association.

Tarakeshwar, N., Pargament, K .I., & Mahoney, A. (2003a). Religious coping and mental health of Hindus in the United States. *Journal of Community Psychology, 31*, 607–628.

Tarakeshwar, N., Pargament, K. I., & Mahoney, A. (2003b). Measures of Hindu path-ways: Development and preliminary evidence of reliability and validity. *Cultural Diversity and Ethnic Minority Journal, 34,* 377–394.

Tarakeshwar, N., Pearce, M. J., & Sikkema, K. J. (2005). Development and imple-mention of a spiritual coping group intervention for adults living with HIV/ AIDS: A pilot study *Mental Health, Religion, and Culture, 8,* 179–190.

Tarakeshwar, N., Swank, A. B., Pargament, K . I., & Mahoney, A. (2001). The sancti-fication of nature and theological conservatism: A study of opposing religious correlates of environmentalism. *Review of Religious Research, 42,* 387–404.

Tepper, L., Rogers, S. A., Coleman, E. M., & Malony, H. N. (2001). The prevalence of religious coping among persons with persistent mental illness. *Psychiatric Ser-vices, 52,* 660–665.

Thurston, N. S. (2000). Psychotherapy with evangelical and fundamentalist Protes-tants. In P. S. Richards & A. E. Bergin (Eds.), *Handbook of religious diversity* (pp. 131–154). Washington, DC: American Psychological Association.

Tillich, P. (1952). *The courage to be.* New Haven, CT: Yale University Press.

Tillich, P. (1957). *Dynamics of faith.* New York: Torchbooks.

Tillich, P. (1967). *My search for absolutes.* New York: Simon & Schuster.

Tisdale, T. C. (2003). Listening and responding to spiritual issues in psychotherapy: An interdisciplinary perspective. *Journal of Psychology and Christianity, 22,* 262–272.

Tisdale, T. C., Keys, T. L., Edwards, K. J., Brokaw, B. F., Kemperman, S. R., Cloud, H., et al. (1997). Impact of treatment on God image and personal adjustment, and correlations of God image to personal adjustment and object relations adjust-ment. *Journal of Psychology and Theology, 25,* 227–239.

Tix, A. P., & Frazier, P. A. (1998). The use of religious coping during stressful life events: Main effects, moderation, and mediation. *Journal of Consulting and Clinical Psychology, 66,* 411–422.

Toh, Y. M., & Tan, S. Y. (1997). The effectiveness of church-based lay counselors: A controlled outcome study. *Journal of Psychology and Christianity, 16,* 260–267.

Trice, P. D., & Bjorck, J. P. (2006). Pentecostal perspectives on causes and cures of de-pression. *Professional Psychology: Research and Practice, 37,* 283–294.

True, G., Phipps, E., Braitman, L. E., Harralson, T., Harris, D., & Tester, W. (2003, April). *Attitudes, behaviors, and preferences at end of life: The role of ethnicity and spiritual coping in cancer patients.* Paper presented at the conference Inte-grating Research on Spirituality and Health and Well-Being into Service Deliv-ery, Bethesda, MD.

Tyler, F. B. (2001). *Cultures, communities, competence, and change.* New York: Kluwer Academic/Plenum Press.

Tyler, F. B., Pargament, K. I., & Gatz, M. (1983). The resource collaborator role: A model for interactions involving psychologists. *American Psychologist, 38,* 388–398.

Upanishads: Breath of the eternal, The (S. Prabhavananda & F. Manchester, Trans.). (1975). New York: Mentor Books.

Van Uden, M. H. F., Pieper, J. Z. T., & Alma, H. A. (2004). "Bridge over troubled wa-ter": Further results regarding the Receptive Coping Scale. *Journal of Empirical Theology, 17,* 101–114.

Wachholtz, A. (2005). *Does spirituality matter?: Effects of meditative content and orientation on migraneurs*. Unpublished doctoral dissertation, Bowling Green State University, Bowling Green, OH.

Wachholtz, A. B., & Pargament, K. I. (2005). Is spirituality a critical ingredient of meditation?: Comparing the effects of spiritual meditation, secular meditation, and relaxation on spiritual, psychological, cardiac, and pain outcomes. *Journal of Behavioral Medicine, 28*, 369–384.

Wade, N. G., Worthington, E. L., Jr., & Vogel, D. L. (2007). Effectiveness of religiously tailored interventions in Christian therapy. *Psychotherapy Research, 17*, 91–105.

Wahass, S., & Kent, G. (1997). The modification of psychological interventions for persistent auditory hallucinations to an Islamic culture. *Behavioral and Cognitive Psychotherapy, 25*, 351–364.

Wallace, B. A., & Shapiro, S. L. (2006). Mental balance and well-being: Building bridges between Buddhism and Western psychology. *American Psychologist, 61*, 690–701.

Walsh, R. (1999). Asian contemplative disciplines: Common practices, clinical applications, and research findings. *Journal of Transpersonal Psychology, 31*, 83–107.

Walters, J., & Neugeboren, B. (1995). Collaboration between mental health organizations and religious institutions. *Psychiatric Rehabilitation Journal, 19*, 51–57.

Warren, R. (2002). *The purpose driven life: What on earth am I here for?* Grand Rapids, MI: Zondervan.

Weaver, A. J., Pargament, K. I., Flannelly, K. J., & Oppenheimer, J. E. (2006). Trends in the scientific study of religion, spirituality, and health: 1965–2000. *Journal of Religion and Health, 45*, 208–214.

Webb, M., & Whitmer, K. J. O. (2003). Parental religiosity, abuse history, and maintenance of beliefs taught in the family. *Mental Health, Religion, and Culture, 6*, 229–239.

Weinborn, M. (1999). *A theoretical approach to the religion–mental health connection: Initial exploration of a religious orienting system*. Unpublished doctoral dissertation, Bowling Green State University, Bowling Green, OH.

Weisbuch-Remington, M., Mendes, W. B., Seery, M. D., & Blascovich, J. (2005). The nonconscious influence of religious symbols in motivated performance situations. *Personality and Social Psychology Bulletin, 31*, 1203–1216.

White, R. W. (1963). Ego and reality in psychoanalytic theory. *Psychological Issues, 3*, 1–210.

Why we pray. (1994, March). *Life*, pp. 54, 57, 59, 60, 62.

Wick, E. (1985). Lost in the no-man's-land between psyche and soul. In E. M. Stern (Ed.), *Psychotherapy and the religiously committed patient* (pp. 13–24). New York: Haworth Press.

Wilson, K. M., & Huff, J. L. (2001). Scaling Satan. *Journal of Psychology, 135*, 292–300.

Wink, P., & Dillon, M. (2001). Religious involvement and health outcomes in late adulthood: Findings from a longitudinal study of women and men. In T. G. Plante & A. C. Sherman (Eds.), *Faith and health: Psychological perspectives* (pp. 75–106). New York: Guilford Press.

Worthington, E. L. Jr. (1986). Religious counseling: A review of published empirical research. *Journal of Counseling and Development, 64,* 421–431.

Worthington, E. L. Jr. (1994). A blueprint for interdisciplinary integration. *Journal of Psychology and Theology, 22,* 79–86.

Worthington, E. L. Jr. (1998). The pyramid model of forgiveness: Some interdisciplinary speculations about unforgiveness and the promotion of forgiveness. In E. L. Worthington Jr. (Ed.), *Dimensions of forgiveness: Psychological research and theological perspectives* (pp. 107–137). Radnor, PA: Templeton Foundation Press.

Worthington, E. L. Jr. (2004). *Experiencing forgiveness: Six practical sessions for becoming a more forgiving Christian.* Unpublished manuscript, Virginia Commonwealth University, Richmond, VA.

Worthington, E. L. Jr. (Ed.). (2005). *Handbook of forgiveness.* New York: Routledge.

Worthington, E. L. Jr., Kurusu, T. A., McCullough, M. E., & Sandage, S. J. (1996). Empirical research on religion and psychotherapeutic processes and outcomes: A 20-year review and research prospectus. *Psychological Bulletin, 119,* 448–487.

Worthington, E. L. Jr., & Sandage, S. (2002). Religion and spirituality. In J. C. Norcross (Ed.), *Psychotherapy relationships that work: Therapist contributions and responsiveness to patients* (pp. 383–400). New York: Oxford University Press.

Wright, S., Pratt, C., & Schmall, V. (1985). Spiritual support for caregivers of dementia patients. *Journal of Religion and Health, 24,* 31–38.

Wulff, D. M. (1997). *Psychology of religion: Classic and contemporary* (2nd ed.). New York: Wiley.

Wuthnow, R. (1998). *After heaven: Spirituality in America since the 1950's.* Berkeley and Los Angeles: University of California Press.

Yalom, I. D. (1980). *Existential psychotherapy.* New York: Basic Books.

Yalom, I. D. (1989). *Love's executioner.* New York: HarperCollins.

Yancey, P. (1977). *Where is God when it hurts?* Grand Rapids, MI: Zondervan.

Yanni, G. M. (2003). *Religious and secular dyadic variables and their relation to parent–child relationships and college students' psychological adjustment.* Unpublished doctoral dissertation, Bowling Green State University, Bowling Green, OH.

Yau, J. (2003). *Neptune's daughter: Journey into oneness.* Laguna Beach, CA: Mystic Hill.

Yeats, W. B. (1920, November). Ten poems. *The Dial,* November, *69,* 455–466.

Zerubavel, J. (1991). *The fine line: Making distinctions in everyday life.* New York: Free Press.

Zimmerman, C. C. (1974). Family influence upon religion. *Journal of Comparative Family Studies, 5,* 1–16.

Zinnbauer, B. J., & Pargament, K. I. (1998). Spiritual conversion: A study of religious change among college students. *Journal for the Scientific Study of Religion, 37,* 161–180.

Zinnbauer, B. J., & Pargament, K. I. (2005). Religiousness and spirituality. In R. F. Paloutzian & C. L. Park (Eds.), *Handbook of the psychology of religion and spirituality* (pp. 21–42). New York: Guilford Press.

Zinnbauer, B. J., Pargament, K. I., Cole, B., Rye, M. S., Butter, E. M., Belavich, T. G., et al. (1997). Religion and spirituality: Unfuzzying the fuzzy. *Journal for the Scientific Study of Religion, 36*, 549–564.

Zinnbauer, B. J., Pargament, K. I., & Scott, A. B. (1999). Emerging meanings of religiousness and spirituality: Problems and prospects. *Journal of Personality, 67*, 889–919.

Zornow, G. B. (2001). *Crying out to God: Prayer in the midst of suffering.* Unpublished manuscript, Evanglical Lutheran Church of America. Leipsic, OH.

Index

Struggles, spiritual (*continued*)
    spiritual coping and, 111–116
    transforming the sacred and, 115, 127
    types of, 112–116
Suicidality, 252–253
Support, spiritual
    helping clients draw on, 264–269
    interpersonal spiritual struggles and, 112
    spiritual coping and, 102–105, 269–272
Supreme Being. *See also* God
    sacred core and, 32–34, 33*f*
    spiritual destinations and, 137–149
Sweat lodge ritual, 118
Symbols, 168–169
Synagogue membership, 84
Systems, social, 308–315

Taoism
    meditation and, 87–88
    pathways to the sacred and, 78
    sacred core and, 33
Texts, religious
    education and, 340
    integrating into psychotherapy, 251–253, 327
    manualized interventions and, 325
    pathways to the sacred and, 79–81, 80, 91–92
    spiritual coping and, 98–99
    spiritual inflexibility and, 301–302
Therapeutic relationship, 268–269, 345
Therapists
    bias of, 332–335
    boundaries of, 244–245
    humor and, 304–306
    pluralism and, 20–21
    spiritual resources of clients and, 244–245
    spiritually integrated psychotherapy and, 177*t*, 186–194
    training and, 332–336, 333*t*, 336*t*
    values and, 22–23
Threat, sacred
    loss of the sacred and, 94–98
    measures of, 235*t*
    spiritual purification and, 105–106
Time, as sacred, 47–49
Timidity, spiritual, 333*t*
Tolerance
    problems of fit and, 310–312
    spiritually integrated therapists and, 191
    therapeutic orientation and, 187–189
Toronto Blessing, 88
Traditions, religious
    discovery of the sacred and, 64–65
    spiritual practices and, 83
Training, professional, 9, 190, 332–336, 333*t*, 336*t*

Transcendence
    discovery of the sacred and, 74
    pathways to the sacred and, 87
    sacred ring and, 39–41
    self-worship and, 43
    sexuality and, 46
Transcendent reality, 32–34, 33*f*
Transformation, spiritual
    assessment and, 218*t*
    centering the sacred and, 121–126
    overview, 126–128
    research on, 126
    revisioning the sacred and, 119–121
    rituals and, 261
    sacred transitions and, 117–119
    spiritual coping and, 116–126
Transitions
    discovery of the sacred and, 66–67
    the sacred and, 48
    spiritual coping and, 117–119
Traumatic events
    as desecration or violation of the sacred, 97
    positive spiritual reappraisals of, 100–102
    revisioning the sacred after, 119–121
    spiritual assessment and, 213–215
    spiritual meaning making and, 10, 274–275
    spiritual struggles and, 114
Triangling, divine, 107, 113–114, 308
Truth-based criteria, 130–131. *See also* Evaluating spirituality
Truths, problems of breadth and depth and, 297
Twelve-step programs, 126

Ultimacy, sacred ring and, 39–41
Upanishads, 80

V code in diagnoses, 176–181
Values
    of author, 23–26
    spiritually integrated psychotherapy and, 22–23
    transforming the sacred and, 122–126
Violation, loss of the sacred and, 12–13, 94–98
Violence
    demonization of self and others and, 146–147
    problem of insufficiency and, 138–139
    spiritual problems and, 151–152, 181
Virtues
    integration of into Western psychology, 11
    intrapsychic spiritual struggles and, 112–113
    self-worship and, 43
Visualization, 198–199

Wisdom, spiritual, 162